Eating Disorders and Obesity: Prevention and Treatment

Eating Disorders and Obesity: Prevention and Treatment

Editor: Carlyle Bennet

AMERICAN
MEDICAL PUBLISHERS
www.americanmedicalpublishers.com

AMERICAN
MEDICAL PUBLISHERS
www.americanmedicalpublishers.com

Cataloging-in-Publication Data

Eating disorders and obesity : prevention and treatment / edited by Carlyle Bennet.
p. cm.
Includes bibliographical references and index.
ISBN 978-1-63927-665-3
1. Eating disorders. 2. Obesity. 3. Eating disorders--Treatment. 4. Eating disorders--Prevention.
5. Weight loss. 6. Nutrition disorders. 7. Reducing diets. I. Bennet, Carlyle.
RC552.E18 E28 2023
616.852 6--dc23

American Medical Publishers,
41 Flatbush Avenue,
1st Floor, New York,
NY 11217, USA

ISBN 978-1-63927-665-3 (Hardback)

Contents

Preface

The main aim of this book is to educate learners and enhance their research focus by presenting diverse topics covering this vast field. This is an advanced book which compiles significant studies by distinguished experts in the area of analysis. This book addresses successive solutions to the challenges arising in the area of application, along with it; the book provides scope for future developments.

Eating disorder is a form of a mental disorder that is characterized by abnormal eating habits. These disorders cause negative effect on an individual's mental or physical health. There are various types of eating disorders such as anorexia nervosa, bulimia nervosa, muscle dysmorphia and binge eating disorder. Obesity is a complex disease caused by an eating disorder in which a person eats too much without enough physical activity. It can be caused by genetic, behavioral, metabolic and hormonal influences on body weight. The most common symptoms of eating disorders include fatigue, weakness and sensitivity to cold. Preventive measures focus on early identification of an eating disorder. Some of the most common treatments of eating disorders are cognitive behavioral therapy, recreation therapy, art therapy, medical nutrition therapy, dialectal behavioral therapy, and family therapy. This book contains some path-breaking studies on eating disorders and obesity. The topics included herein are of utmost significance and bound to provide incredible insights on the prevention and treatment of these medical conditions. The extensive content of this book provides the readers with a thorough understanding of the subject.

It was a great honour to edit this book, though there were challenges, as it involved a lot of communication and networking between me and the editorial team. However, the end result was this all-inclusive book covering diverse themes in the field.

Finally, it is important to acknowledge the efforts of the contributors for their excellent chapters, through which a wide variety of issues have been addressed. I would also like to thank my colleagues for their valuable feedback during the making of this book.

Editor

1

Child Trauma Experiences and Dissociative Symptoms in Women with Eating Disorders

María F. Rabito-Alcón [1,*], José I. Baile [1] and Johan Vanderlinden [2]

1 Department of Psychology, Open University of Madrid (UDIMA), 28400 Madrid, Spain; ignaciobaile@hotmail.com
2 Campus Kortenberg, Universitair Psychiatrisch (Centrum KU Leuven), 3070 Kortenberg, Belgium; johan.vanderlinden@upckuleuven.be
* Correspondence: mariafrenzi.rabito@udima.es

Abstract: Background: many people with different diagnoses, including eating disorders, have suffered traumatic experiences in childhood. Method: a case-control study was performed. The objective of this study was to evaluate the presence of child trauma and dissociative symptoms in people with eating disorders and compare the results obtained with a control group. Participants were administered the Mini International Neuropsychiatric Interview (MINI) and the Structured Clinical Interview for Personality Disorders (SCID-II) to confirm diagnostic criteria and explore possible comorbidities. Traumatic experiences in childhood were evaluated with the Child Trauma Questionnaire in its abbreviated version (CTQ-SF), psychoform dissociation was measured with the Scale of Dissociative Experiences (DES-II) and somatoform dissociation with the Somatoform Dissociation Scale (SDQ-20). Results: women with eating disorders reported a greater severity and higher prevalence of child trauma than the control group. Significant differences were found by groups in dissociative symptoms. Conclusions: our results, in a Spanish sample, confirm the findings of previous studies.

Keywords: somatoform; psychoform; trauma; dissociation; eating disorders

---

1. Introduction

Early exposure to traumatic events, such as repeated sexual and physical abuse during childhood, has a profound negative effect on people's lives [1]. The consequences of undergoing a traumatic event are complex and may affect individuals by increasing the risk for many health conditions as drug abuse, diabetes, cancer, heart and respiratory diseases and obesity among others [2–4] as well as the individual's relationship with their own body [5,6]. In their study on the link between childhood trauma and dissociation, Scheffers et al. (2017) concluded that childhood trauma seriously affected the patient's relationship with their body (body attitude, body satisfaction and body awareness). Consequently, traumatized people can find it difficult to detect internal sensations and perceptions, and sometimes even deny any somatic awareness [5,6].

Furthermore, memories of traumatic events, which are often related to the body, can lead to the rejection and loss of contact with the body [5,7]. Previous studies have suggested the link between eating disorders and traumatic events during childhood [2,8–12]. Palmisano et al. (2016) carried out a systematic review of studies which tied trauma with obesity and a binge-eating disorder. Out of the studies analyzed, 87% showed that trauma was a risk factor for the development of obesity and binge-eating disorder (BED). In their systematic review, Caslini et al. (2016) concluded that sexual abuse is linked to the development of bulimia nervosa (BN) and BED, but the results for anorexia nervosa (AN) were not conclusive. Another systematic review on neglect during childhood and eating disorders [13] confirmed the high prevalence of emotional and physical neglect in people with eating disorders when compared with the general population.

Other researchers have tried to explore the mediating variables between traumatic events and the development of eating disorders. According to such studies, some of the possible related factors are lack of emotional self-regulation, self-denigration, borderline personality organization and the presence of dissociative symptoms [14–17]. In this vein, results from previous researchers have suggested that dissociation plays a significant mediating role in cases of childhood trauma and the development of eating disorders [10,18,19]. Such patients might have "learnt" to dissociate and to resort to behavior such as purging or compulsive eating to avoid or escape trauma-related feelings, sensations, memories and cognition. Or, maybe, they are trying to achieve a less attractive body, even an infertile one in AN patients with a history of sexual abuse. Moreover, vomiting is often linked to feelings of disgust and the quest for purity that come as a result of abuse. In many cases, there might also be a need to punish oneself due to self-blame for the abuse [10,14–19].

Mental dissociation would thus emerge as a secondary reaction to trauma. On a behavioral level, this covers numbness, freezing, avoidance, submission and detachment to allow for a state of energy conservation [14]. Some authors have argued that sexual abuse during childhood could trigger a type of dissociative coping mechanism, which results in low self-esteem, poor regulation of emotions and, in some patients, feeling as if life is out of their control. This leads to the need to exert control through disordered self-starvation behaviors [12,14]. Some researchers found a positive relation between early traumatic experiences, dissociation and binge eating behaviors [20–22].

Nijenhuis (2000) wrote that "somatoform dissociation" is the result of sexual abuse during childhood. It is defined as a lack of integration of sensorimotor experiences and the mental functions and reactions of the individual. Somatoform dissociation is a somatic manifestation of dissociation, including somatic symptoms which cannot be explained by a medical condition (anesthesia or analgesia, pain, mobility loss...) [23,24]. Researchers on this topic [11,23,25] concluded that psychoform and somatoform dissociation are strongly correlated with early trauma. Some authors found a positive relation between somatoform dissociation and eating disorders [26], and purging [27]. Psychoform dissociation includes amnesia, depersonalization, derealization and identity alteration and confusion in response to traumatic events, especially those which involve physical contact such as physical or sexual abuse [23,24].

Previous studies [11,19,23] have demonstrated this link between traumatic experiences, dissociative symptoms and eating disorders, showing that both past traumatic events and dissociation play a significant role in the etiology and development of eating disorders. In Belgium, Sweden, Italy and Australia [8,11,19,28,29], similar studies have been developed which confirm the link between traumatic events during childhood, dissociation and eating disorders. However, all of these papers concluded that it was necessary to continue research on this topic due to the potential implications for treating people with eating disorders in the future and due to the inconclusive results of other studies regarding the link between these variables [5,9].

In Spain, there is only one published work on the topic [30]: a doctoral thesis. The subject of this paper was to study the link between eating disorders and dissociative disorders, connecting these to the possibility of having suffered early sexual abuse. However, it does not consider other types of abuse, such as physical abuse, emotional abuse, emotional neglect and physical neglect. These researchers concluded that the sample of people with eating disorders presented with higher comorbidity with dissociative disorders than the control group. They also found that BN sufferers had a greater history of sexual abuse than other subtypes of eating disorders included in the study.

A review of the published works on the topic seems to show a connection between trauma, dissociation and eating disorders, but this relationship is not yet clear [10,18,19]. Thus, the objective of our study was to examine the link between (psychoform and somatoform) dissociative symptoms and childhood trauma (sexual abuse, emotional abuse, physical abuse, emotional neglect and physical neglect) in Spanish patients with eating disorders and to compare the results with a Spanish control group.

The following hypotheses will be used in this study:

1. We expected greater (somatoform and psychoform) dissociation in the group of participants with eating disorders than in the control group;
2. We expected greater dissociation amongst the compulsive eating disorder subtypes than amongst the restrictive types;
3. We expected a greater severity/prevalence of traumatic events in the group of participants with eating disorders than in the control group;
4. We expected a greater severity/prevalence of traumatic events amongst the compulsive eating disorder subtypes than amongst the restrictive types.

2. Method

2.1. Participants

This is a case-control study. We recruited 22 patients: Spanish women from various hospitals and psychological centers who were diagnosed with eating disorders in line with DSM-IV-TR (Diagnostic and Statistical Manual of Mental Disorders) [31] or DSM-5 [32] criteria. In our sample, 68.18% of patients were diagnosed with AN, 13.6% with BN, 9.09% with BED and 9.09% were diagnosed with an eating disorder not otherwise specified (EDNOS). The sample of the group of participants with eating disorders was reflected in the age and gender in the control group, which was made up of 21 women from the general population. Due to the scarce number of men diagnosed with eating disorders in the participating centers, we decided to only include women in this study. Each participant voluntarily consented to take part in the study, after being informed of its objectives.

All the participants signed informed consent forms. The eligibility criteria for the group of participants with eating disorders were: women over the age of 18 with a current diagnosis of an eating disorder. For the control group, the eligibility criteria were: women over the age of 18 with no known psychiatric diagnosis before inclusion in the study. The study was approved by the Committee on Ethics, Research and Teaching of Madrid Open University meeting the declaration of Helsinki.

2.2. Procedure

Each participant in the group with eating disorders had been previously diagnosed by their psychiatrist. To confirm the diagnostic criteria, participants took the Mini International Neuropsychiatric Interview (MINI). We collected sociodemographic data in a data set elaborated for the study. The variables included were age, gender, expected weight, actual weight, expected height, actual height, marital status, eating disorder diagnosis, age of onset of the disorder and the duration of the disorder in years.

2.3. Measuring Instruments

We used the following questionnaires: Clinical Global Impressions severity scale (CGI-S), Mini International Neuropsychiatric Interview (MINI), Structured Clinical Interview for Personality Disorders (SCID II), Dissociative Experiences Scale (DES-II), Somatoform Dissociation Questionnaire (SDQ 20) and the Childhood Trauma Questionnaire (CTQ).

CGI-S [33] is a scale which evaluates the clinical global impression of the severity of the patient's illness at the time of assessment. There are eight items which range from 0 ("not evaluated") to 7 ("amongst the most extremely ill patients").

MINI [34] is a short structured diagnostic interview. It explores the main diagnoses of DSM-IV Axis I and ICD 10 (International Classification of Diseases) for detection and diagnosis purposes.

The MINI is divided into 16 modules, identified by letters, which each correspond to a diagnostic category. At the beginning of each module (except the module on psychotic disorders), one or several 'filter' questions are set out in a grey box. These correspond to the main diagnostic criteria of the disorder. At the end of each module, one or several diagnostic check boxes allow the clinic to indicate whether the patient meets the diagnostic criteria. The questions asked throughout the test were closed and must be answered by the interviewer, who responds regarding the presence or absence of the symptom. For this study, we used the Spanish version of the interview [35].

SCID-II [36,37] is an interview which categorically or dimensionally evaluates personality disorders. The questionnaire includes an interview section made up of 119 questions, in addition to others on antisocial disorder. It contains open, closed and yes/no questions to evaluate personality disorders of the DSM-IV Axis II, as well as depressive and passive-aggressive personality disorder. This includes a detection questionnaire of 119 items. For this study, we used the Spanish version of the interview [37].

DES-II [38,39] is a scale with 28 items to be filled out by the patients themselves. It is used to measure a wide range of dissociative experiences, including memory, identity, absorption, depersonalization and derealization problems. Each item is marked in a range of 0–100. Scores over 30 indicate a dissociative disorder. The questionnaire is based on three factors: dissociative amnesia, absorption and depersonalization/derealization. For this study, we used the Spanish version of DES-II, made by Icarán et al. [40,41]. The Spanish version is valid and reliable (Cronbach's alpha = 0.91) [40,41].

SDQ-20 [42,43] is a questionnaire of 20 items filled in by the patients themselves. It evaluates the presence of somatoform dissociation. These items include symptoms of analgesia, anesthesia, motor problems, altered taste and smell, pain and loss of consciousness. Answers to the items are chosen on a 5-point Likert-type scale, ranging from 1 ("never") to 5 ("almost always or always"). The sum of these answers equals a total score between 20 and 100. The items include positive and negative dissociative symptoms. For this study, we used the Spanish version of SDQ-20 made by Holm in 2002 and has good psychometric properties [25]. The internal consistency is very high (Cronbach's alpha = 0.95) [42,43].

CTQ-SF [44] is made up of 28 items, adapted and translated into Spanish by Hernández et al. 2013. The scale measures five types of childhood trauma: emotional abuse during childhood, physical abuse during childhood, sexual abuse during childhood, emotional neglect during childhood and physical neglect during childhood. Answers to the items are chosen on a 5-point Likert-type frequency scale, with scores ranging from 1 ("never") to 5 ("always"). The CTQ-SF gives both dimensional and categorical levels of abuse. To obtain the categorical level, cut points are used for each of the scales on the questionnaire. To calculate the dimensional level, all of the scores are added together. CTQ-SF is valid and reliable. The Spanish version, used in this study, is valid and internally consistent (Cronbach's alpha coefficients ranged from 0.66 for emotional neglect to 0.94 for sexual abuse) [45].

2.4. Statistical Analysis

For all continuous variables, data was shown as the mean (M) and standard deviation (SD). On the other hand, all categorical variables were expressed as number percentage (%). The data were analyzed with nonparametric tests, because the sample did not fulfil the criteria for normalization. The SPSS program for Windows version 24.0 (IBM Corporation, Armonk, NY, USA) was used to analyze the data. It calculated the descriptive statistics of the variables. The Kruskal–Wallis H test was used to compare the subtypes of eating disorders in the group of participants with a disorder. The Mann–Whitney U test was used to compare the group of participants with eating disorders with the control group. Statistical significance was maintained at p-value ≤ 0.050.

3. Results

Socio-Demographic Data

The average age of women in the group of participants with eating disorders was 30.64 (SD = 10.18) with age in the range of 20–54. The average age of women in the control group was 34.29 (SD = 7.72) with an age range between 20 and 49. The average expected weight in the group of participants with eating disorders was 55.86 kg (SD = 22.25), while the average actual weight was 55.8 kg (SD = 26.96). The expected weight in the control group was 61.75 kg (SD = 9.64), while the actual weight was 62.36 kg (SD = 9.83). The averages for expected height and actual height in the group of participants with eating disorders were 164.63 cm (SD = 5.88) and 164.28 cm (SD = 6.43), respectively. The expected height in the control group was 164.38 cm (SD = 5.02), while the actual height was 163.71 cm (SD = 2.62).

In the group of participants with eating disorders, the average age of onset of the disorder was 21.62 (SD = 10.28), and the average duration of the disorder was 9.19 years (SD = 7.18).

Different subtypes of eating disorders and their correlation with trauma, psychoform and somatoform dissociation.

In order to study the link between different subtypes of eating disorders and trauma severity, we conducted a Kruskal–Wallis H test, which allowed us to establish that the asymptotic significance was 0.530 ($\chi^2 = 2.208$; $df = 3$; $p = 0.530$). This led us to conclude that there were no statistically significant differences between different subtypes of eating disorders as regards trauma severity (0.530 > 0.005). Using the same test, we analyzed the potential correlation between different subtypes of eating disorders and symptoms of psychoform and somatoform dissociation. Again, no statistically significant differences were found between different subtypes of eating disorders as regards symptoms of psychoform dissociation ($\chi^2 = 2.691$; $df = 3$; $p = 0.442$), nor as regards symptoms of somatoform dissociation ($\chi^2 = 4.064$; $df = 3$; $p = 0.255$), and some clear differences were found, however these were not statistically significant. For example, the DES score for the BN group was double that of the AN group (28 versus 14). Therefore, these results do not confirm two of the preliminary hypotheses of this study. On the one hand the one that which put forward the possibility that compulsive subtypes of eating disorders might correlate with higher levels of dissociation. On the other hand, we had expected a higher severity/prevalence of traumatic events in compulsive subtypes of eating disorders. Despite these expectations, the results did not show any statistically significant links between such variables.

Table 1 does, however, show that the averages for all variables were higher in patients with a diagnosis of BN than in patients with a diagnosis of AN. Amongst the former, dissociative symptoms were more prevalent, and there were more cases of traumatic childhood events, or those cases were more severe than amongst the patients with a diagnosis of AN. This was not the case for patients with a diagnosis of BED, who showed lower average values than patients with a diagnosis of AN across all variables, except for amnesia, where they scored the highest of all subtypes of eating disorders. Table 1 provides a summary of all differences found between such different subtypes as regards the following variables: childhood trauma, psychoform dissociation and somatoform dissociation.

Table 1. Differences between the subtypes of eating disorders as regards the variables: childhood trauma, psychoform dissociation and somatoform dissociation.

Variables	AN	BN	BED	EDNOS	*p*
	Average (SD)	Average (SD)	Average (SD)	Average (SD)	
DES—amnesia	5.75 (5.96)	22.5 (20.11)	26.25 (24.75)	0.62 (0.88)	0.082
DES—absorption	21.68 (13.03)	38.33 (26.16)	12 (8.48)	23 (8.48)	0.459
DES—depersonalization/derealization	12 (14.47)	15 (7.26)	2.5 (3.53)	3.33 (4.72)	0.474
DES—total	14.43 (11.85)	28.02 (17.67)	13.57 (11.11)	9.29 (3.52)	0.442
SDQ-20—total	26.6 (7.92)	39 (19)	21 (1.41)	25.5 (7.77)	0.255
CTQ—emotional abuse	11.4 (5.3)	14.33 (8.14)	6 (0)	13 (2.82)	0.556

Table 1. *Cont.*

Variables	AN	BN	BED	EDNOS	*p*
	Average (SD)	Average (SD)	Average (SD)	Average (SD)	
CTQ—physical abuse	6.6 (2.13)	12.33 (6.35)	6.5 (2.12)	7 (2.82)	0.563
CTQ—sexual abuse	8.4 (3.56)	8.67 (4.72)	5 (0)	7.5 (2.12)	0.385
CTQ—emotional neglect	11.57 (4.65)	18 (2.64)	7 (0)	17.5 (6.36)	0.059
CTQ—physical neglect	7.64 (3.67)	11.33 (5.86)	6 (1.41)	9.5 (2.12)	0.180
CTQ—total	54.71 (17.14)	69 (24.74)	50 (14.14)	66.5 (12.02)	0.530

Note. AN = anorexia nervosa group, BN = bulimia nervosa group, BED = binge-eating disorder group, EDNOS = eating disorder not otherwise specified, SD = standard deviation, DES = Dissociative Experiences Scale, SDQ-20 = Somatoform Dissociation, CTQ = Child Trauma Questionnaire.

Differences between the control group and the group of participants with eating disorders regarding trauma, psychoform dissociation and somatoform dissociation.

In order to test our hypothesis that the group of participants with eating disorders would have more, and more serious, traumatic childhood experiences, we carried out a Mann–Whitney U test compared with the control group. This time, the test concluded that the bilateral asymptotic significance was 0.000, which enabled us to determine that traumatic childhood events were more prevalent/severe in the group of participants with eating disorders than in the control group. We applied the same test across all five different types of abuse. The two groups scored quite differently for emotional abuse, physical abuse, emotional neglect and physical neglect, for which members of the group of participants with eating disorders scored significantly higher. However, the results showed no statistically significant differences between groups regarding sexual abuse.

We also conducted a set of Mann–Whitney U tests in order to test the hypothesis whereby we had expected higher levels of psychoform and somatoform dissociation in the group of participants with eating disorders. On this occasion, the results showed higher levels of psychoform dissociation in the group of participants with eating disorders, in particular for the depersonalization/derealization factor (0.001 < 0.005). For the rest of psychoform dissociation factors, as well as for the DES-II and SDQ-20 total scores, significant differences were found between the groups, which enabled us to conclude that these hypotheses are confirmed. Table 2 provides a summary of all differences found between the group of participants with eating disorders and the control group as regards the following variables: childhood trauma, psychoform dissociation and somatoform dissociation.

Table 2. Differences between the group of participants with eating disorders and the control group as regards the variables: childhood trauma, psychoform dissociation and somatoform dissociation.

Variables	Group with Eating Disorders	Control Group	*p*
	Average (SD)	Average (SD)	
DES—amnesia	9.43 (12.64)	2.32 (4.85)	**0.007**
DES—absorption	23.19 (15.21)	14.04 (8.65)	**0.015**
DES—depersonalization/derealization	10.75 (12.72)	1.98 (7.33)	**0.001**
DES—total	15.74 (12.53)	8.59 (7.65)	**0.026**
SDQ-20—total	27.68 (10.15)	21.73 (2.16)	**0.024**
CTQ—emotional abuse	11.45 (5.44)	6.09 (1.17)	**0.001**
CTQ—physical abuse	7.4 (3.39)	5.42 (0.87)	**0.016**
CTQ—sexual abuse	8.04 (3.44)	6.33 (2.43)	0.063
CTQ—emotional neglect	12.61 (5.23)	8.88 (2.99)	**0.012**
CTQ—physical neglect	8.19 (3,85)	5.38 (0,66)	**0.001**
CTQ—total	57.42 (17.09)	38.42 (6.73)	**0.000**

Note. SD = standard deviation, DES = Dissociative Experiences Scale, SDQ-20 = Significant results marked in boldface, $p < 0.05$. The statistically significant are in boldface.

4. Discussion

This study had two main initial purposes. Firstly, it attempted to provide an overview of the differences that may exist regarding childhood trauma, psychoform dissociation and somatoform dissociation in a group of women which had been diagnosed with different subtypes of an eating disorder (subtypes: AN, BN, EDNOS and BED). Secondly, it aimed to compare the results for these variables between a group of women which had been diagnosed with an eating disorder and a control group composed of healthy women with a similar age and the same sex. Our results were similar to those from previous research on this matter [11,29], which showed that trauma was more prevalent/serious amongst participants with eating disorders. Significant differences between groups were found, as regards symptoms of psychoform dissociation and somatoform dissociation.

Our results are similar from those in the study by Vanderlinden et al. (1996), in which participants with eating disorders showed greater dissociation levels than the individuals in the control group. Incidentally, the results of our research regarding childhood trauma and dissociation of both a psychoform and a somatoform nature for different subtypes of eating disorders were not statistically significant, which was also the case in some previous research in this field of study [8,11]. Despite these similar results, other pieces of research did find statistically significant differences between different subtypes of eating disorders in terms of the prevalence/severity of traumatic events and dissociative symptoms [14,29,46].

An overview of the average scores for all the variables enabled us to notice that average scores tended to be higher in BN cases, a result that is similar to that of a recent study by Palmisano et al. (2018), where there were higher dissociation levels in BN, BED and AN (purging type) sufferers [11]. Carretero et al. (2012) found that trauma exposure had been an on-going occurrence during childhood and most purging subtypes of AN, which might be explained by a more acute need to induce dissociation through impulsive behavior in patients whose condition appears to be more serious. It stands to reason that repeated abuse/trauma will have a greater psychological impact than isolated traumatic abuse/events [47].

Some authors have concluded that post-traumatic stress disorder-related symptoms, such as dissociative symptoms, are frequent in eating disorders, but that there is no correlation between the type or seriousness of the eating disorder and those symptoms [30,48]. However, Vanderlinden and Vandereycken (1999) concluded that, as far as correlation with trauma is concerned, up to 50% of women with an eating disorder suffered sexual abuse in their childhood [49]. This history of sexual abuse was found to be particularly prevalent amongst women with BN. Indeed, sexual abuse in childhood and/or adolescence is a risk factor for the development of eating disorders [30].

It should be noted, however, as a limitation, that traumatic events are not always disclosed by the patient with an eating disorder. Thus, these experiences could be dissociated and may result in false negatives (in cases where patients do not reveal a traumatic event which did, indeed, happen), or false positives (where patients report traumatic events which never happened) [23]. The seriousness of the abuse or abuses reported by the patient, as well as the length of time over which the abuse took place, should also be considered, even though this study did not provide us with any information in that regard. In addition, this study suffered, to some extent, from the limited size of both groups of participants. Many of the results found in this study might change if the number of participants increased including more participants suffering from each specific type of eating disorder, for this would enable researchers to establish relevant comparisons.

In conclusion, traumatic events during childhood as well as psychoform and somatoform dissociative symptoms are all relevant factors in the development of an eating disorder. These factors should be taken into account, and the type of correlation between different variables should be studied in more detail in future research on the topic. Current treatments for eating disorders are largely insufficient in many cases. In this respect, childhood trauma (including sexual, physical and emotional abuse as well as physical and emotional neglect) and dissociation could play a major role in improving success rates for treatments, and as such, they must not be disregarded. As early as 1994, Rosen and Petty outlined the potential correlation between eating disorders and dissociation and called for the inclusion of an educational element to treatment, whereby professionals would teach patients to recognize their own ability to dissociate. Moreover, high levels of dissociation in eating disorders have been proven to hinder the effectiveness of therapies such as cognitive behavioral therapy [18].

This study's findings, as well as those from previous studies, enable us to better grasp the reason why patients who suffered childhood abuse/trauma and who show dissociation symptoms find it extremely difficult to put a stop to the symptoms of their eating disorder.

In conclusion, we must take into account the fact that eating disorder symptoms may be used by patients as a means to fight the emotional consequences of trauma. Indeed, they are, for many patients, nothing but coping mechanisms aimed at enabling survival.

Author Contributions: Conceptualization, methodology, investigation, resources, writing—original draft preparation, writing—review and editing, visualization, supervision: M.F.R.-A., J.I.B. and J.V. All authors have read and agreed to the published version of the manuscript.

Acknowledgments: To the Open University of Madrid (support).

References

1. Lanius, R.A.; Vermetten, E.; Pain, C. *The Impact of Early Life Trauma on Health and Dissease. The Hidden Epedemic*; Cambridge University Press: Cambridge, UK, 2010.
2. Felitti, V.J.; Anda, R.F.; Nordenberg, D.; Williamson, D.F.; Spitz, A.M.; Edwards, V.; Koss, M.P.; Marks, J.S. Reprint of: Relationship of Childhood Abuse and Household Dysfunction to Many of the Leading Causes of Death in Adults: The Adverse Childhood Experiences (ACE) Study. *Am. J. Prev. Med.* **2019**, *56*, 774–786. [CrossRef] [PubMed]
3. Hughes, K.; Bellis, M.A.; Hardcastle, K.A.; Sethi, D.; Butchart, A.; Mikton, C.; Jones, L.; Dunne, M.P. The effect of multiple adverse childhood experiences on health: A systematic review and meta-analysis. *Lancet Public Health* **2017**, *2*, e356–e366. [CrossRef]
4. Felitti, V.J. Childhood sexual abuse, depression, and family dysfunction in adult obese patients: A case control study. *South. Med. J.* **1993**, *86*, 732–736. [CrossRef]
5. Scheffers, M.; Hoek, M.; Bosscher, R.J.; Van Duijin, M.A.J.; Schoevers, R.A.; Van Busschbach, J.T. Negative body experience in women with early childhood trauma: Associations with trauma severity and dissociation. *Eur. J. Psychotraumatol.* **2017**, *8*, 1322892. [CrossRef] [PubMed]
6. Van der Kolk, B.A. Clinical implications of neuroscience research in PTSD. *Ann. N. Y. Acad. Sci.* **2006**, *1071*, 277–293. [CrossRef] [PubMed]
7. Petzold, H.G. *Integrative Movement and Living Body Based Therapy. A Holistic Path of Living Body Based Psychotherapy*; Junfermann: Paderborn, Germany, 1996.
8. Backhlom, K.; Isomaa, R.; Birgegard, A. The prevalence and impact of trauma history in eating disorders patients. *Eur. J. Psychotraumatol.* **2013**, *4*, 1–8. [CrossRef] [PubMed]
9. Caslini, M.; Bartoli, F.; Crocamo, C.; Dakanalis, A.; Clerici, M.; Carrà, G. Disentangling the association between child abuse and eating disorders: A systematic review and meta-analysis. *Psychosom. Med.* **2016**, *78*, 79–90. [CrossRef] [PubMed]
10. Palmisano, G.L.; Innamorati, M.; Vanderlinden, J. Life adverse experiences in relation with obesity and binge eating disorder: A systematic review. *J. Behav. Addict.* **2016**, *5*, 11–31. [CrossRef]
11. Palmisano, G.L.; Innamorati, M.; Susca, G.; Traetta, D.; Sarracino, D.; Vanderlinden, J. Childhood traumatic experiences and dissociative phenomena in eating disorders: Level and disociation with the severity of binge eating symptoms. *J. Trauma Dissociation* **2018**, *10*, 1–20. [CrossRef]
12. Smolak, L.; Murnen, S. A meta- analytic examination of the relationship between child sexual abuse and eating disorders. *Int. J. Eat. Disord.* **2002**, *31*, 136–150. [CrossRef]
13. Pignatelli, A.M.; Wampers, M.; Loriedo, C.; Biondi, M.; Vanderlinden, J. Childhood neglect in eating disorders: A systematic review and meta- analysis. *J. Trauma Dissociation* **2017**, *18*, 100–115. [CrossRef] [PubMed]
14. Behar, R.; Arancibia, M.; Sepúlveda, E.; Muga, A. Child sexual abuse as risk factor in eating disorders. In *Eating Disorders*; Morton, N., Ed.; Nova Science Publishers: Hauppauge, NY, USA, 2016; pp. 149–172.
15. Moulton, S.J.; Newman, E.; Power, K.; Swanson, V.; Day, K. Chilhood trauma and eating psychopatology: A mediating role for dissociation and emotion dysregulation. *Child. Abuse Negl.* **2015**, *39*, 167–174. [CrossRef] [PubMed]

16. Racine, S.E.; Wildes, J.E. Emotion dysregulation and anorexia nervosa: An exploration of the role of childhood abuse. *Int. J. Eat. Disord.* **2015**, *48*, 55–58. [CrossRef] [PubMed]
17. Vanderlinden, J.; Claes, L.; De Cuyper, K.; Vrieze, E. Dissociation and dissociative disorders. In *Encyclopedia of Feeding and Eating Disorders*; Wade, T., Ed.; Springer: Singapore, 2015.
18. Beato, L.; Rodríguez; T. ; Belmonte, A. Relationship of dissociative experiences to body shape concerns in eating disorders. *Eur. Eat. Disord. Rev.* **2003**, *11*, 38–45. [CrossRef]
19. Vanderlinden, J.; Vanderreycken, W.; Van Dyck, R.; Vertommen, H. Dissociative experiences and trauma in eating disorders. *Int. J. Eat. Disord.* **1993**, *13*, 187–193. [CrossRef]
20. La Mela, C.; Maglietta, M.; Castellini, G.; Amoroso, L.; Lucarelli, S. Dissociation in eating disorders: Relationship between dissociative experiences and binge-eating episodes. *Compr. Psychiatry* **2010**, *51*, 339–400. [CrossRef]
21. Lyubomirsky, S.; Casper, R.C.; Sousa, L. What triggers abnormal eating in bulimic and non-bulimic women? The role of dissociative experiences, negative affect, and psychopathology. *Psychol. Women Q.* **2001**, *25*, 223–232. [CrossRef]
22. Rodriguez-Srednicki, O. Childhood sexual abuse, dissociation and adult self-destructive behavior. *J. Child Sex Abuse* **2001**, *10*, 75–90. [CrossRef]
23. Nijenhuis, E.R.S.; Spinhoven, P.; Van Dyck, R.; Van der Hart, O.; Vanderlinden, J. Degree of somatoform and psychological dissociation in dissociative disorder is correlated with reported trauma. *J. Trauma Stress* **1998**, *11*, 711–730. [CrossRef]
24. Nijenhuis, E. Somatoform dissociation: Major symptoms of dissociative disorders. *J. Trauma Dissociation* **2000**, *1*, 7–32. [CrossRef]
25. González-Vázquez, A.; Río-Casanova, L.; Seijo-Almendros, N.; Cabaleiro-Fernández, P.; Seoane-Pillado, T.; Justo-Alonso, A.; Santed-Germán, M.A. Validity and reliability of the Spanish version of the Somatoform Dissociation Questionnaire (SDQ-20). *Psicothema* **2017**, *29*, 275–280. [PubMed]
26. Fuller-Tyszkiewicz, M.; Mussap, A. Examining the dissociative basis for body image disturbances. *Int. J. Psychol. Stud.* **2011**, *3*, 3–13. [CrossRef]
27. Fuller-Tyszkiewicz, M.; Mussap, A. The relationship between dissociation and binge eating. *J. Trauma Dissociation* **2008**, *9*, 445–462. [CrossRef] [PubMed]
28. Brown, L.; Russell, J.; Thornton, C.; Dunn, S. Dissociation, abuse and the eating disorders: Evidence from an Australian population. *Aust. N. Z. J. Psychiatry* **1999**, *33*, 521–528. [CrossRef]
29. Dalle Grave, R.; Oliosi, M.; Todisco, P.; Bartocci, C. Trauma and dissociative experiences in eating disorders. *Dissociation Prog. Dissociative Disord.* **1996**, *9*, 274–281.
30. Oberst, U.; Baltà, M.; Sánchez, L.; Rangil, T. Trastornos disociativos en mujeres con trastornos alimentarios. *Rev. Psiqu. Facult. Med. Barc.* **2001**, *28*, 284–290.
31. American Psychiatric Association. *Diagnostic and Statistical Manual of Mental Disorders*, 4th ed.; American Psychiatric Association: Washington, DC, USA, 2000.
32. American Psychiatric Association. *Diagnostic and Statistical Manual of Mental Disorders (DSM-5TM)*; American Psychiatric Association: Arlington, VA, USA, 2013.
33. Guy, W. *Clinical Global Impression*; Department of Health, Education and Welfare: Rockville, MD, USA, 1976.
34. Sheehan, D.V.; Lecrubier, Y.; Harnett-Sheehan, K.; Janavs, J.; Weiller, E.; Bonora, L.I.; Keskiner, A.; Schinka, J.; Knapp, E.; Sheehan, M.F.; et al. Reliability and Validity of the MINI International Neuropsychiatric Interview (mini): According to the SCID-P. *Eur. Psychiatry* **1997**, *12*, 232–241. [CrossRef]
35. Ferrando, L.; Bobes, J.; Gibert, M.; Soto, M.; Soto, O. *Mini International Neuropsychiatric Interview. Versión en Español 5.0.0.DSM-IV*; Instituto IAP: Madrid, Spain, 1998.
36. First, M.B.; Gibbon, M.; Spitzer, R.L.; Williams, J.B.W.; Benjamin, L.S. *User's Guide for the Structured Clinical Interview for DSM-IV Axis II Personality Disorders*; American Psychiatric Press, Inc.: Washington, DC, USA, 1997.
37. First, M.B.; Gibbon, M.; Spitzer, R.L.; Williams, J.B.W.; Benjamin, L.S. *Entrevista Clínica Estructurada para los Trastornos de Personalidad del Eje II del DSM-IV*; Masson: Barcelona, Spain, 1999.
38. Bernstein, E.M.; Putnam, F.W. Development, reliability, and validity of a dissociation scale. *J. Nerv. Mental Dis.* **1986**, *174*, 121–130. [CrossRef]
39. Carlson, E.B.; Putnam, M.D. An update on the Dissociative Experiences Scale. *Dissociation Prog. Dissociative Disord.* **1993**, *6*, 16–25.

40. Icarán, E.; Colom, R.; Orengo, F. Experiencias disociativas: Una escala de medida. *Annu. Psicol.* **1996**, *70*, 69–84.
41. Icarán, E.; Colom, R.; Orengo, F. Estudio de validación de la escala de experiencias disociativas con muestra de población española. *Actas Luso Esp. Neurol. Psiquiatr. Cienc. Afines* **1996**, *24*, 7–10.
42. Nijenhuis, E.R.S.; Spinhoven, P.; Van Dyck, R.; Van der Hart, O.; Vanderlinden, J. The development and psychometric characteristics os the somatoform dissociation questionnaire (SDQ-20). *J. Nerv. Mental Dis.* **1996**, *184*, 688–694. [CrossRef]
43. Nijenhuis, E.R.R.; Spinhoven, P.; Vanderlinden, J.; Van Dyck, R.; Van der Hart, O. Somatoform dissociative symptoms as related to animal defensive reactions to predatory imminence and injury. *J. Abnor. Psychol.* **1998**, *107*, 63–73. [CrossRef]
44. Bernstein, D.P.; Fink, L. *Childhood Trauma Questionnaire: A Retrospective Self-Report Manual*; The Psychological Corporation: San Antonio, TX, USA, 1998.
45. Hernández, A.; Gallardo-Pujol, D.; Pereda, N.; Arntz, A.; Bernstein, D.P.; Gaviria, A.M.; Labal, A.; Valero, J.; Gutiérrez-Zotes, A. Initial validation of Spanish childhood trauma questionnaire-short form: Factor structure, reliability and association with parenting. *J. Interpers. Violence* **2013**, *20*, 1–21. [CrossRef] [PubMed]
46. Brewerton, T.D. Eating disorders, trauma and comorbidity: Focus on PTSD. *Eat. Disord.* **2007**, *15*, 285–304. [CrossRef] [PubMed]
47. Carretero-García, A.; Sánchez, L.; Doval, E.; Rusiñol, J.; Raich, R.; Vanderlinden, J. Repeated traumatic experiences in eating disorders and their association with eating symptoms. *Eat. Weight Disord.* **2012**, *17*, e267–e273. [CrossRef]
48. Gleaves, D.H.; Eberenz, K.P. Assessing dissociative symptoms in eating disordered patients: Construct validation of two self-report measures. *Int. J. Eat. Disord.* **1995**, *18*, 99–102. [CrossRef]
49. Vanderlinden, J.; Vandereycken, W. *Trauma, Disociación y Descontrol de los Impulsos en los Trastornos Alimentarios*; Granica: Barcelona, Spain, 1999.

2

Arts Therapies Interventions and their Outcomes in the Treatment of Eating Disorders

Monika Bucharová [1,*], Andrea Malá [1], Jiří Kantor [1] and Zuzana Svobodová [2]

1 Palacky University Evidence-Based Education Working Team: Mentee Centre, and Institute of Special Education Studies, Faculty of Education, Palacky University, 779 00 Olomouc, Czech Republic; maladmp@gmail.com (A.M.); jiri.kantor@upol.cz (J.K.)

2 Czech National Centre for Evidence-Based Healthcare and Knowledge Translation (Cochrane Czech Republic, Czech Evidence-Based Healthcare Centre: Joanna Briggs Institute Centre of Excellence, Masaryk University GRADE Centre), Institute of Biostatistics and Analyses, Faculty of Medicine, Masaryk University, Kamenice 3, 625 00 Brno, Czech Republic; zuzana.kelnarova@gmail.com

* Correspondence: monika.bucharova01@upol.cz

Abstract: Arts therapies (AsTs) are considered a valuable intervention for people with eating disorders, however the range of research studies and the comparison between the types of arts therapies are unknown. The goal of the future scoping review is to explore the therapeutic outcomes addressed by arts therapists in research studies on people with eating disorders and compare the different types of arts-based interventions. This scoping review will be conducted in accordance with the Joanna Briggs Institute methodology. Included will be research studies and sources oriented towards people with eating disorders of all ages and AsTs of any type (art therapy, drama therapy, music therapy, dance/movement therapy, and expressive therapies). There is no language/publication period limitation. The following databases will be searched: CINAHL Plus, EMBASE, MEDLINE (OvidSP), ProQuest Central, PsycINFO, PubMed, Scopus, and Web of Science. Sources of unpublished studies and grey literature will include Google Scholar, MedNar, clinical trials, and current controlled trials. Titles/abstracts and full texts of studies will be assessed against the inclusion criteria, and the data extracted by two independent reviewers. Based on the results, we will compare the types of AsTs according to the research designs, country/settings, intervention methods/materials, adverse effects reported, and therapeutic outcomes related to AsTs.

Keywords: arts therapies; music therapy; art therapy; drama therapy; dance/movement therapy; dance movement psychotherapy; dance therapy; eating disorder; anorexia; bulimia

---

1. Introduction

Eating disorders (EDs) are mental illnesses that cause serious disturbances to people's everyday diet. Since EDs are on the rise throughout the world, healthcare policies and practitioners need to research different treatment options and their affectivity, value for patients, and cost effectiveness, in order to make any substantial change to the growth of this disease. The goal of this paper is to explore the contribution arts therapies (AsTs) bring to the treatment of patients with EDs, based on the analysis of AsTs interventions and possible outcomes of the treatment. In the introduction section of this protocol, the theoretical framework including different aspects of EDs; their prevalence, definition, and treatment, plus the unique features of different AsTs modalities, will be presented, followed by the justification and objectives of this review proposal.

1.1. Eating Disorders and Their Clinical Aspects

Once seen as a westernized condition, the shift of EDs into the global population is accelerating [1–3]. Erskine et al. [4] states that the inclusion of EDs in the Global Burden of Disease Study (GBD) is a milestone in the recognition of the wider health issue affecting the global community. The Smink et al. [5] review of the worldwide epidemiology of eating disorders states that anorexia nervosa (AN), bulimia nervosa (BN), and binge eating disorder (BED), combined, ranked as the 12th leading cause of disability-adjusted life years (DALYs) in females between the ages of 15–19. Epidemiological studies show a clear increase in the prevalence of EDs over a study period, from 3.5% for the 2000–2006 period to 7.8% for the 2013–2018 period, which seems alarming [6]. According to the National Eating Disorder Association (NEDA) [7] up to 30 million people in the United States alone suffer from an ED. Furthermore, Qian et al. [8] found that EDs are more common in Western countries compared to Asian countries [8].

Currently there are many discussions as to why we are experiencing such a growth in ED cases. Grave [9] suggests there are various and combined causal factors such as psychological, sociocultural, biological, or family factors. People of all ages and genders, as well as cultural backgrounds, can be affected by an eating disorder [10]. On one hand, experts are partly attributing the increase to a greater awareness of the wide range of disorders and the changes in diagnostic criteria [8]. On the other hand, shifts in populations and cultural influences, the advances in technology with the surge in social media and the focus on body shape and gender roles, combined with the questioning of traditional family and work structures are contributing to changes in what is seen as healthy eating and a healthy body image.

EDs can manifest as eating extremely small amounts of food or severely overeating. The National Health Service (NHS) [11] terms EDs as an unhealthy attitude to food; an attitude by which the focal point of a person´s life is their relationship to food. In addition to maladaptive eating patterns are concerns, even obsessions, around weight and body shape/image. These behaviors are classified as mental health illnesses not because of the significant impact on the body's ability to get appropriate nutrition, but because of the psychological distress, fear of gaining weight, distorted body image, and excessive exercise, which then categorizes the ED as a biologically-influenced medical illness [12]. Further evidence shows that eating behaviors are affected by emotional regulation. Specifically, higher levels of alexithymia, a personality trait characterized by an inability to modulate and identify one's feelings and body sensations, were found in overweight persons [13]. Alexithymia frequently co-occurs with depression, anxiety, social phobia, and substance abuse, all of which are disorders which often overlap with an ED.

Eating disorders have their own specific diagnostic criteria according to both major diagnostic manuals. The American Psychiatric Association's fifth edition of Diagnostic and Statistical Manual of Mental Disorders (DSM-5) provides diagnostic criteria for pica, rumination syndrome, avoidant/restrictive food intake disorder, AN, BN, and BED [14]. The tenth revision of the International Statistical Classification of Diseases and Related Health Problems (ICD-10) by the World Health Organization provides slightly different diagnostic criteria for EDs [15]. ICD-10 recognizes diagnostic criteria for AN, atypical AN, BN, atypical BN, overeating associated with other psychological disturbances, vomiting associated with other psychological disturbances, and other eating disorders. It is common to observe migration between ED diagnoses as well as frequent use of unspecified eating disorder diagnoses [9], however, AN and BN are known as the most predominant eating disorders.

Studies point out that EDs have, in recent years, had the highest mortality risk among other psychiatric diagnoses [5], however the exact mechanism for how a person's susceptibility to an ED might work is not fully understood. Research in general concurs that a combination of genetic, biological, behavioral, psychological, and social factors can raise a person's risk [9]. Although an ED can be developed at any age, the National Institute for Health and Care Excellence (NICE) reminds us that the highest risk of development is seen in young women and men between 13 and 17 years of age [2]. Certain psychological factors and personality traits which develop during these adolescent years may predispose a person to an eating disorder [14]. Neuroticism, obsessiveness, and perfectionism can play a large role in facilitating EDs, particularly AN and BN. Individuals with these personality features are prone to anxiety and depression, and display perfectionistic and self-critical tendencies, all of which are factors that may contribute to their difficulty managing their weight and eating in a healthy manner [7,14]. Fassino et al. [16], in their controlled study of the temperament and personality of eating disorder patients, state that those diagnosed with AN tend to have high levels of harm avoidance, characterized by worrying and pessimism, and low levels of novelty seeking, characterized by a rigidity in thinking and an unwillingness towards new experiences. Individuals diagnosed with BN also show high levels of harm avoidance, but instead is it combined with high levels of novelty seeking, which is linked to the lack of impulse control associated with binge–purge behaviors [16].

For some years now it has been suggested that a developmental understanding of disordered eating would be greatly enhanced if we were to look through the lens of developmental psychopathology, more specifically the clarity and distortions that emerge from primary relationships [17]. An insecure attachment is the key risk factor to developing an ED. Attachment theory, originating from the work of Bowlby [18], offers a comprehensive framework for understanding the potential individual and family characteristics which contribute to the development of an ED. Furthermore, it provides an insight into a range of different psychological functions like emotion regulation and interpersonal functioning, which are associated with EDs [19]. Mantillia et al. [20] and Gander et al. [19] extend this point by arguing that the relationship a person has with their eating disorder is shaped by that person's understanding of what meaningful relationships should look like, this in turn has important consequences on the severity of their disorder.

Mantillia et al. [20] uses "attachment theory" to establish a link between the attachment to a significant other and the attachment to an ED. The study group researched consisted of 148 women with EDs aged from 16–25 in an outpatient setting in Sweden. ED behaviors were measured by questions looking at the regularity and the relationship of the ED to the patient. The findings showed that the less securely attached individuals experienced their ED as more in control, and themselves as less autonomous [20]. Findings from Gander et al.'s [19] study of research and literature that used a narrative-based methodology in the field of EDs in adolescences, showed a high prevalence of unresolved attachment status caused by possible abuse. So instead of choosing to be close to someone consistently, this adult attachment behavior in the patient escapes consistently into the ED in order to overcome the emotional/physical injury. A plausible link can therefore be made from this data which suggests that insecure and unresolved (disorganized) attachment types produce a tendency to internalize unexpressed emotions and the expectation of a controlling relationship which in turn produces disordered eating symptoms as a means to survive and manage the unhealthy relationship.

The treatment of EDs is one of the most difficult among other psychiatric disorders. Currently there is a large spectrum of therapeutic approaches and a strong therapeutic alliance between therapist and patient is emphasized [21]. Various forms of cognitive behavioral therapy (CBT) are widely used [21,22]. Enhanced cognitive behavioral therapy (CBT-E) was specifically developed to maintain eating disorder psychopathology and studies support its efficacy and effectiveness [23,24]. Another approach offers cognitive remediation therapy (CRT) which focuses on core cognitive processes [25]. Some of the newer approaches in the treatment of EDs are the Maudsley Anorexia Nervosa Treatment for Adults (MANTRA), as well as specialist supportive clinical management (SSCM). SSCM combines features of clinical management and supportive psychotherapy [26]. After unsuccessful application of CBT, MANTRA, or SSCM, eating-disorder-focused focal psychodynamic therapy (FPT) is applied [2]. A family-based approach for children and young people with EDs which shows promising results especially at follow-up care, and according to given evidence may be more beneficial than individual therapy [25,27]. Medication should not be offered as a sole treatment for AN, BN, or BED [2]. However pharmacotherapy is frequently prescribed in combination with CBT or other psychotherapy as a means to help decrease other psychological symptoms such as anxiety or depression [25,28]. At this stage it is challenging to describe the efficacy of each treatment approach. Outcomes of residential care in various studies reported positive results of in-patient treatment, however the difficulty remains in identifying which approach provides the most efficient outcomes since each program combines them differently [29].

1.2. Arts Therapies and Their Modalities in the Treatment of Eating Disorders

Arts therapy (AsT) disciplines which have been developed as the result of multidisciplinary efforts between artists, psychotherapists, educators, and social/health workers share common characteristics, namely the value they each place upon creativity. They each share an appreciation of the non-verbal aspect of communication and understand the use of imagery, symbolism, and metaphor as a link to psychological/emotional states. They acknowledge the need to work safely in the presence of a secure therapeutic relationship, guided with interventions that are based on the therapeutic aims of the specific individual as well as the client population [30].

A central premise of the AsTs is that any individual regardless of ability, disability, illness, or health can engage creatively in the arts and use them to help restore health and well-being. It is this open position to engage creatively that gives AsTs a unique contribution to the treatment of EDs. AsTs (also creative therapies (CTs), or creative arts therapies (CAsTs)) are defined as "the creative use of the artistic media (visual art, music, drama, and dance/movement) as vehicles for non-verbal and/or symbolic communication, within a holding environment, encouraged by a well-defined client–therapist relationship, in order to achieve personal and/or social therapeutic goals appropriate for the individual" [30] (p. 46). Apart from the main four types/specializations of AsTs (namely art therapy, music therapy, drama therapy, and dance/movement therapy), there is also an intermodal approach defined by Knill [31] called expressive arts therapies. Comparative research focusing on the unique contribution of every artistic media is needed for the further development of AsTs as a treatment intervention in the field of EDs.

EDs are present in both genders and in those with a more fluid understanding of gender, however to date EDs are more prevalent in the female population. To address gender aspects in the AsTs it is perhaps timely to mention the influence of feminist and post-feminist theories on the work with the female population in AsT practice. Approaches that lean towards exploring the social and cultural context of a person with an ED often have their roots in feminist theories as a way to gauge a broader perspective of issues that are directly linked to women. For instance Dokter [32] in her drama therapy (DT) practice identified that patients with an ED using DT as a treatment intervention are more likely to be female, and thus interventions/methods should reflect gender differences.

Compared to traditional verbal treatments, AsTs are described as non-verbal, creative, expressive, and experiential (action oriented). The creative process on a non-verbal level may lessen defense mechanisms, rationalization, intellectualization, and persuasion tendencies that are frequently used by patients with EDs when describing their symptoms and feelings on a verbal level [33]. The same defense mechanisms used by the patient to protect the self and provide a sense of control are often replicated in verbal psychotherapy. Reliance on rationalism, intellectualization, or arguments about the patients' intimate relationships with food can slow the verbal psychotherapy process and stop patients from processing their emotions on a deeper level [34]. AsTs allow patients to work with other parts of their bodies through various methods and techniques such as playing music, painting, movement, or role-play. The shift to a more "right brain" creative approach which facilitates the psychotherapeutic use of music, art, movement, and drama opens the door for the patient to shift from explaining their feelings into actually feeling them. Alternative means of expression such as metaphors can build a bridge into a deep awareness that may be missed in a more verbal treatment. Plus the engagement of other body parts in the treatment of EDs can be crucial for patients' reconnection with their bodies, as well as facilitating a better understanding and expression of emotions [10]. Although the argument for the use of creativity and non-verbal expression is both a valuable and practical resource that offers countless applications and interventions, there must also be a clear understanding of the possible risks. Physical activity as a compensation mechanism is a clear risk factor for patients who use exercise to lose weight, and therefore dance/movement therapy could be a more detrimental than helpful treatment path for the patient. As with all AsTs the therapeutic aim and intervention of the treatment must reflect the not just the ED but the individual.

As mentioned earlier, music therapy (MT), art therapy (AT), dance/movement therapy (D/MT), and drama therapy (DT) are the main four types of AsTs. Each approach has its own definition, specifics, methodology, and techniques. Since the careful description of each type of art therapy is required in more detail, the overview with specifications of each of these therapies can be found in Appendix C.

1.3. Justification of This Review Proposal and Its Objectives

There is a considerable lack of evidence-based research and outcome-focused studies in the field of AsTs and EDs [35]. While the AsTs have been clinically used as a treatment intervention in EDs, much of the published work in this area consists of case studies rather than the more robust method of randomized control trials [30,35].

The intention of the scoping review is to investigate and synthesize research evidence, aiming to map out the literature in the area of AsT interventions and their outcomes in their treatment of EDs. We will examine the scope, extent, and range of research activity undertaken in this area in order to determine the value and potential of AsTs as an intervention, and the outcomes of the treatment. Our objective is to be able to identity key concepts in the practice of AsTs and EDs, such as the therapeutic relationship, and categorize particular interventions and methods within each of the modalities: art therapy, music therapy, dance/movement therapy, and drama therapy. Although there is some primary research on AsTs and EDs, a search of Epistemonikos, Cochrane Reviews, JBI Evidence Synthesis, and Prospero showed no current or ongoing scoping review on this topic. The PCC format (P—participants/population, C—context, C—concept) was used to formulate two review questions [36]:

- What types of arts-related interventions are used in the treatment of persons with eating disorders?
- What therapeutic outcomes are addressed in research studies on persons with eating disorders related to arts therapies?

2. Materials and Methods

The proposed scoping review will be conducted in accordance with the Joanna Briggs Institute (JBI) methodology for scoping reviews [36] and according to PRISMA extension for scoping review [37] or its updates. Any deviation from this prospectively published protocol will be recorded and referred to in the full text of the scoping review.

Inclusion criteria:

- Participants: the review will consider studies that included persons of any age with eating disorders, including persons with various comorbidities such as other mental disorders (schizophrenia, schizotypal and delusional disorders, mood disorders, neurotic and stress-related disorders, disorders of adult personality and behavior, and mental disability).
- Concept: the review will consider any studies on AsTs, namely art therapy, music therapy, drama therapy, dance/movement therapy, as well as their combinations and expressive arts therapies. Excluded will be studies using arts for non-therapeutic objectives, e.g., for educational, personal, artistic, and other purposes.
- Context: the review will consider studies conducted in a broad geographical context or therapeutic setting without limitations.
- Types of sources: the review will consider all quantitative and qualitative research studies as well as systematic reviews, diploma thesis, and conference papers. Text, opinion papers, all types of non-systematic reviews, pre-conference abstracts, and bachelor theses will be excluded. There will be no time limit or language limit as long as the abstract of the paper is available in English.

The search databases will be: CINAHL Plus, EMBASE, MEDLINE (OvidSP), ProQuest Central, PsycINFO, PubMed, Scopus, and Web of Science. Sources of unpublished studies and grey literature will include Google Scholar, MedNar, clinical trials, and current controlled trials. An adapted search strategy will be used for grey literature in order to avoid an extremely high number of irrelevant results. An initial search was made in PubMed and PsycINFO (Appendix A). A manual search will be carried out in the selected books and chapters [33,34,38–40]. The reference list of all relevant studies will be screened for additional studies. The full search strategy for each database will be described in the full text of the scoping review.

Following the completion of the search, and to allow for the completion of a Preferred Reporting Items for Systematic Reviews and Meta-Analyses for Scoping Reviews (PRISMA-ScR) flow diagram [27], a full set of results will be exported from the sources into Zotero V5.0.85. Additional information, database name, export date, search terms used, number of results, grey literature sources searched, other search techniques, limitations, and duplicates will be recorded, alongside a customized field to provide comments. After the removal of duplicates, articles will then be selected in a two-step process by two reviewers working independently at each step:

- In step 1, two reviewers (MB and JK) will independently screen all the titles and abstracts returned for potential relevance. Each reviewer will assess the article against the inclusion and exclusion criteria. The proposed abstracts for full-text review will be compared between the two reviewers.
- Step 2 will be undertaken for each abstract selected. The full version of the article will be retrieved and imported into Zotero-5.0.85. Two reviewers (MB and JK) will independently undertake full-text analyses. Reasons for exclusion of full-text articles will be noted in Zotero-5.0.85 by each reviewer and provided as an appendix in the full review. The proposed full-text articles for the review will be compared between the two reviewers until a final set is agreed upon by both. The final set will be held in a Zotero-5.0.85 library. Where there is a disagreement between the two reviewers in either step, the final agreement will be sought by mutual consensus with input from a third reviewer (AM).

Data will be extracted from papers using a data extraction tool, which was developed by the authors (Appendix B: data extraction instrument). Two reviewers (MB and AM) will independently extract study data as per JBI scoping review methodology [36]. Data to be extracted from selected studies will include information about author and year, study design (quantitative studies will be described according to JBI levels of quantitative evidence), country, settings, population (number of participants, age, gender, comorbidities), methodology (data collection, analysis, description of experimental and control interventions), other therapeutic interventions (referred to in the study), type of AsTs, characteristics of arts-based interventions (materials, forms, methods/techniques, procedures/stages of therapy, length of treatment), and therapeutic outcomes related to AsTs.

3. Expected Results and Discussion

The extracted data will be presented in tabular form and as a narrative summary that aligns with the objective of the review. The table will report the following: author and year, study design (code according to JBI levels of evidence for quantitative studies), country, settings, population (number of participants, age, gender, presence of any comorbidities), methodology (measurements and any other methods used for data collection, methods of data analysis, and description of experimental and control interventions), other therapeutic interventions (referred to in the study), type of AsTs, and characteristics of arts-based interventions (therapeutic approach, materials, forms, methods/techniques, procedures/stages of therapy, length of treatment). This table may be further refined after data extraction and accompanied by graphic representations such as bar charts and diagrams. Any deviation from this protocol will be clearly detailed and justified.

In the proposed review we will compare arts/creative interventions according to different types of artistic media. This analysis may offer important information for AsT practitioners and their potential collaboration. The analysis of therapeutic outcomes related to AsTs will be important considering any potential future goals of AsT treatment of persons with EDs. The review will also offer a special comparison of therapeutic outcomes according to the type of AsTs. Furthermore, we will analyze the outcomes according to the type of research and study designs. We expect each type and design of empirical research to produce a special type of evidence that may concern the affectivity of treatment, the analysis of factors influencing the treatment, the patients' lived experience with treatment, and the personal relevance of different kinds of treatment for every patient. Based on these findings (e.g., number of quantitative and qualitative studies), it will be possible to offer recommendations for future research that would motivate future advancements in the treatment of EDs through the invention of AsTs.

4. Conclusions

This is a protocol which is prospectively designed towards a scoping review of arts therapy interventions and their outcomes in the treatment of eating disorders. It can offer essential information for practitioners and researchers, and it will provide data for the development of future protocols of systematic reviews. Furthermore, it will offer a comparison of therapeutic interventions based on different arts' medias used within each AsTs, which may potentially support the co-operation among arts therapists and stimulate a more systematic development of AsTs in the future.

Author Contributions: Conceptualization, M.B., A.M., and J.K.; methodology, J.K. and Z.S.; software, M.B.; validation, M.B., A.M., and J.K.; formal analysis, M.B. and A.M.; investigation, M.B. and A.M.; resources, J.K.; data curation; writing—original draft preparation, M.B., A.M., and J.K.; writing—review and editing, A.M. and J.K.; visualization, M.B.; supervision, A.M. and J.K.; project administration, J.K.; funding acquisition, J.K. All authors have read and agreed to the published version of the manuscript.

Acknowledgments: The first author would like to thank Hana Prikrylova Kucerova for her expertise and additional support.

Appendix A Search Formula and Preliminary Search in Databases

Search formula: eating disorder * OR anorexia OR bulimia OR anorexia nervosa OR bulimia nervosa OR binge eating disorder * (binge-eating disorder * or binge-eating syndrome * could be used as preferred term in the database) OR pica OR hyperorexia OR night eating syndrome * (night eating disorder * could be used as preferred term in the database) OR overeating OR orthorexia nervosa OR food intake disorder * and art therapy * OR art psychotherapy * OR music therapy * OR music medicine OR dramatherapy * OR drama therapy * OR psychodrama OR dance therapy * OR dance/movement therapy * OR dance/movement psychotherapy * OR arts therapy * OR expressive therapy *.

Appendix B

Table A1. Data extraction table.

Scoping Review Details	
Scoping review title:	Arts Therapies Interventions and their Outcomes in the Treatment of Eating Disorders
Review objective/s:	The aim of the prepared scoping review is to analyze the research studies on AsTs in the treatment of eating disorders.
Review question/s:	What types of arts-related interventions are used in the treatment of persons with eating disorders? What therapeutic outcomes are addressed in research studies on persons with eating disorders related to arts therapies?
Author	
Year	
Study design	
Country and settings	
Population	
Methodology	
Other therapeutic interventions	
Type of AsTs	
Characteristics of arts-based interventions	
Therapeutic outcomes related to AsTs	

Appendix C

Music therapy (MT) uses music and its unique qualities, together with a strong therapeutic relationship, to address individual goals. The American Music Therapy Association [41] defines MT as the clinical and evidence-based use of music interventions to accomplish individualized goals within a therapeutic relationship by a credentialed professional who has completed an approved music therapy training program. The AMTA definition emphasizes the importance of evidence-based music interventions. MT can address and engage with specific characteristics exhibited by clients with EDs in different ways, depending on the music therapy approach used, and framework for understanding the illness.

When working with patients who have EDs, music therapists mostly use musical improvisation (with or without structure, role-plays), receptive methods (relaxation, guided imagery to music, song lyric discussion, responding to music through art, movement, or writing), and composing (songwriting) [10,42]. MT techniques can be applied in individual as well as in group settings, however there are arguments against group work for adolescents suffering from AN. Working with those patients separately prevents them from sharing strategies and behaviors supporting their restrictive practices and it also eliminates competitive factors within the group [10].

Playing music creates an opportunity for the client to be heard and acknowledged by the therapist without having to do anything about it. Music improvisation may enable clients to reconnect with other parts of themselves as well as with others, and may encourage the client to accept their current needs. This can be a challenging concept since patients with an ED often find it difficult to both experience and tolerate emotions. However, the benefits of a client expressing themselves through music can not only support the integration of thoughts and emotions, but build a base from which patients may learn to relax and create the capacity for self-soothing techniques [10].

Art therapy (AT) integrates psychotherapeutic techniques through a creative process which involves the use of painting, drawing, sculpturing, collage, and coloring. The American Art Therapy Association [43] characterizes art therapy as an approach to mental health that utilizes the process of creating art to improve mental, physical, and emotional wellness. AT is founded upon the belief that expression through artistic means has therapeutic value, and as clients create art they may interpret what they have made and how it makes them feel. It is through a process of exploring their art that clients can look for themes that might be affecting their thoughts, emotions, and behaviors [38].

Hinz [34] suggests the use of images in AT can bypass language-based defenses and go more directly to the core of the issue with an ED patient. Since most ED suffers have a highly developed rhetoric for their ED they are less likely to censor themselves in the artistic process and argue about what they see in the final image [34,44]. Both the art product and the creative process of the AT session give insights into understanding a person's ED struggle. The art product/image can convey directly or indirectly how the patient represents themselves, their relationships, and their environment. A direct image of a patient´s family, for example, can be understood through the size, color, shape, and placement of figures on the page. Figures which are small and surrounded by space may indicate feeling lost and lonely. Images can also speak indirectly through metaphors which AT describes as the "unconscious (the part involved in creating), speaking to the conscious (the part involved in perceiving the finished product)" [34] (p. 15). As a result, the patient who consciously sees "safety" in the eating disorder may be faced with an unconscious self-revealing image that opposes the conscious rationalizing of the disease.

The process of creating art can be just as important as the image produced. Purposely chosen colors, shapes, and paper may provide an insight into the patient's likes and dislikes. The exploration of certain combinations, whether complimentary or clashing, can show the patient in a clearer way than if they had been explaining likes and dislikes in verbal psychotherapy [34,44]. Therefore, the use of art allows the patient to participate in therapy and recovery without having to reveal themselves verbally earlier than is comfortable. In summary, AT expression is able to provide information from three sources: (1) the person, (2) the process of creating, and (3) the final product [34]. Additionally, the therapeutic art images chronicle the progression of the ED recovery which may otherwise be lost or elusive in verbal psychotherapy.

Dance/movement therapy (D/MT) recognizes body movement as an implicit form of expression. The Association for Dance Movement Psychotherapy (ADMP, UK) [45] defines the field as a "relational process in which client/s and therapist engage in an empathic creative process using body movement and dance to assist integration of emotional, cognitive, physical, social, and spiritual aspects of self". As a treatment intervention, D/MT is practiced through individual or group sessions in wide range of health, education, social care, and private practice settings. The role of D/MT as an intervention in mental health continues to be explored and researched worldwide especially in the UK, USA, and Germany. Moreover, there is evidence-based research in the field of D/MT in the treatment of EDs [46,47] which indicates that D/MT can assist the patient with an ED through re-connection to feelings, improve mood states, and increased self-awareness [48]. The most recent findings from the Savidaki et al.'s [48] pilot study on the effects of dance/movement therapy on body image and alexithymia in eating disorders state that the participants of the study received the D/MT intervention positively, and appreciated the movement relationship with the therapist and the group. The ability D/MT has to address body-related issues means it has the potential to be more effective than the current verbal therapies when the crux of the psychological state is manifested in the body.

The body is the central battleground in EDs and as individuals focus on their thoughts, feelings are ignored. Ignoring feelings with processes that include and directly affect the body such as starvation, bingeing, and purging, amounts to burying the feelings through self-controlled physical sensation, the burial site being the body itself [49]. Subsequently D/MT can be seen as a promising, but potent treatment intervention, which may not be applicable for all patients. The dance/movement therapists' role is to assist a patient with an ED to experience feelings and express them through their body language, with the aim of identifying connections between what they experience in the D/MT session and how it might reflect their lives [46,47]. For this reason, the therapeutic alliance is a crucial feature as dance/movement therapists use the signals from their own bodies to respond to the expression of the patient. Developing a therapeutic relationship involves the resonance (attunement) between patient and therapist and can lead to the exploration of deeper, unconscious feelings that have been buried in the body.

Kleinman [46], alongside Ressler [50], in her extensive work with D/MT and the recovery of patients with ED suggests there are three key concepts that underline the D/MT process as building blocks for recovery: rhythmic synchrony, kinesthetic awareness, and kinesthetic empathy. When a therapist is in tune or attuned to the rhythm of the patient, through rhythmic synchrony they sharpen their somatic awareness to their own feeling states as a way of understanding possible feelings present in the patient and how they respond to them, demonstrating kinesthetic awareness. From this information the therapist can make interventions based on the deeper understanding of the patients' feelings. This capacity to experience the other is known as kinesthetic empathy, such as experiencing another's body tension, and is significant to the conjoint journey that the patient and therapist share towards recovery. The intentions of D/MT is to encourage patients to gain a more realistic perception of their feelings around food and body image, by seeing themselves mirrored/reflected in the therapists' movement [35].

Drama therapy (DT) is an embodied practice which the British Association of Dramatherapists' [51] term as a "form of psychological therapy in which all of the performance arts are utilized within the therapeutic relationship". Through the use of drama techniques such as role-play, storytelling, exploration of metaphors, empathy, distancing, witnessing, performance, and improvisation, drama therapy can support people by exploring painful and difficult life experiences in an indirect way [51–53].

A large percentage of the research on DT and EDs state that as an intervention DT often includes a level of psychodrama [32,54–56] in its application, especially in group sessions. Psychodrama founded by Moreno is a deep action method in which individuals and groups enact scenes from their lives, dreams, or fantasies in an effort to externalize unexpressed feelings, gain new insights, and practice new and more satisfying ways of being in the world. However DT literature does suggest that the experiential format of psychodrama, whereby the individual experiences the roles of protagonist, auxiliary ego, director, and observing group member, could uncover an underlying psychosis, or problem which may exacerbate an already fragile ED patient [32,57]. It seems the combination of psychodrama with the framework of DT and DT-focused methods has the potential to raise unsettling issues but provides structure and a clear technique for the expression of actions, emotions, and relationships. Since most patients with an ED may be anxious and easily frightened, it is clinically appropriate to provide predictability, structure, support, and clear explanations about each exercise [54].

The purpose of each method in DT is to better understand what the patient is trying to communicate and to offer a variety of channels in which to externalize the inner state, in order to assist psychological growth and behavioral change. As Rubin (in Brooke 2008) [54] says "dramatic enactment can create a bridge between human limitation and human aspirations, between who we are and who we want to become" (p. 174). Additionally, DT exercises according to Brooke [54] can evoke positive feelings and positive qualities in ED patients who have a rigidity about how they hold themselves and how they express themselves. For many patients the access to playfulness, spontaneity, resourcefulness, imagination, humor, and empathy represent the very qualities that have been frozen inside themselves [32,54].

There are six common DT concepts which lay down the psychological foundations of the DT intervention: transitional space, dramatic metaphor, embodiment, dramatic distancing, dramatic projection, and incorporation of additional modalities [51,52]. Each concept is aimed at concentrating either directly or indirectly on achieving integration of the mind and body, whilst encouraging the individual to see themselves as separate from their ED. The externalization and dramatic distancing assists patients in feeling they can safely analyze their attitude and behaviors within a safe transitional space, where anything can be imagined and therefore exist and potentially become reality [56].

References

1. WHO. Mental Health. Available online: http://www.who.int/mental_health/en/ (accessed on 12 August 2020).
2. NICE. Eating Disorders: Recognition and Treatment. Available online: https://www.nice.org.uk/guidance/ng69 (accessed on 9 October 2020).
3. National Association of Anorexia Nervosa and Associated Disorders. *Eating Disorder Statistics. General & Minority Stats|ANAD*. Available online: https://anad.org/education-and-awareness/about-eating-disorders/eating-disorders-statistics/ (accessed on 9 October 2020).
4. Erskine, H.E.; Whiteford, H.A.; Pike, K.M. The Global Burden of Eating Disorders. *Curr. Opin. Psychiatry* **2016**, *29*, 346–353. [CrossRef] [PubMed]
5. Smink, F.R.E.; van Hoeken, D.; Hoek, H.W. Epidemiology of Eating Disorders: Incidence, Prevalence and Mortality Rates. *Curr. Psychiatry Rep.* **2012**, *14*, 406–414. [CrossRef] [PubMed]
6. Galmiche, M.; Déchelotte, P.; Lambert, G.; Tavolacci, M.P. Prevalence of Eating Disorders over the 2000-2018 Period: A Systematic Literature Review. *Am. J. Clin. Nutr.* **2019**, *109*, 1402–1413. [CrossRef] [PubMed]
7. NEDA. Available online: https://www.nationaleatingdisorders.org/about-us/our-work (accessed on 9 October 2020).
8. Qian, J.; Hu, Q.; Wan, Y.; Li, T.; Wu, M.; Ren, Z.; Yu, D. Prevalence of Eating Disorders in the General Population: A Systematic Review. *Shanghai Arch. Psychiatry* **2013**, *25*, 212–223. [CrossRef]
9. Grave, R.D. Eating Disorders: Progress and Challenges. *Eur. J. Intern. Med.* **2011**, *22*, 153–160. [CrossRef] [PubMed]
10. Edwards, J. *The Oxford Handbook of Music Therapy*; Oxford University Press: Oxford, UK, 2016. [CrossRef]
11. National Health Service (NHS). Eating Disorders. Available online: https://www.nhs.uk/conditions/eating-disorders/ (accessed on 9 October 2020).
12. National Institute of Mental Health (NIMH). NIMH Eating Disorders: About More Than Food. Available online: https://www.nimh.nih.gov/health/publications/eating-disorders/index.shtml (accessed on 9 October 2020).
13. Casagrande, M.; Boncompagni, I.; Forte, G.; Guarino, A.; Favieri, F. Emotion and Overeating Behavior: Effects of Alexithymia and Emotional Regulation on Overweight and Obesity. *Eat. Weight Disord. Stud. Anorex. Bulim. Obes.* **2020**, *25*, 1333–1345. [CrossRef]
14. American Psychiatric Association. *Diagnostic and Statistical Manual of Mental Disorders*, 5th ed.; American Psychiatric Association: Washington, DC, USA, 2013.
15. *International Statistical Classification of Diseases and Related Health Problems*, 10th revision, 2nd ed.; World Health Organization (Ed.) World Health Organization: Geneva, Switzerland, 2004.
16. Fassino, S.; Abbate-Daga, G.; Amianto, F.; Leombruni, P.; Boggio, S.; Rovera, G.G. Temperament and Character Profile of Eating Disorders: A Controlled Study with the Temperament and Character Inventory. *Int. J. Eat. Disord.* **2002**, *32*, 412–425. [CrossRef]
17. Attie, I.; Brooks-Gunn, J.; Petersen, A.C. A Developmental Perspective on Eating Disorders and Eating Problems. In *Handbook of Developmental Psychopathology*; Lewis, M., Miller, S.M., Eds.; Springer US: Boston, MA, USA, 1990; pp. 409–420. [CrossRef]
18. Bowlby, J. Attachment and Loss: Volume II: Separation, Anxiety and Anger. In *Attachment and Loss: Volume II: Separation, Anxiety and Anger*; The Hogarth Press and the Institute of Psycho-Analysis: London, UK, 1973; pp. 1–429.
19. Gander, M.; Sevecke, K.; Buchheim, A. Eating Disorders in Adolescence: Attachment Issues from a Developmental Perspective. *Front. Psychol.* **2015**, *6*. [CrossRef]
20. Forsén Mantilla, E.; Clinton, D.; Birgegård, A. The Unsafe Haven: Eating Disorders as Attachment Relationships. *Psychol. Psychother.* **2019**, *92*, 379–393. [CrossRef]
21. Allen, S.; Dalton, W.T. Treatment of Eating Disorders in Primary Care: A Systematic Review. *J. Health Psychol.* **2011**, *16*, 1165–1176. [CrossRef]
22. Grilo, C.M.; Mitchell, J.E. *The Treatment of Eating Disorders: A Clinical Handbook*; Guilford Publications: New York, NY, USA, 2009.

23. Atwood, M.E.; Friedman, A. A Systematic Review of Enhanced Cognitive Behavioral Therapy (CBT-E) for Eating Disorders. *Int. J. Eat. Disord.* **2019**, *53*, 311–330. [CrossRef] [PubMed]
24. Murphy, R.; Straebler, S.; Cooper, Z.; Fairburn, C.G. Cognitive Behavioral Therapy for Eating Disorders. *Psychiatr. Clin. N. Am.* **2010**, *33*, 611–627. [CrossRef] [PubMed]
25. Agras, W.S.; Robinson, A. *The Oxford Handbook of Eating Disorders*; Oxford University Press: Oxford, UK, 2018. [CrossRef]
26. McIntosh, V.V.W.; Jordan, J.; Luty, S.E.; Carter, F.A.; McKenzie, J.M.; Bulik, C.M.; Joyce, P.R. Specialist Supportive Clinical Management for Anorexia Nervosa. *Int. J. Eat. Disord.* **2006**, *39*, 625–632. [CrossRef] [PubMed]
27. Couturier, J.; Kimber, M.; Szatmari, P. Efficacy of Family-Based Treatment for Adolescents with Eating Disorders: A Systematic Review and Meta-Analysis. *Int. J. Eat. Disord.* **2013**, *46*, 3–11. [CrossRef] [PubMed]
28. Svaldi, J.; Schmitz, F.; Baur, J.; Hartmann, A.S.; Legenbauer, T.; Thaler, C.; von Wietersheim, J.; de Zwaan, M.; Tuschen-Caffier, B. Efficacy of Psychotherapies and Pharmacotherapies for Bulimia Nervosa. *Psychol. Med.* **2019**, *49*, 898–910. [CrossRef] [PubMed]
29. Peckmezian, T.; Paxton, S.J. A Systematic Review of Outcomes Following Residential Treatment for Eating Disorders. *Eur. Eat. Disord. Rev.* **2020**, *28*, 246–259. [CrossRef]
30. Karkou, V.; Sanderson, P. *Arts Therapies: A Research-Based Map of the Field*; Elsevier Churchill Livingstone: Edinburgh, UK; New York, NY, USA, 2006.
31. Estrella, K. Expressive Therapy: An Integrated Arts Approach. In *Expressive Therapies*; Guilford Publications: New York, NY, USA, 2007.
32. Dokter, D. (Ed.) *Arts Therapies and Clients with Eating Disorders: Fragile Board*; Jessica Kingsley: London, UK; Bristol, UK, 1994.
33. Levens, M. *Eating Disorders and Magical Control of the Body*, 1st ed.; Routledge: London, UK; New York, NY, USA, 1995.
34. Hinz, L.D. *Drawing from Within: Using Art to Treat Eating Disorders*; Jessica Kingsley Publishers: London, UK, 2006.
35. Frisch, M.J.; Franko, D.L.; Herzog, D.B. Arts-Based Therapies in the Treatment of Eating Disorders. *Eat. Disord.* **2006**, *14*, 131–142. [CrossRef]
36. Peters, M.; Godfrey, C.; McInerney, P.; Munn, Z.; Trico, A.; Khalil, H. Chapter 11: Scoping Reviews (2020 version). In *JBI Manual for Evidence Synthesis*; Aromataris, E., Munn, Z., Eds.; JBI: Adelaide, Australia, 2020; Available online: https://synthesismanual.jbi.global (accessed on 11 October 2020). [CrossRef]
37. Page, M.J.; McKenzie, J.; Bossuyt, P.; Boutron, I.; Hoffmann, T.; Mulrow, C.; Shamseer, L.; Tetzlaff, J.; Akl, E.; Brennan, S.E.; et al. The PRISMA 2020 Statement: An Updated Guideline for Reporting Systematic Reviews. *Meta ArXiv* **2020**. [CrossRef]
38. Gussak, D.E.; Rosal, M.L. (Eds.) *The Wiley Handbook of Art Therapy: Gussak/The Wiley Handbook of Art Therapy*; John Wiley & Sons, Ltd: Chichester, UK, 2015. [CrossRef]
39. Heiderscheit, A. (Ed.) *Creative Arts Therapies and Clients with Eating Disorders*; Jessica Kingsley Publishers: London, UK; Philadelphia, PA, USA, 2016.
40. Rabin, M. *Art Therapy and Eating Disorders: The Self as Significant Form*; Columbia University Press: New York, NY, USA, 2003.
41. American Music Therapy Association (AMTA). Available online: https://www.musictherapy.org/ (accessed on 11 October 2020).
42. Tileston, P. Adults and Adolescents with Eating Disorders. In *Guidelines for Music Therapy Practice in Mental Health*; Eyre, L., Ed.; Barcelona Publishers: New Braunfels, TX, USA, 2013; p. 968.
43. American Art Therapy Association. Available online: https://arttherapy.org/ (accessed on 11 October 2020).
44. Hunter, M. Art Therapy and Eating Disorders. In *The Wiley Handbook of Art Therapy*; John Wiley & Sons: Chichester, UK, 2016; p. 387.
45. Association for Dance Movement Psychotherapy. Available online: https://admp.org.uk/ (accessed on 11 October 2020).
46. Kleinman, S. Becoming Whole Again; Dance/Movement Therapy for Those Who Suffer from Eating Disorders. In *The Art and Science of Dance/Movement Therapy: Life Is Dance*; Chaiklin, S., Wengrower, H., Eds.; Routledge: London, UK, 2009.

47. Meekums, B.; Vaverniece, I.; Majore-Dusele, I.; Rasnacs, O. Dance Movement Therapy for Obese Women with Emotional Eating: A Controlled Pilot Study. *Arts Psychother.* **2012**, *39*, 126–133. [CrossRef]
48. Savidaki, M.; Demirtoka, S.; Rodríguez-Jiménez, R.-M. Re-Inhabiting One's Body: A Pilot Study on the Effects of Dance Movement Therapy on Body Image and Alexithymia in Eating Disorders. *J. Eat. Disord.* **2020**, *8*, 22. [CrossRef]
49. Ressler, A.; Kleinman, S.; Mott, E. The Use of Holistic Methods to Integrate the Shattered Self. In *Treatment of Eating Disorders*; Elsevier: Amsterdam, The Netherlands, 2010; pp. 405–423. [CrossRef]
50. Ressler, A.; Kleinman, S. Experiential and Somatopsychic Approaches to Body Image Change. In *Encyclopedia of Body Image and Human Appearance*; Cash, T., Ed.; Academic Press: San Diego, CA, USA, 2012; pp. 418–424.
51. The British Association of Dramatherapists. Available online: https://badth.org.uk/ (accessed on 11 October 2020).
52. North American Drama Therapy Association. Available online: https://www.nadta.org/ (accessed on 11 October 2020).
53. Olejníčková, J.; Kantor, J.; Maštalíř, J.; Valenta, M.; Růžička, M. Trust in Dramatherapy Intervention in Patients with a Neurotic Disorder. *Rehabilitacia* **2020**, *57*, 21–30.
54. Brooke, S.L. (Ed.) *The Creative Therapies and Eating Disorders*; Charles C. Thomas: Springfield, IL, USA, 2008.
55. Pellicciari, A.; Rossi, F.; Iero, L.; Di Pietro, E.; Verrotti, A.; Franzoni, E. Drama Therapy and Eating Disorders: A Historical Perspective and an Overview of a Bolognese Project for Adolescents. *J. Altern. Complement. Med. N. Y.* **2013**, *19*. [CrossRef] [PubMed]
56. Wood, L.L.; Schneider, C. Setting the Stage for Self-Attunement: Drama Therapy as a Guide for Neural Integration in the Treatment of Eating Disorders. *Drama Ther. Rev.* **2015**, *1*, 55–70. [CrossRef]
57. Pramann, R. Benefits, Limitations, and Potential Harm in Psychodrama. Available online: http://cccutah.org/blph.pdf (accessed on 11 October 2020).

3

Food Addiction, Binge Eating Disorder and Obesity: Is there a Relationship?

Tracy Burrows [1,2,*], Janelle Skinner [1,2], Rebecca McKenna [1,2] and Megan Rollo [1,2]

1 School of Health Sciences, Faculty of Health and Medicine, University of Newcastle, Callaghan 2308, Australia; Janelle.skinner@uon.edu.au (J.S.); Rebecca.Mckenna@uon.edu.au (R.M.); megan.rollo@newcastle.edu.au (M.R.)

2 Priority Research Centre for Physical Activity and Nutrition, University of Newcastle, Callaghan 2308, Australia

* Correspondence: tracy.burrows@newcastle.edu.au

Abstract: Existing research suggests that there is an overlap between binge eating disorder (BED) and the construct of 'food addiction' (FA). The objective of this study was to determine the overlapping features of BED and FA through a comparison of the individual scales of commonly used tools including the Binge Eating Scale (BES) and the Yale Food Addiction Scale (YFAS) in a sample of Australian adults. Adults (>18 years of age) were invited to complete an anonymous online survey on FA. Binge eating was assessed through the BES and addictive eating behaviours were assessed through the YFAS ($n = 1344$). The prevalence and severity of both FA and binge eating increased across weight categories. The overall correlation between the total score from the BES and FA symptoms was $r = 0.76$, $p < 0.001$; for females it was $r = 0.77$, $p < 0.001$, and for males it was $r = 0.65$, $p < 0.001$. Total BES score and the BES emotion factor were most often associated with FA symptoms, as was demonstrated to produce stronger correlations with FA symptoms. In contrast, the BES behaviour factor was less strongly associated to FA with the majority of correlations <0.6. This study demonstrates the overlap between BED and FA, and highlights the possible unique differences between the forms of disordered eating.

Keywords: binge eating; food addiction

---

1. Introduction

'Food addiction' (FA) presents as a contentious construct, which has yet to gain scientific acceptance due to an overall lack of high quality research [1]. There is scientific debate about the appropriateness of terminology, with 'eating addiction' previously proposed to be more reflective rather than 'food addiction', given the uncertainty of whether addictive eating behaviours more closely align to substance-based addictions, like drug and alcohol addictions, or with behavioural addictions, such as gambling addiction [2]. Addictions to drugs, alcohol, and gambling are formally recognised in the Diagnostic Statistics Manual, version 5 (DSM-5) [2]. However, FA is currently not a recognised condition in DSM and instead is characterised through the assessment and endorsement of addiction-like symptoms through self-report tools or surveys. The most commonly used tool is the Yale Food Addiction Scale (YFAS). Originally developed in 2009 and revised in 2016, the YFAS 2.0 maps to the criteria used to classify substance dependence [3]. The YFAS tool assesses 11 symptoms of addiction, as well the level of distress associated with them, which parallel other addiction symptoms in DSM such as tolerance and craving. In addition, the tool can determine the level of severity of addiction ranging from mild to severe [4].

There has been previous suggestion that FA may be a sub-type of disordered eating, and that the FA construct is an indicator of higher eating disorder severity [5]. Research suggests that FA does show overlap with several disordered eating phenotypes, with the majority of existing research investigating binge eating disorder (BED) and bulimia nervosa rather than other disordered eating categories such as anorexia nervosa [6,7].

BED is classified by the DSM-5 as the recurrent, periodic, and uncontrolled consumption of large quantities of food without compensatory behaviours (e.g., purging, laxative use) to control weight [8]. It has been estimated that BED affects approximately 2% of the global population [9], while FA affects approximately 20%, with both conditions found to be more common in females [1,10]. The prevalence of FA in two existing studies of individuals with diagnosed BED was 41.5% and 56.8% [11,12]. The prevalence of FA in individuals with a current diagnosis of bulimia nervosa was 83.6% and 100%, and 30% of individuals with a history of bulimia nervosa met the diagnostic criteria for FA [13,14]. In a more recent study of individuals with clinical BED assessed through an objective clinical interview rather than self-report, those with BED were also identified with FA (33.8%). Existing research suggests an overlap between these conditions, often through cross-sectional studies, which show that the overlap between BED and FA varies between 0.59 and 0.78) [1]. The overlap between BED and FA however is not 100%, and while binge eating is a key eating disorder feature, the association between FA and disordered eating behaviour is unclear. It is acknowledged that the symptoms of general psychological distress found to be associated with FA are strongly associated with binge eating and other eating disorder symptoms [15,16].

Similarities in symptomology that exist between FA and BED include the consumption of larger amounts of food than intended, reduced control over eating and continued use despite negative consequences [13,17], intense cravings [18], emotional dysregulation, and increased impulsivity [5,6,19]. Due to these similarities, it is not unusual that BED and FA are often highly correlated. A meta-analysis also reported that YFAS symptom scores were positively associated with binge eating behaviours [1].

Existing research has investigated FA specifically in binge eating populations and individuals seeking bariatric surgery, and identified similarities in the specific characteristics of both conditions when assessed by validated surveys [20,21]. In addition, recent research highlights the associations between patterns of compulsive overeating, including binge eating with 'food addiction' [22]. However, these conditions have not been investigated at the scale, factor, or item level of common assessment scales. Instead previous research has explored associations in absolute scores that indicate the overall severity of FA or BED. Investigating factor levels for these constructs may provide important information about where the overlapping features exist and whether there are factors which separate these conditions. Strong correlations would be expected between subscales that may map to the same attribute, and lower correlations between subscales from different attributes. Therefore, the current study aims to determine the overlapping features of BED and FA through a comparison of the individual constructs of the Binge Eating Scale (BES) and YFAS in a sample of Australian adults.

2. Materials and Methods

Participants aged 18 years or above and living in Australia were invited to complete an anonymous online survey on FA. The survey took approximately 20 min to complete. Exclusion criteria included being pregnant/currently lactating and being unable to comprehend English. Recruitment was undertaken over a three month period in 2016. The study was advertised through University of Newcastle media releases and promoted via a variety of social media platforms (i.e., Facebook, Twitter). The advertisements contained a link to the survey, and participants provided informed consent before completing the survey. Survey completers were invited to enter a prize draw to win 1 of 10 shopping vouchers ($50 value). This study was approved by The University of Newcastle Ethics Committee.

The survey comprehensively assessed a range of measures relating to diet and mental health which has been previously reported [15]. The current study is a secondary analysis relating specifically to FA and BED status. Demographic information was assessed through 10 items and included information on gender, age, ethnicity, marital status, postcode, highest level of education, height, and weight, which was converted into body mass index (BMI) using standardised equations. Participants' BMI was then classified according to World Health Organisation classifications [23]. Postcode was used to determine the Index of Relative Socioeconomic Advantage and Disadvantage (ISRAD), where postcode is rated from one (most disadvantage/least advantage) to 10 (least disadvantaged/most advantaged).

FA was assessed using the 35-item YFAS 2.0 [4]. Each question offers a participant an option of eight responses ranging from 'never' to 'every day'. Each symptom is considered met when one or more of the relevant questions for each criteria meet a predefined threshold. It provides a 'diagnosis' of FA which, depending on the number of symptoms endorsed, can be classified as 'mild', 'moderate' or 'severe'. A mild diagnosis score is given when 2–3 symptoms are reported, moderate when 4–5 symptoms are present, and severe when 6 or more symptoms. Symptoms include tolerance, withdrawal, and loss of control with respect to eating behaviour. The YFAS 2.0 asks participants to think of specific foods such as highly processed foods; however, participants in this study were asked to consider all food. In the current study, the Cronbach alpha for this tool was 0.95, indicating acceptable internal consistency.

Binge eating was assessed through the standardised BES, which comprises 16 questions. Each question requires a response consisting of three to four possible responses, reflecting a range of severity. The total score is tallied to give a score out of 46, with higher scores representing increased binge status. Based on the total score, individuals can be classified as 'no binge eating' if the score is ≤17, 'mild to moderate binge eating' if the score is 18–26, and 'severe binge eating' if the score is >27. The BES has been previously shown to have a two-factor structure, which was originally demonstrated by Gormally et al. [24] and confirmed more recently by Kelly et al. [25]. These factors relate to (1) behavioural manifestations (eight items) including factors such as eating large amounts of food, and (2) feelings and cognitions (eight items) surrounding a binge eating episode including guilt, fear of not being able to stop eating, and preoccupation with eating. For the current study, in addition to the total score, the two-factor scores were also determined according to author instructions. The BES is not designed as a direct measure of BED [26]. In the current, study the Cronbach alpha for this tool was 0.92, indicating acceptable internal consistency.

Statistics: Descriptive statistics were undertaken, *t*-tests were used to examine differences between groups (food addicted vs. non-food addicted or females vs. males). ANOVA were used to determine differences in addiction severity (mild, moderate, severe). Correlation matrices for the scales for both YFAS and BES were undertaken. Also, Spearman and Pearson correlations were determined in the cases where data distribution was not normal. Both correlations produced similar results; associations between factors of the BES and between symptoms of the YFAS are presented using Pearson correlations. Correlations were determined as small (0.1–0.2), medium (0.3–0.5), or large (>0.6). The correlation analysis between scales used for this study has been undertaken in previous health research [27]. The results presented are for complete cases, with 869 of the 1344 respondents who started the survey having answered all questions. A missing value analysis was undertaken, and the demographics of those with missing values were compared, with no patterns identified. Therefore, there was no imputation of data for missing values. Due to the multiple statistical tests completed as part of this analysis, data were adjusted using a Bonferroni correction with a lower statistical threshold, and a statistical significance of $p < 0.01$. Data was analysed using SPSS version 22.0 (SPSS Inc., Chicago, IL, USA).

3. Results

3.1. Participants

The survey recruited $n = 1344$ individual; 80.7% were female and 19.3% were male. The demographic details can be found in Table 1. The mean ISRAD score was 6.2 ± 2.9, reflecting a moderate socioeconomic status; however, this value varied from 1–10, reflecting a moderately diverse population group. A total of 44.3% of the sample were married, 27% were never married, and 14.5% had been married but were without a current partner. The population comprised 1.6% with a trade/apprenticeship, 20% with a certificate/diploma, 36% with a university degree, and 31% with a higher education including masters, Ph.D.

3.2. Food Addiction and Binge Eating

Across the whole sample, the prevalence of FA was found to be 22.2% ($n = 228$). This differed significantly by gender, with females (24.4%) having a higher prevalence than males (13.3%; $p < 0.001$). According to the YFAS 2.0 categorisations of severity, the majority of individuals classified as severely food addicted 18.9% ($n = 194$), while 2.6% ($n = 27$) were moderately addicted, and <1% were classified as mild. The prevalence and severity of both FA and binge eating increased across weight categories (Table 2).

Table 1. Demographic details of samples according to food addiction status.

Demographic	NFA Male ($n = 176$)	FA Male ($n = 27$)	p Value	NFA Female ($n = 624$)	FA Female ($n = 201$)	p Value
	Mean ± SD	Mean ± SD		Mean ± SD	Mean ± SD	
Age (years)	42.0 ± 13.2	46.0 ± 16.4	0.531	39.6 ± 13.1	40.1 ± 13.0	0.407
Height (cm)	178.8 ± 0.1	179.7 ± 0.1	0.629	166.0 ± 0.1	165.9 ± 0.1	0.935
Weight (kg)	87.4 ± 15.4	113.7 ± 28.3	<0.01	70.0 ± 16.7	88.4 ± 22.9	<0.01
BMI * (kg/m^2)	27.4 ± 4.8	35.4 ± 8.8	<0.01	25.5 ± 6.0	32.7 ± 13.1	<0.01
	$n = 149$	$n = 22$		$n = 517$	$n = 183$	
BES total	7.4 ± 5.8	20.1 ± 6.1	<0.01	8.5 ± 6.5	22.8 ± 8.1	<0.01

Note: Statistically significant differences between sex determined by t-tests. NFA, non-food addicted; FA, food addicted; BES, Binge Eating Survey. BMI body mass index

Table 2. Comparison of food addiction (FA) and Binge Eating (BE) according to BMI category [a].

Condition	Underweight ($n = 14$)	Healthy ($n = 439$)	Overweight ($n = 263$)	Obese ($n = 286$)	p Value
Food Addiction (FA)	%	%	%	%	
NFA	85.7	92.5	78.7	53.8	<0.001
Mild FA	0.0	0.9	0.4	0.7	0.368
Moderate FA	7.1	1.6	3.4	3.5	0.07
Severe FA	7.1	5.0	17.5	42.0	<0.001
Binge Eating (BE)					
Non-bingeing	90.0	89.3	74.8	50.6	<0.001
Moderate	10.0	7.5	19.5	30.4	<0.001
Severe	0.0	3.2	5.8	19.0	<0.001

Note: Data are shown as percentages within each group. Statistical significance was determined using ANOVA between weight categories [a] BMI categories (kg/m^2): Underweight ≤18.50, Healthy = 18.50–24.99, Overweight = 25.00–29.99, Obese ≥30.00. FA, food addiction; NFA, non-food addicted.

For those who had completed the BES, the mean BES score was 11.9 ± 9.3 (range 0–42). For males the mean BES scores was 9.2 ± 7.4 (range 0–36), and for females the mean score was 12.6 ± 9.6 (range 0–42). The mean values for each sex were significantly different ($p < 0.01$). For the BES, severity for the total group was determined, with 74% of individuals classified as non-binge eaters ($n = 660$), 17.4% ($n = 155$) moderate binge eaters, and 8.7% ($n = 78$) severe binge eaters. Differences in BES severity were determined by sex, and significant differences were found between males and females. Among non-binge eaters, males accounted for 86.2% vs. females 70.9%, among moderate binge eaters it was males 12.1% vs. females 18.6%, and among severe binge eaters it was males 1.7% vs. females 10.4%, all $p < 0.01$. Individuals with FA reported significantly higher on the BES total, emotions, and behavioural scales than those who were non-food addicted (Table 3). Of those with FA, 72.7% reported scores of either moderate (41%) or severe (31.7%) bingeing compared with only 9.9% in the non-food addicted group. A significant correlation was found between the two-factor scores of behaviours and emotions of the BES: $r = 0.82$, $p < 0.001$ (Table 4).

Table 3. Comparison of BES scores and categories according to food addiction status.

Condition	NFA (n = 666)	FA (n = 205)	p Value
	Mean ± SD	Mean ± SD	
BES total	8.23 ± 6.35	22.56 ± 7.93	<0.001
BES emotions	4.05 ± 3.71	12.76 ± 4.44	<0.001
BES behaviours	4.72 ± 3.66	11.56 ± 4.75	<0.001
	%	%	
Non-bingeing	90.1	27.3	<0.001
Moderate bingeing	9.0	41.0	0.046
Severe bingeing	0.9	31.7	<0.001
Total	100.0	100.0	

Note: BES, Binge Eating Survey; NFA, Non-food addicted; FA, food addicted. Differences in BES scores determined by independent samples t-tests, differences in proportions for BES category determined by chi squares.

Table 4. Pearson correlation coefficients between the BES factors and YFAS symptoms (n = 953).

Measure	**BES Total**	**BES Emotions**	**BES Behaviours**
Binge Eating			
1. BES total	-		
2. BES emotions	0.95 ***	-	
3. BES behaviours	0.96 ***	0.82 ***	-
Food Addiction			
4. Total FA symptoms	0.76 ***	0.75 ***	0.71 ***
5. Consumed more than planned	0.24 ***	0.21 ***	0.25 ***
6. Unable to cut down or stop	0.61 ***	0.62 ***	0.55 ***
7. Great deal of time spent	0.58 ***	0.55 ***	0.56 ***
8. Activities given up or reduced	0.61 ***	0.61 ***	0.56 ***
9. Continued use despite physical/emotional consequences	0.67 ***	0.67 ***	0.60 ***
10. Tolerance	0.54 ***	0.54 ***	0.50 ***
11. Withdrawal	0.52 ***	0.52 ***	0.48 ***
12. Continued use despite social consequences	0.52 ***	0.51 ***	0.48 ***
13. Fail to fulfil roles and obligations	0.53 ***	0.53 ***	0.48 ***
14. Use in physically hazardous situations	−0.49 ***	−0.50 ***	−0.44 ***
15. Craving	0.65 ***	0.64 ***	0.59 ***
16. Impairment or distress	0.68 ***	0.70 ***	0.61 ***

*** $p < 0.001$. Shading indicates correlations that are > r = 0.6, BES, Binge Eating Survey; YFAS, Yale Food Addiction Scale.

3.3. *Relationships between Food Addiction and Binge Eating*

The overall correlation between the total score from the BES and FA symptoms was $r = 0.76$, $p < 0.001$; for females it was $r = 0.77$, $p < 0.001$, and for males it was $r = 0.65$, $p < 0.001$ (Figure 1). Total BES score and BES emotion factor were more strongly associated with FA symptoms, as evidenced by the majority of correlations ($n = 7$) with values >0.6. In contrast, the BES behaviour factor was less strongly associated to FA, as evidenced by smaller correlation values, with only three correlations classified as large ($r > 0.6$, $p < 0.001$). Of the 11 individual FA symptoms and clinical impairments, correlations with BES factors and the FA symptoms 'consumed more than planned' were small, with the majority being <0.3, while 'use in physically hazardous situations' produced significant negative correlations.

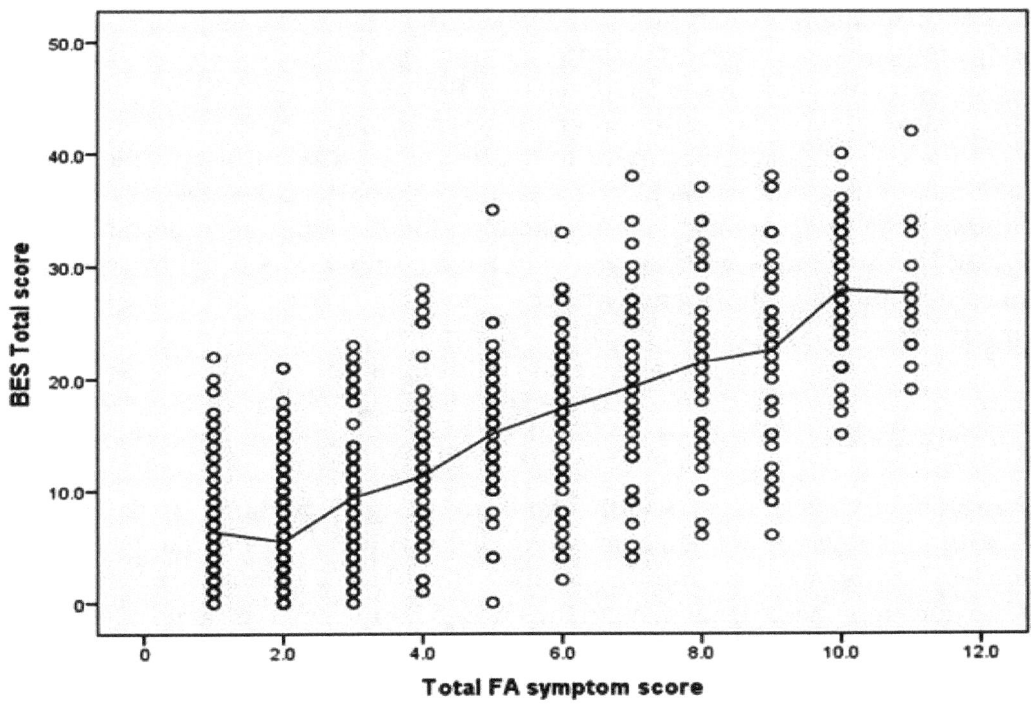

Figure 1. Correlation between BES total scores and YFAS symptom scores.

4. Discussion

This study investigated the overlap in symptoms of FA and BED as measured by the YFAS 2.0 and the BES's emotional and behavioural factors. It was found that substantial overlap (r = 0.76) exists between the commonly used assessment tools in a sample of Australian adults from a wide age range, which concurs with existing research [28,29]. However, this is the first study to demonstrate that the strongest overlap occurred with the BES emotion factor, while less overlap was observed with the BES behaviour factor. This was evidenced by larger correlation values with the BES emotion factor, compared with very few strong correlations (greater than 0.6) with the BES behaviour factor. The behaviour factor relates to behavioural expressions surrounding a binge eating episode which showed small to moderate correlations with the majority of the 11 symptoms assessed by the YFAS 2.0 tool. These correlations are not unexpected, as previous findings indicate that individuals with co-existing FA and BED experience significantly higher levels of depression, negative affect, poorer emotion dysregulation, and lower self-esteem [11]. This would seem to indicate that high levels of emotional and psychosocial distress accompany both eating pathologies. Research has demonstrated that, in the context of binge eating, emotions and behaviour rarely occur exclusively [30] and are correlated as shown in this study. For this reason, it would be expected that both features be present and it is unsurprising that these symptoms would co-occur in FA. However, strong evidence for the cognitive and behavioural aspects of BED is lacking, and further investigations into BED and behaviour are warranted.

It is important to attempt to articulate the unique features that may set the construct of FA apart from BED, given that previous overlaps have been shown, although these are not in entirety or not 100% overlapping. In this study, it appears that several symptoms are unique to FA, as evidenced by lower correlation valueswith BES. Specifically, small associations were found with FA symptoms of 'consumed more than planned' or 'use in physically hazardous situations'; the latter symptom in this study actually showed significant negative relationships. The symptom of 'use in physically hazardous situations' has previously been debated as a difficult factor to interpret in relation to food, given that food in its true sense is needed for survival. Recent studies assessing FA using the YFAS 2.0 tool have found the endorsement of 'use in physically hazardous situations' symptom in three non-clinical samples (n = 1900) to have low endorsement rates ranging from 9.1% to 24.8%; with two of the studies reporting the endorsement rate in FA individuals (n = 109) as 37.0% and 68.3%, respectively [4,28,31]. However, in the context of FA, this symptom can be described as causing impairment to performance, such as eating while driving, or impairment to health that is hazardous. In the context of obesity and related metabolic syndrome risk factors, this could include the consequences of individuals with diabetes, dyslipidaemia, or hypertension overconsuming foods containing excessive amounts of sugar, fat, or sodium [32]. However, this symptom may not have been well-reported by participants with this rationale in mind nor understood in terms of addiction by the participants completing the surveys, thus influencing the results because the questions did not ask participants to consider this aspect of the symptom. Existing public views suggest that individuals believe some foods are addictive and that addiction can cause obesity [33]. Future qualitative work on FA is warranted to better understand how the symptoms are experienced and if they differ for each individual, particularly as this field is still emerging.

The FA symptom of "loss of control with respect to eating behaviour" overlaps with that of "loss of control over eating", the latter being a core eating disorder behaviour and a diagnostic criterion for the eating disorders bulimia nervosa and binge eating disorder [32]. The symptoms of FA as assessed by the YFAS were determined with mapping to the DSM–5. However, it is noted that when considering some of these symptoms at a broader population level, with increasing prevalence rates of overweight and obesity, some symptoms or traits presently being assessed overlap with general dieting practices undertaken by many individuals. FA symptoms measured by the YFAS, specifically 'repeated attempts to cut down food', may not be unique to FA, but apply to the population in general.

In the current analysis of those individuals with FA, 72.7% also had reported BES scores which related to either moderate or severe bingeing. While not directly comparable due to the use of different tools and methods to assess the disordered eating status, the value in the current study is higher than that previously reported by Gearhardt et al., who found in a sample of overweight individuals with BED, determined by clinical interview, that 57% met the classification for FA [11]. In a more racially diverse sample of obese, treatment-seeking adults with BED (n = 96) as assessed by an alternate tool, The Eating Disorder Examination Questionnaire (EDEQ), the findings were similar, with 42% of participants meeting the classification for FA [12]. In both studies, YFAS scores were also significant predictors of binge eating frequency. In an additional study, Ivezaj et al. [34] examined the eating and health-related behaviours of overweight/obese adults (n = 502), and found that 61.7% of adults meeting BED criteria as assessed by the EDEQ also met FA criteria. Adults with co-occurring BED and FA had significantly higher BMI and depression scores, combined with greater disturbances on most impulsivity and self-control measures relative to the control group [35]. A strong association between FA and BE severity (r = 0.78, p = 0.0045) as well as a moderate association between FA and measures of general psychopathology were reported. A similar relationship between FA and BE has also been shown to exist in younger adolescent populations [35].

Rates of FA among those with BED is higher in individuals with obesity than in those who are not obese [36]; this was also shown in the current study across increasing weight status of healthy, overweight, and obese participants. Individuals who meet the criteria for both BED and FA tend to exhibit more frequent binge eating episodes, experience stronger cravings for food, and elevated levels of impulsivity and depressive symptoms than those with only BED [5,12,13]. It has been suggested the co-occurrence of BED and FA may represent a more severe BED subgroup characterised by greater eating disorder psychopathology and associated pathology [11].

Recent evidence suggests altered reward sensitivity may contribute to the pathophysiology of disordered eating behaviours. A review of neuroimaging studies (n = 15) in BED found that the alterations in corticostriatal circuitry were similar to those observed in substance abuse, including altered function of prefrontal, insular, and orbitofrontal cortices and the striatum [37]. Preliminary evidence by Gearhardt et al. suggests that reward dysfunction may also be a relevant mechanism in the FA construct [38]. Human genetics and animal studies suggest that changes in neurotransmitter networks, including dopaminergic and opioidergic systems, are associated with compulsive-eating behaviours [37,39].

This study has several limitations which should be considered when interpreting the findings: the survey was collected online and is based on self-report measures and was analysed using correlation analysis only. However, it is noted that for food addiction and binge eating, the majority of measures used for these eating behaviours are based on self-report, and self-reported height and weight have been shown previously to be a valid measure of weight status [40]. It could be likely that individuals who are motivated by food may have been more likely to complete the survey. The study sample had a majority of participants who were female, so results may not be generalisable to the broader population or to other ethnicities. The findings of this study have some clinical implications, as they provide a further understanding of the underlying aetiology of co-occurring FA and BED, to progress and tailor treatment options as FA appears to be more physiological than behavioural in nature.

5. Conclusions

This is one of the first studies to investigate the potential overlap between the common tools used to assess BED and FA and their individual constructs, particularly with reference to the YFAS 2.0 tool which maps to current DSM criteria. This study demonstrates the overlap between BED and FA, and highlights the possible unique differences between the forms of disordered eating.

Acknowledgments: T.B. is supported by a UON Brawn research fellowship.

Author Contributions: T.B. conceived, designed and conducted the study; T.B. analysed the data; T.B. developed initial draft of paper, and J.S., R.M. and M.R. contributed to and approved the final version of the manuscript.

References

1. Pursey, K.M.; Stanwell, P.; Gearhardt, A.N.; Collins, C.E.; Burrows, T.L. The Prevalence of Food Addiction as Assessed by the Yale Food Addiction Scale: A Systematic Review. *Nutrients* **2014**, *6*, 4552–4590. [CrossRef] [PubMed]
2. Hebebrand, J.; Albayrak, Ö.; Adan, R.; Antel, J.; Dieguez, C.; de Jong, J.; Leng, G.; Menzies, J.; Mercer, J.G.; Murphy, M.; et al. "Eating addcition" rather than "food addcition" better captures addictive like eating behaviour. *Neurosci. Biobehav. Rev.* **2014**, *47*, 295–306. [CrossRef] [PubMed]
3. Gearhardt, A.; Corbin, W.; Brownwell, K.D. Preliminary validation of the Yale Food Addiction Scale. *Appetite* **2009**, *52*, 32–36. [CrossRef] [PubMed]
4. Gearhardt, A.N; Corbin, W.R; Brownwell, K.D. Development of the Yale Food Addiction Scale Version 2.0. *Psychol. Addict. Behav.* **2016**, *30*, 113–121. [CrossRef] [PubMed]
5. Davis, C. From Passive Overeating to "Food Addiction": A Spectrum of Compulsion and Severity. *ISRN Obes.* **2013**, 1–20. [CrossRef] [PubMed]
6. Schulte, E.M.; Grilo, C.M.; Gearhardt, A.N. Shared and unique mechanisms underlying binge eating disorder and addictive disorders. *Clin. Psychol. Rev.* **2016**, *44*, 125–139. [CrossRef] [PubMed]
7. Hilker, I.; Sánchez, I.; Steward, T.; Jiménez-Murcia, S.; Granero, R.; Gearhardt, A.N.; Rodríguez-Muñoz, R.C.; Dieguez, C.; Crujeiras, A.B.; Tolosa-Sola, I.; et al. Food Addiction in Bulimia Nervosa: Clinical Correlates and Association with Response to a Brief Psychoeducational Intervention. *Eur. Eat. Disord. Rev.* **2016**, *24*, 482–488. [CrossRef] [PubMed]
8. American Psychiatric Association. *Diagnostic and Statistical Manual of Mental Disorders*, 5th ed.; American Psychiatric Publishing: Arlington, TX, USA, 2013.
9. Kessler, R.; Berglund, P.A.; Chiu, W.T.; Deitz, A.C.; Hudson, J.I.; Shahly, V.; Aguilar-Gaxiola, S.; Alonso, J.; Angermeyer, M.C.; Benjet, C.; Bruffaerts, R.; et al. The Prevalence and Correlates of Binge Eating Disorder in the World Health Organization World Mental Health Surveys. *Biol. Psychiatry* **2013**, *73*, 904–914. [CrossRef] [PubMed]

10. Preti, A.; de Girolamo, G.; Vilagut, G.; Alonso, J.; de Graaf, R.; Bruffaerts, R.; Demyttenaere, K.; Pinto-Meza, A.; Haro, J.M.; Morosini, P.; et al. The epidemiology of eating disorders in six European countries: Results of the ESEMeD-WMH project RSS. *J. Psychiatr. Res.* **2009**, *43*, 1125–1132. [CrossRef] [PubMed]
11. Gearhardt, A.N.; White, M.A.; Masheb, R.M.; Morgan, P.T.; Crosby, R.D.; Grilo, C.M. An Examination of the food addcition construct in obese patients with binge eating disorder. *Int. J. Eat. Disord.* **2012**, *45*, 657–663. [CrossRef] [PubMed]
12. Gearhardt, A.; White, M.A.; Masheb, R.M.; Grilo, C.M. An examination of food addiction in a racially diverse sample of obese patients with binge eating disorder in primary care settings. *Compr. Psychiatr.* **2013**, *54*, 500–505. [CrossRef] [PubMed]
13. Gearhardt, A.N.; Boswell, R.G.; White, M.A. The association of "food addiction" with disordered eating and body mass index. *Eat. Behav.* **2014**, *15*, 427–433. [CrossRef] [PubMed]
14. Meule, A.; von Rezori, V.; Blechert, J. Food addiction and bulimia nervosa. *Eur. Eat. Disord. Rev.* **2014**, *5*, 33. [CrossRef] [PubMed]
15. Burrows, T.; Hides, L.; Brown, R.; Dayas, C.V.; Kay-Lambkin, F. Differences in Dietary Preferences, Personality and Mental Health in Australian Adults with and without Food Addiction. *Nutrients* **2017**, *9*, 285. [CrossRef] [PubMed]
16. Heatherton, T.; Baumeister, R. Binge eating as escape from self-awareness. *Psychol. Bull.* **1991**, *110*, 86–108. [CrossRef] [PubMed]
17. Gearhardt, A.; White, M.; Potenza, M. Binge Eating Disorder and Food Addiction. *Curr. Drug Abuse Rev.* **2011**, *43*, 201–207. [CrossRef]
18. Potenza, M.N.; Grilo, C.M. How relevant is food craving to obesity and its treatment? *Front. Psychiatry* **2014**, *5*, 164. [CrossRef] [PubMed]
19. Pivarunas, B.; Conner, B.T. Impulsivity and emotion dysregulation as predictors of food addiction. *Eat. Behav.* **2015**, *19*, 9–14. [CrossRef] [PubMed]
20. Clark, S.; Saules, K. Validation of the yale Food Addiction Scale among a weight loss surgery population. *Eat. Behav.* **2013**, *14*, 216–219. [CrossRef] [PubMed]
21. Meule, A.; Heckel, D. Correlates of food addiction in obese individuals seeking bariatric surgery. *Clin. Obes.* **2014**, *4*, 228–236. [CrossRef] [PubMed]
22. Davis, C. A commentary on the associations among 'food addiction', binge eating disorder, and obesity: Overlapping conditions with idiosyncratic clinical features. *Appetite* **2017**, *115*, 3–8. [CrossRef] [PubMed]
23. WHO (The World Health Organisation). BMI Classifcation. Available online: http://apps.who.int/bmi/index.jsp?introPage=intro_3.htm (accessed on 25 July 2017).
24. Gormally, J.; Black, S.; Daston, S.; Rardin, D. The assessment of Binge Eating Severity among obese. *Addict. Behav.* **1982**, *7*, 47–55. [CrossRef]
25. Kelly, N.R.; Mitchell, K.S.; Gow, R.W.; Trace, S.E.; Lydecker, J.A.; Bair, C.E.; Mazzeo, S. An evaluation of the reliability and construct validity of eating disorder measures in white and black women. *Psychol. Assess.* **2012**, *24*, 608–617. [CrossRef] [PubMed]
26. Grupski, A.E.; Hood, M.M.; Hall, B.J.; Azarbad, L.; Fitzpatrick, S.L.; Corsica, J.A. Examining the binge eating scale in screening for binge eating disorder with bariatric surgery candidates. *Obes. Surg.* **2013**, *23*, 1–6. [CrossRef] [PubMed]
27. Santor, D.A.; Haggerty, J.L.; Lévesque, J.-F.; Burge, F.; Beaulieu, M.-D.; Gass, D.; Pineault, R. An Overview of Confirmatory Factor Analysis and Item Response Analysis Applied to Instruments to Evaluate Primary Healthcare. *Healthc. Policy* **2011**, *7*, 79–92. [CrossRef] [PubMed]
28. Brunault, P.; Courtois, R.; Gearhardt, A.N.; Gaillard, P.; Journiac, K.; Cathelain, S.; Réveillère, C.; Ballon, N. Validation of the French Version of the DSM-5 Yale Food Addiction Scale in a Nonclinical Sample. *Can. J. Psychiatry* **2017**, *62*, 199–210. [CrossRef] [PubMed]
29. Imperatori, C.; Fabbricatore, M.; Vumbaca, V.; Innamorati, M.; Contardi, A.; Farina, B. Food Addiction: definition, measurement and prevalence in healthy subjects and in patients with eating disorders. *Riv. Psichiatr.* **2016**, *51*, 60–65. [PubMed]
30. Kittel, R.; Brauhardt, A.; Hilbert, A. Hilbert A. Cognitive and emotional functioning in binge-eating disorder: A systematic review. *Int. J. Eat. Disord.* **2015**, *48*, 535–554. [CrossRef] [PubMed]

31. Hauck, C.; Weiß, A.; Schulte, E.M.; Meule, A.; Ellrott, T. Prevalence of 'Food Addiction' as Measured with the Yale Food Addiction Scale 2.0 in a Representative German Sample and Its Association with Sex, Age and Weight Categories. *Eur. J. Obes.* **2017**, *10*, 12–24. [CrossRef] [PubMed]
32. Meule, A.; Gearhardt, A.N. Food addiction in the light of DSM-5. *Nutrients* **2014**, *6*, 3653–3671. [CrossRef] [PubMed]
33. Ruddock, H.; Hardman, C. Food Addiction Beliefs Amongst the Lay Public: What Are the Consequences for Eating Behaviour? *Curr. Addict. Rep.* **2017**, *4*, 110–115. [CrossRef] [PubMed]
34. Ivezaj, V.; White, M.A.; Grilo, C.M. Examining binge-eating disorder and food addiction in adults with overweight and obesity. *Obesity* **2016**, *24*, 2064–2069. [CrossRef] [PubMed]
35. Ahmed, A.Y.; Sayed, A.M.; Alshahat, A.A.; Abd Elaziza, E.A. Can food addiction replace binge eating assessment in obesity clinics? *Egypt. J. Med. Hum. Genet.* **2017**, *18*, 181–185. [CrossRef]
36. Long, C.; Blundell, J.; Finlayson, G. A Systematic Review of the Application and Correlates of YFAS-Diagnosed 'Food Addiction' in Humans: Are Eating-Related 'Addictions' a Cause for Concern or Empty Concepts? *Obes. Facts* **2015**, *8*, 386–401. [CrossRef] [PubMed]
37. Kessler, R.M.; Hutson, P.H.; Herman, B.K.; Potenza, M.N. The neurobiological basis of binge-eating disorder. *Neurosci. Biobehav. Rev.* **2016**, *63*, 223–238. [CrossRef] [PubMed]
38. Gearhardt, A.N.; Yokum, S.; Orr, P.T.; Stice, E.; Corbin, W.R.; Brownell, K.D. Neural correlates of food addiction. *Arch. Gen. Psychiatry* **2011**, *68*, 808–816. [CrossRef] [PubMed]
39. Schrieber, L.; Odlaug, B.; Grant, J. The overlap between binge eating disorder and substance use disorders: Diagnosis and neurobiology. *J. Behav. Addict.* **2013**, *2*, 191–198. [CrossRef] [PubMed]
40. Pursey, K.; Burrows, T.L.; Stanwell, P.; Collins, C.E. How accurate is web-based self-reported height, weight and body mass index in young adults? *J. Med. Internet Res.* **2014**, *16*, e4. [CrossRef] [PubMed]

4

Dietary Interventions and Changes in Cardio-Metabolic Parameters in Metabolically Healthy Obese Subjects

Marta Stelmach-Mardas [1,2,*] and Jarosław Walkowiak [2]

1 Department of Epidemiology, German Institute of Human Nutrition, Potsdam-Rehbruecke, Arthur-Scheunert-Allee 114-116, Nuthetal 14558, Germany

2 Department of Pediatric Gastroenterology and Metabolic Diseases, Poznan University of Medical Sciences, Szpitalna Str 27/33, Poznan 60-572, Poland; jarwalk@ump.edu.pl

* Correspondence: stelmach@dife.de

Abstract: The aim of this systematic review was to assess the effect of diet on changes in parameters describing the body size phenotype of metabolically healthy obese subjects. The databases Medline, Scopus, Web of Knowledge and Embase were searched for clinical studies carried out between 1958 and June 2016 that reported the effect of dietary intervention on BMI, blood pressure, concentration of fasting triglyceride (TG), high density lipoprotein cholesterol (HDL-C), fasting glucose level, the homoeostatic model assessment of insulin resistance (HOMA-IR) and high sensitivity C-Reactive Protein (hsCRP) in metabolically healthy, obese subjects. Twelve clinical studies met inclusion criteria. The combined analyzed population consists of 1827 subjects aged 34.4 to 61.1 with a BMI > 30 kg/m^2. Time of intervention ranged from eight to 104 weeks. The baseline characteristics related to lipid profile were more favorable for metabolically healthy obese than for metabolically unhealthy obese. The meta-analyses revealed a significant associations between restricted energy diet and BMI (95% confidence interval (CI): −0.88, −0.19), blood pressure (systolic blood pressure (SBP): −4.73 mmHg; 95% CI: −7.12, −2.33; and diastolic blood pressure (DBP): −2.75 mmHg; 95% CI: −4.30, −1.21) and TG (−0.11 mmol/l; 95% CI: −0.16, −0.06). Changes in fasting glucose, HOMA-IR and hsCRP did not show significant changes. Sufficient evidence was not found to support the use of specific diets in metabolically healthy obese subjects. This analysis suggests that the effect of caloric restriction exerts its effects through a reduction in BMI, blood pressure and triglycerides in metabolically healthy obese (MHO) patients.

Keywords: metabolically healthy obese; diet; biomarkers

---

1. Introduction

The prevalence of obesity is increasing worldwide with prognoses expected to affect more than one billion people by 2030 [1]. An association between obesity and increased risk of co-morbidities, i.e., metabolic syndrome (MetS) and cardiovascular disease (CVD) leading to significantly higher all-causes of mortality, has been observed [2]. However, the metabolically healthy obese (MHO) phenotype was described in the early 1980s [3], and, to date, there is no single consistent definition that covers "the metabolic health" approach in relation to differentiated dietary habits in obese subjects [4–6].

So far, the direct mechanism, which contributes to the different effects of weight loss in MHO and metabolically unhealthy obese (MUHO) subjects is not known, though it seems that it may vary as a function of different baseline metabolic profiles in MHO and MUHO groups. Only limited data are available with regards to dietary behaviors in MHO [7]. The prevalence of MHO is predicted to be 30%–40% of the obese population, with higher rates in younger subjects and in females [4,8]. Nevertheless, it should be taken under consideration that MHO subjects can shift to the metabolically unhealthy phenotype, a change confirmed by Schröder et al. [9] in a 10 years follow-up study.

Due to the fact that the effectiveness of dietary interventions in MHO is not very well known, we aimed to describe the influence of applied diet from intervention studies on changes in parameters describing the body size phenotype (body mass index—BMI, blood pressure—BP and concentration of selected biomarkers) of MHO.

2. Experimental Section

2.1. Search Strategy

The databases Medline, Scopus, Web of Knowledge and Embase were searched for clinical studies carried out between 1958 and June 2016 that reported the effect of dietary intervention on BMI and selected cardio-metabolic parameters (blood pressure and concentration of selected biomarkers) as primary or secondary outcomes in MHO. Search strategy was restricted to humans, English language and full length, original articles. The search based upon the listed below following index terms and title: #1 "Benign Obesity, Metabolically" OR "Metabolically Healthy Obesity" OR "Healthy Obesity, Metabolically" OR "Obesity, Metabolically Healthy" OR "Metabolically Benign Obesity" OR "Metabolically normal" OR "Metabolic syndrome" AND #2 "Diet" OR "Diet, carbohydrate-restricted" OR "Diet, fat-restricted" OR "Diet, protein-restricted" OR "Ketogenic diet" OR "Diet, high-fat" OR "Diet, reducing" OR "Weight reduction programs" OR "Caloric restriction" OR "Lifestyle intervention" NOT "Animals". The Preferred Reporting Items for Systematic Reviews and Meta-Analyses (PRISMA) Statement was followed [10].

2.2. Metabolically Healthy Obese—Definition

The criteria for MHO used in the studies include: absence of abdominal obesity on the basis of waist circumference, absence of metabolic syndrome components, e.g., normal blood pressure, normal lipid values, normal fasting glucose concentrations (at times also including normal C-reactive protein concentrations), insulin sensitivity determined on the basis of the homoeostatic model assessment of insulin resistance (HOMA-IR) and a high level of cardiorespiratory fitness [11]. All features were also used in the long-term prognosis of cardiovascular disease and all-cause mortality for MHO by Bo et al. [12], Calori et al., [13] and Hammer et al. [14].

Specifically, the criteria for the body size phenotype of MHO subjects include: a BMI $\geqslant$ 30 kg/m^2 and <2 cardio-metabolic abnormalities (systolic/diastolic blood pressure (SBP/DBP) $\geqslant$ 130/85 mmHg or antihypertensive medication use; fasting triglyceride (TG) level $\geqslant$ 150 mg/dL (1.693 mmol/L)); decreased high density lipoprotein cholesterol (HDL-C) level < 40 mg/dL (1.0344 mmol/L) in men and <50 mg/dL (1.293 mmol/L) in women or lipid-lowering medication use; fasting glucose (Glc) level $\geqslant$ 100 mg/dL (5.55 mmol/L) or antidiabetic medication use; insulin resistance: HOMA-IR > 5.13, i.e., the 90th percentile; systemic inflammation: high sensitivity C-Reactive Protein (hsCRP) level > 0.1 mg/L, i.e., the 90th percentile) [6]. Similar criteria were proposed by Meigs et al. [5] including the addition of waist circumference (WC) (>102 cm in men and >88 cm in women) and expanding the definition to include up to <3 cardio-metabolic abnormalities.

2.3. Inclusion and Exclusion Criteria

Only studies conducted with subjects described as metabolically healthy obese subjects, indicating the changes in BMI, blood pressure and selected blood parameters after various dietary interventions, were included. The intervention studies (randomized controlled trial and non-randomized trial) were taken into consideration. The articles that did not meet inclusion criteria (animal studies, other than the type of documents mentioned above, articles in any other language than English) were excluded.

2.4. Data Extraction and Analysis

Relevant articles were identified by screening the abstracts, titles and full-texts. The study selection process was performed by two independent researchers (M.S.-M. and J.W.) in parallel for each database. In every step of assessment, all disagreements between researchers were resolved after consultation. In the case of disagreement during the title assessment process, the paper was included in the next step. The process outline and workflow is presented in Figure 1.

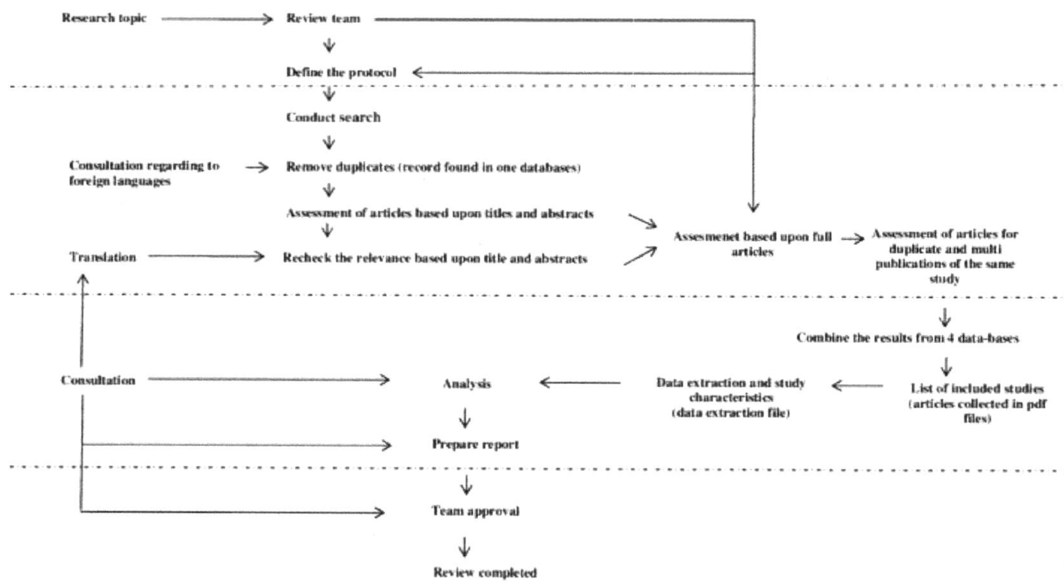

Figure 1. Process flow sheet.

Eligible studies were evaluated according to: the number of participants, study design, type of dietary intervention, changes in BMI (defined as body mass divided by the square of the height), and criteria for body size phenotype of MHO defined according to Third Report of the National Cholesterol Education Program Adult Treatment Panel (NCEP ATP III) [6]. To assess the study quality, a nine-point scoring system according to the Newcastle-Ottawa Scale was used. The maximum score was nine, with a high-quality study defined by a threshold of $\geqslant$7 points [15].

The recorded biomarkers concentrations were converted to mmol/L (fasting glucose, Triglycerides, HDL-Cholesterol) and mg/L (hsCRP) in order to standardize results. A meta-analysis was performed to combine the results of individual studies. Data were analyzed using a random-effects model. The effect size of a study was investigated by calculating the standardized mean difference with a 95% confidence interval (CI). The heterogeneity of the sum of studies was tested for significance. As a measure for quantifying inconsistency, I^2 was selected [16]. Although included studies in our analysis were heterogeneous, careful inclusion of the suited arms (MHO group) in different interventions allowed us to combine the collected papers and run our analyses. The results of the meta-analysis were visualized using a forest plot which illustrates the results of the individual studies and the summary effect. The analysis was performed with Review Manager (RevMan, V5.3, The Nordic Cochrane Centre, the Cochrane Collaboration, Copenhagen, Denmark, 2014).

3. Results

3.1. Search Results

Using wide terms to describe the metabolically healthy obese patients, we end up with more than 14,000 articles that were screened. After initial exclusion criteria, 135 papers were assigned for full-text review with 12 articles included for data extraction and analysis [17–28] (Figure 2).

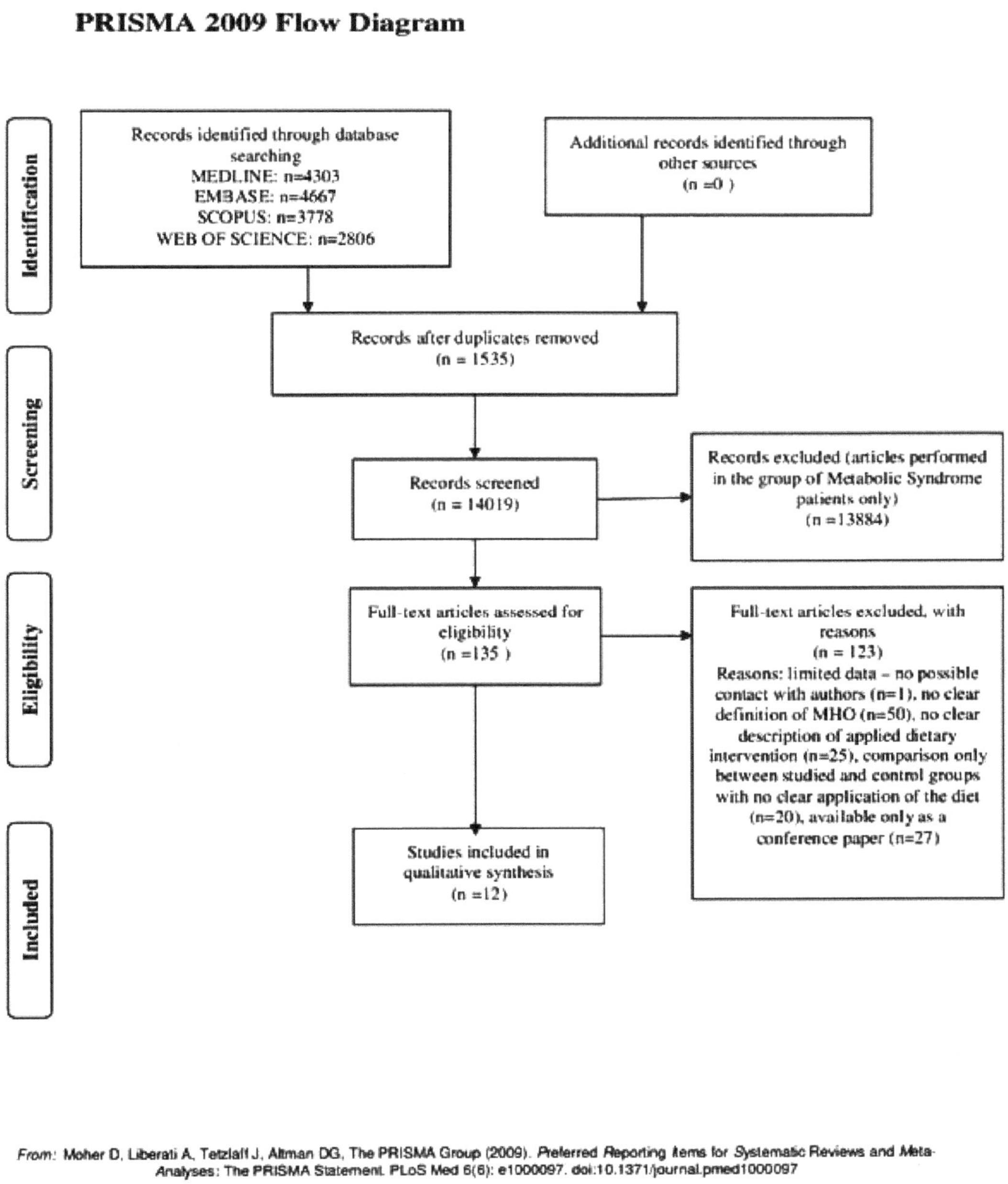

Figure 2. Process of literature search on the association between diet and selected cardio-metabolic parameters in metabolically healthy obese.

3.2. Studies and Populations Characteristics

The characteristics of clinical studies (randomized and non-randomized) and populations are presented in Table 1. The population consists of 1827 subjects and was characterized by a baseline BMI > 30 kg/m^2, a mean age from 34.4 [18] to 61.1 [20], and representing Caucasian and Asian ethnicities. Time of interventions ranged from 12 to 104 weeks and were based on diet only [18,21–27] or diet with combination of light to moderate physical activity (PA) [19,20,28] that supported the daily energy deficit.

Table 1. Characteristics of the included studies and study populations.

Study	Country	Total Number (Number of MHO)	Age (Years) Mean ± SD	Study Design	Intervention	Time of Intervention	Study Quality (Newcastle-Ottawa Scale)
Rondanelli et al., 2015 [17]	Italy	MHO: 103	MHO: 42.2 ± 9.2	Clinical study: non-RCT	Low-energy mix, well-balanced (55% carbohydrates, 30% lipids and 15% proteins) diet providing 600 kcal less than individually estimated energy requirements based on the measured Resting Energy Expenditure	8-week	7
Ruiz et al., 2013 [18]	Spain	78 (MHO: 25)	MHO: 34.4 ± 6.8 MUHO: 37.8 ± 6.9	Clinical study: non-RCT	Low-energy mixed diet (55% carbohydrates, 30% lipids and 15% proteins) providing 600 kcal less than individually estimated energy requirements based on measured resting metabolic rate (RMR) and multiplied by a factor of 1.3, corresponding to a low physical activity level	12-week	8
Kantartzis et al., 2011 [19]	Germany	262 (MHO: 26)	MHO: 46.8 ± 2.2 MUHO: 47.1 ± 1.3	Clinical study: non-RCT	Lifestyle intervention program with aim to reduce body weight by ≥5%, to reduce the intake of energy from fat to <30% and particularly the intake of saturated fat to ≤10% of energy consumed and to increase the intake of dietary fiber to at least 15 g/4184 kJ (1000 kcal). Moderate sports per week: at least 3 h	36-week	7
Janiszewski & Ross, 2010 [20]	Canada	106 (MHO: 63)	MHO a. women: 61.1 ± 12.0 b. men: 61.4 ± 11.8 MUHO a. women: 46.5 ± 10.7 b. men: 53.1 ± 14.8	Clinical study: RCT	Men: program (diet or exercise) designed to induce a daily 700-kcal energy deficit Women: program (diet or exercise) designed to induce a daily 500-kcal energy deficit	Men: 12-week Women: 14-week	7
Shin et al., 2006 [21]	Korea	129 (MHO: 23)	MHO: 36.4 ± 11.2 MUHO: 39.8 ± 13.3	Clinical study: non-RCT	Weight loss program consisting of a 300 kcal/day reduction of usual caloric intakes to achieve the goal of losing a minimum of 3% of initial body weight	12-week	7
Liu et al., 2012 [22]	Canada	392 (MHO: 83)	53.6 ± 12.3	Clinical study: non-RCT	Calorie restricted meal plan of approximately 500–1000 calories below the patient's baseline daily caloric requirement to achieve the goal of losing a 5% of initial body weight	>12-week	8
Sesti et al., 2011 [23]	Italy	190	MHO: 38 ± 10 MUHO: 40 ± 10	Clinical study: non-RCT	Diet applied after Laparoscopic Adjustable Gastric Banding First month: a semiliquid diet of 800 and 950 kcal/day in women and men, respectively (33% proteins, 19% lipids, 48% carbohydrates). Second month: a solid diet was reintroduced. Third month: the suggested diet was 970 and 1090 kcal/day in women and men, respectively (diet included 48% carbohydrates (starch or bread), 33% proteins (fat-free parts of different animals and fish), and 19% lipids (olive oil)	>12-week	7

Table 1. *Cont.*

Study	Country	Total Number (Number of MHO)	Age (Years) Mean ± SD	Study Design	Intervention	Time of Intervention	Study Quality (Newcastle-Ottawa Scale)
Haro et al., 2015 [24]	Spain	MHO: 20	The LFHCC diet (a low-fat, high-complex carbohydrate diet) 61.4 ± 2.6 The Med diet (Mediterranean diet) 65.2 ± 3.2	Clinical study: RCT	The LFHCC diet contained 28% fat (12% monounsaturated; 8% polyunsaturated and 8% saturated) The Med diet contained 35% fat (22% monounsaturated; 6% polyunsaturated and 7% saturated)	52-week	8
Madero et al., 2011 [25]	Mexico	MHO: 131	The low-fructose diet 37.56 ± 1.14 The moderate natural fructose diet 40.15 ± 1.01	Clinical study: RCT	Energy-restricted diets: I. The low-fructose diet: first 2-week period of less than 10 g of fructose per day followed by a 4-week period of less than 20 g of fructose per day. II. The moderate natural fructose diet: consisted of 50 to 70 g of fructose consisting of mostly natural fructose from fruits.	6-week	7
Foster et al., 2010 [26]	US	MHO: 307	A low-carbohydrate diet 46.2 ± 9.2 A low-fat diet 44.9 ± 10.2	Clinical study: RCT	A low-carbohydrate diet which consisted of limited carbohydrate intake (20 g/day for 3 months) in the form of low-glycemic index vegetables with unrestricted consumption of fat and protein. After 3 months, participants in the low-carbohydrate diet group increased their carbohydrate intake (5 g per week) until a stable and desired weight was achieved A low-fat diet consisted of limited energy intake (1200 to 1800 kcal/day; ⩽30% calories from fat)	104-week	8
Hermsdorff et al., 2011 [27]	Spain	MHO: 30	36.0 ± 8.0	Clinical study: RCT	The macronutrient-balanced diets (control and legume-based dietary approaches) were designed to provide a similar macronutrients distribution: 53% of energy as carbohydrates, 17% as proteins and 30% as fat	4-week	6
Christiansen et al., 2011 [28]	Denmark	MHO: 79	DIO group: 35.6 ± 7.0 DEX group: 37.5 ± 8.0	Clinical study: RCT	A liquid, very low energy diet of 600 and 800 kcal/day, respectively (proteins 41 g, carbohydrates 29 g, fat 5.6 g per 100 g), for 8 week followed by a weight maintenance diet for 4 week. In Diet-induced weight loss using a very low energy diet (DIO) and exercise and diet-induced weight-loss combined (DEX) groups the subjects should obtain similar weight losses to observe the possible specific, weight-independent effect of exercise. Thus, the subjects in the DEX group were allowed to consume 150–200 kcal more per day than the DIO group, reflecting the estimated extra energy expenditure of 1500 kcal/week during exercise activity. The supervised aerobic exercise three times per week with duration of 60–75 min per training session, with an estimated energy expenditure of 500–600 kcal per session	8-week	7

MHO: metabolically healthy obese; MUHO: metabolically unhealthy obese; non-RCT: non randomized control trial; LFHCC diet: a low-fat, high-complex carbohydrate diet; the Med diet: Mediterranean diet; DIO: a very low energy diet; DEX: exercise and diet-induced weight-loss combined.

3.3. Changes in Body Mass Index and Selected Cardio-Metabolic Outcomes during Dietary Interventions

The changes in BMI and selected cardio-metabolic outcomes during dietary interventions are presented in Table 2. Reduction in BMI, from baseline to the final day of intervention, ranged from 1.1 to 2.9 kg/m^2 in MHO, and were statistically significant in seven of twelve studies [18,20,22,23,25,27,28] within the study group. Kantartizis et al. [19], Haro et al. [24], and Foster et al. [26] failed to report exact values of baseline BMIs. The quantitative meta-analysis revealed a significant association between the restricted energy diets ($p < 0.0001$, $I^2 = 99\%$) and change in BMI (-2.70 kg/m^2; 95% CI: -4.01, -1.39) (Figure 3). The changes in systolic and diastolic blood pressure during the dietary interventions were measured only in six studies [20,22,25–28]. However, the meta-analysis showed statistically significant reduction in SBP (-4.73 mmHg; 95% CI: -7.12, -2.33; $p = 0.0001$, $I^2 = 87\%$) and DBP (-2.75 mmHg; 95% CI: -4.30, -1.21; $p = 0.0005$, $I^2 = 86\%$) within MHO group after applied dietary interventions, clinical relevance cannot be considered (Figure 4). The concentrations of TG and HDL-C were reported in all selected studies, where the baseline characteristic with regards to blood lipids was mostly more favorable for MHO than for metabolically unhealthy obese (MUHO) [19,21,23]. Nevertheless, the statistically significant association was observed only between energy restricted diets and the reduction in TG concentration (-0.11 mmol/L; 95% CI: -0.16, -0.06; $p < 0.0001$, $I^2 = 59\%$) (Figure 5). Fasting glucose was assessed in ten studies [15–18,20–23,25,26] with no significant decrease (-0.05 mmol/L; 95% CI: -0.14, 0.03; $p = 0.21$, $I^2 = 81\%$). Additionally, in the meta-analysis of studies reporting changes in HOMA-IR [17–19,21,25,27,28] in relation to dietary intervention, no significant reduction was observed within MHO group (-0.08; 95% CI: -0.31, 0.14; $p = 0.47$, $I^2 = 85\%$) (Figure 6). The reduction in hsCRP concentration were reported in only four studies [17,18,21,27] with no significant association with dietary intervention found (-0.19 mg/L; 95% CI: -1.35, 0.97; $p = 0.75$, $I^2 = 98\%$) (Figure 7). The funnel plot did not reveal asymmetry despite selected studies being outliers, suggesting no real evidence of a publication bias (Figure S1).

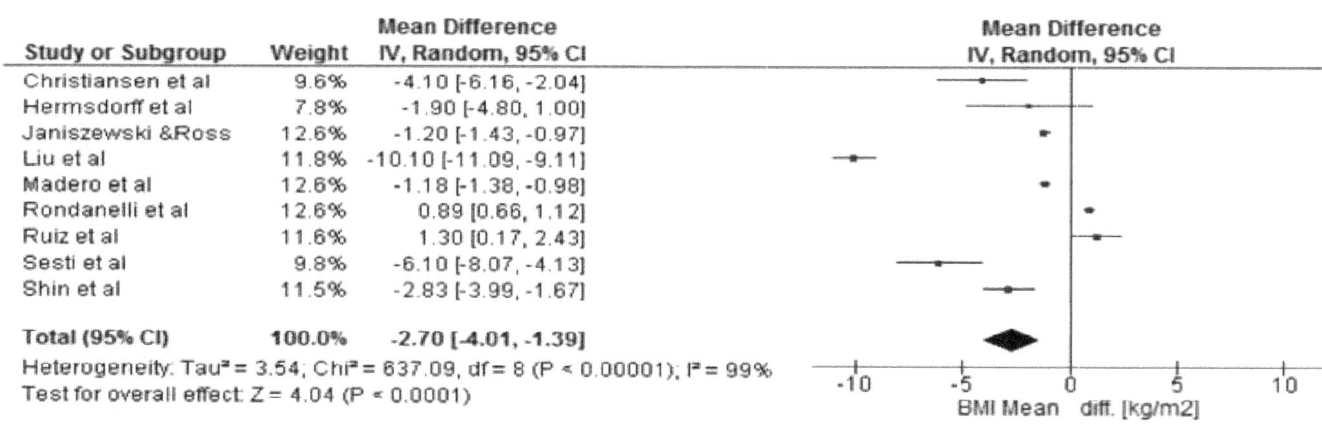

Figure 3. Forest plot of the random-effects meta-analysis of changes in BMI according to reduction in energy intake shown as polled standard differences in the means with 95% Cis and in randomized and non-randomized trials. * For each study, the square represents the point estimate of the intervention effect. Horizontal lines join the lower and upper limits of the 95% CI of this effect. The area of shaded squares reflects the relative weight of the study in the meta-analysis. Diamonds represent the subgroup mean difference and pooled mean differences. CI indicates confidence interval.

Table 2. Changes in Body Mass Index and parameters describing cardio-metabolic outcomes in metabolically healthy obese.

Study	Intervention	Groups	BMI (kg/m^2) Mean ± SD		Systolic/Diastolic Blood Pressure (mmHg) Mean ± SD		TG (mmol/L) Mean ± SD		HDL-C (mmol/L) Mean ± SD		Fasting Glucose (mmol/L) Mean ± SD		HOMA-IR Mean ± SD		hsCRP (mg/L) Mean ± SD	
			B′	I″	B′	I″	B′	I″	B′	I″	B′	I″	B′	I″	B′	I″
Rondanelli et al., 2015 [17]	Diet ONLY	MHO	0.89 (0.66 to 1.12)		-		0.03 (−0.21 to 0.27) *		−0.06 (−0.10 to 0.02) *		−0.06 (−0.17 to 0.05) *		−0.18 (−0.33 to 0.52) *		−4.00 (−6.00 to −1.00) *	
Ruiz et al., 2013 [18]	Diet ONLY	MHO:	+2.88 ± 1.3 *		-		−0.03 ± 0.9 *		+0.14 ± 0.3 *		+1.2 ± 5.6 *		+0.56 ± 0.7 *		+1.51 ± 0.15 *	
		MUHO:	+3.08 ± 1.1 *				+0.31 ± 0.79 *		+0.20 ± 0.28 *		+2.1 ± 6.4 *		+0.59 ± 0.66 *		+0.38 ± 1.88	
Kantartzis et al., 2011 [19]	Diet AND exercise	MHO:	>30		-		1.71 ± 0.41	1.62 ± 0.44	1.37 ± 0.08	1.30 ± 0.05	5.07 ± 0.08	5.17 ± 0.10	1.16 ± 0.06	1.23 ± 0.08	-	
		MUHO:					1.56 ± 0.12	1.49 ± 0.08	1.27 ± 0.03	1.22 ± 0.03	5.42 ± 0.06	5.26 ± 0.06	2.98 ± 0.13	2.44 ± 0.14		
Janiszewski & Ross, 2010 [20]	Diet OR exercise	MHO:											-		-	
		Men	−1.3 ± 1.0 *		−3.0 ± 11.0 */−2.1 ± 6.4 *		−0.2 ± 0.4 *		+0.1 ± 0.1 *		−0.1 ± 0.4 *					
		Women	−1.1 ± 0.8 *		−0.1 ± 11.3 */−1.5 ± 7.1 *		0.0 ± 0.3 *		0.0 ± 0.2 *		0.0 ± 0.4					
		MUHO:														
		Men	−1.9 ± 0.9 *		−2.1 ± 11.9 */−2.9 ± 10.4 *		−0.5 ± 0.7 *		+0.1 ± 0.1 *		−0.6 ± 0.7 *					
		Women	−1.8 ± 1.0 *		−1.9 ± 18.0 */0.3 ± 9.9 *		−0.3 ± 0.5 *		−0.0 ± 0.1 *		−0.3 ± 0.8 *					
Shin et al., 2006 [21]	Diet ONLY	MHO:	−2.83 ± 2 .74 **		-		1.09 ± 0.37	1.25 ± 0.54	1.33 ± 0.24	1.32 ± 0.25	-		1.80 ± 1.27	1.68 ± 0.76	0.74 ± 0.41	0.82 ± 0.45
		MUHO:	−3.16 ± 4.08 **				1.72 ± 0.73	1.54 ± 0.78	1.09 ± 0.26	1.16 ± 0.26			2.60 ± 1.61	2.40 ± 2.3	1.9 ± 1.98	1.50 ± 1.3
Liu et al., 2012 [22]	Diet AND Supporting education	MHO:														
		<5% BW loss	−0.2 ± 3.4		−8.0 ± 1.0		−0.03 ± 0.07		0.08 ± 0.03		0.1 ± 0.15					
		>5% BW loss	−10.1 ± 4.6		−4.0 ± 1.0		−0.14 ± 0.07		−0.015 ± 0.03		0.0 ±0.15					
		MUHO:														
		<5% BW loss	−1.1 ± 3.1		−4.0 ± 1.0		−0.19 ± 0.05		0.05 ± 0.01		−0.16 ± 0.09					
		>5% BW loss	−11.4 ± 5.6		−2.0 ± 1.0		−0.02 ± 0.05		0.02 ± 0.01		−0.07 ± 0.09					
Sesti et al., 2011 [23]	Diet Applied after LAGB ‴	MHO:	41.1 ± 5.5	35.0 ± 5.3	-		1.34 ± 0.60	1.13 ± 0.52	1.24 ± 0.31	1.34 ± 0.31	5.2 ± 0.7	4.9 ± 0.7	-		-	
		MUHO:	44.0 ± 6.4	38.2 ± 5.6			1.58 ± 0.78	1.30 ± 0.55	1.27 ± 0.31	1.32 ± 0.34	5.7 ± 0.8	5.3 ± 0.7				
Haro et al., 2015 [24]	Diet ONLY	MHO:											-		-	
		LFHCC diet #	31.6 ± 0.8	-	129 ± 9.4	-	1.16 ± 0.09	1.11 ± 0.09	1.04 ± 0.06	1.03 ± 0.05	5.2 ± 0.2	5.1 ± 0.2				
		Med diet §	32.8 ± 0.5		136 ± 3.7		1.18 ± 0.13	0.97 ± 0.13	1.09 ± 0.06	1.16 ± 0.05	5.1 ± 0.2	5.4 ± 0.2				

Table 2. *Cont.*

Study	Intervention	Groups	BMI (kg/m^2) Mean ± SD		Systolic/Diastolic Blood Pressure (mmHg) Mean ± SD		TG (mmol/L) Mean ± SD		HDL-C (mmol/L) Mean ± SD		Fasting Glucose (mmol/L) Mean ± SD		HOMA-IR Mean ± SD		hsCRP (mg/L) Mean ± SD	
			B′	I″	B′	I″	B′	I″	B′	I″	B′	I″	B′	I″	B′	I″
Madero et al., 2011 [25]	Diet ONLY	MHO:														
		A low-fructose diet	−1.18 ± 0.82		−9.46 ± 7.77/−5.17 ± 4.69		−0.26 ± 0.78		0.0 ± 0.49		−0.30 ± 1.70		−0.29 ± 0.93		-	
		A moderate natural fructose diet	−1.57 ± 1.08		−7.85 ± 8.73/−6.04 ± 5.40		−0.35 ± 0.62		0.0 ± 0.31		−0.4 ± 0.5		−0.37 ± 0.57			
Foster et al., 2010 [26]	Diet AND Supporting education	MHO:														
		A low-carbohydrate diet	-		−2.68 (−5.08 to −0.27)/ −3.19 (−4.66 to −1.73)		−0.13 (−0.25 to −0.01)		0.20 (0.15 to 0.25)		-		-		-	
		A low-fat diet			−2.59 (−5.07 to −0.12)/ −0.50 (−2.13 to 1.13)		−0.16 (−0.28 to −0.03)		0.10 (0.08 to 0.16)							
Hermsdorff et al., 2011 [27]	Diet ONLY	MHO:														
		Calorie-restricted legume-free diet	31.3 ± 4.0	29.4 ± 4.1	115 ± 9/ 76 ± 9	111 ± 12/ 72 ± 10	1.17 ± 0.32	1.17 ± 0.57	1.50 ± 0.26	1.27 ± 0.31	5.1 ± 0.5	5.0 ± 0.4	2.1 ± 1.7	1.6 ± 1.0	2.0 ± 1.0	1.9 ± 0.8
		Calorie-restricted legume-based diet	33.7 ± 4.7	31.7 ± 3.9	115 ± 13/ 76 ± 6	106 ± 10/ 70 ± 6	1.11 ± 0.43	1.09 ± 0.42	1.27 ± 0.26	1.14 ± 0.18	5.2 ± 0.3	5.1 ± 0.3	1.8 ± 0.9	1.6 ± 0.9	2.7 ± 2.4	1.6 ± 0.9
Christiansen et al., 2011 [28]	Diet OR Exercise OR Diet with Exercise	Exercise only (EXO)	33.3 ± 4	32.2 ± 4	126 ± 15/ 76 ± 12	118 ± 8/ 68 ±9	1.6 ± 0.7	1.5 ± 0.4	1.3 ± 0.4	1.3 ± 0.5	5.6 ± 0.4	5.6 ± 5	2.3 ± 1.0	1.8 ± 1.0	-	
		Diet-induced weight loss using a very low energy diet (DIO)	35.3 ± 4	31.2 ± 4	129 ± 10/ 78 ± 12	122 ± 12/ 82 ± 12	1.5 ± 0.5	1.1 ± 0.3	1.2 ± 0.3	1.2 ± 0.3	5.5 ± 0.6	5.1 ± 0.5	3.1 ± 2.0	2.1 ± 1.0		
		Exercise and diet-induced weight-loss combined (DEX)	34.2 ± 3	30.3 ± 3	140 ± 17/ 82 ± 12	129 ± 18/ 72 ± 13	1.8 ± 0.6	1.2 ± 0.5	1.2 ± 0.3	1.3 ± 0.3	5.6 ± 0.4	5.4 ± 0.5	3.2 ± 2.0	2.0 ± 1.0		

′ B—Baseline; ″ I—Intervention; * absolute changes; ** percent changes, statistically significant $p < 0.05$; MHO: metabolically healthy obese; MUHO: metabolically unhealthy obese; BMI: Body Mass Index; TG: triglycerides; HDL-C: high density lipoprotein cholesterol; HOMA-IR: homeostatic model assessment of insulin resistance; hsCRP: high-sensitivity C-reactive protein; BW—body weight changes; ‴ LAGB: Laparoscopic Adjustable Gastric Banding; # The LFHCC diet (a low-fat, high-complex carbohydrate diet); § The Med diet (Mediterranean diet) 65.2 ± 3.2.

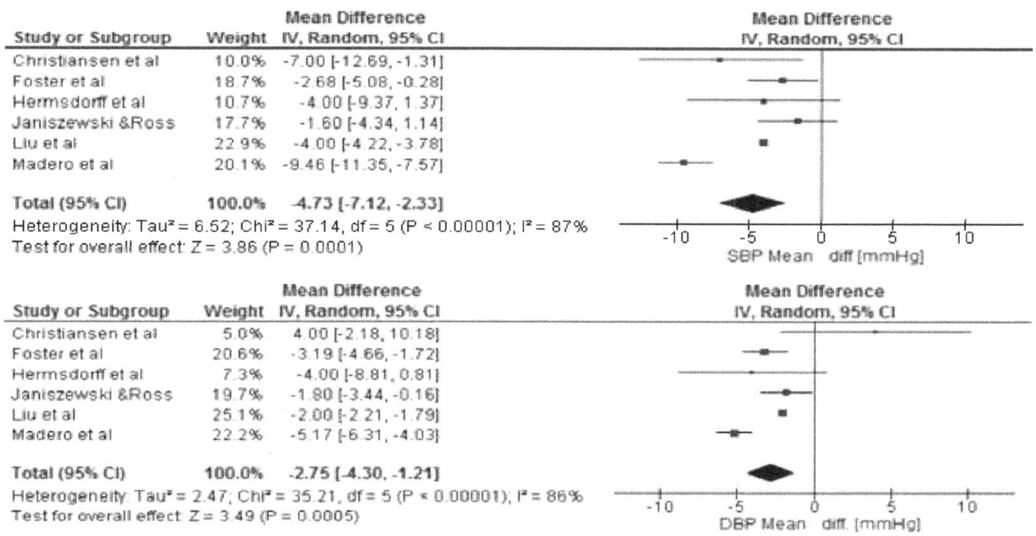

Figure 4. Forest plot of the random-effects meta-analysis of changes in Systolic and Diastolic Blood Pressure according to reduction in energy intake shown as polled standard differences in the means with 95% Cis and in randomized and non-randomized trials. * For each study, the square represents the point estimate of the intervention effect. Horizontal lines join the lower and upper limits of the 95% CI of this effect. The area of shaded squares reflects the relative weight of the study in the meta-analysis. Diamonds represent the subgroup mean difference and pooled mean differences. CI indicates confidence interval.

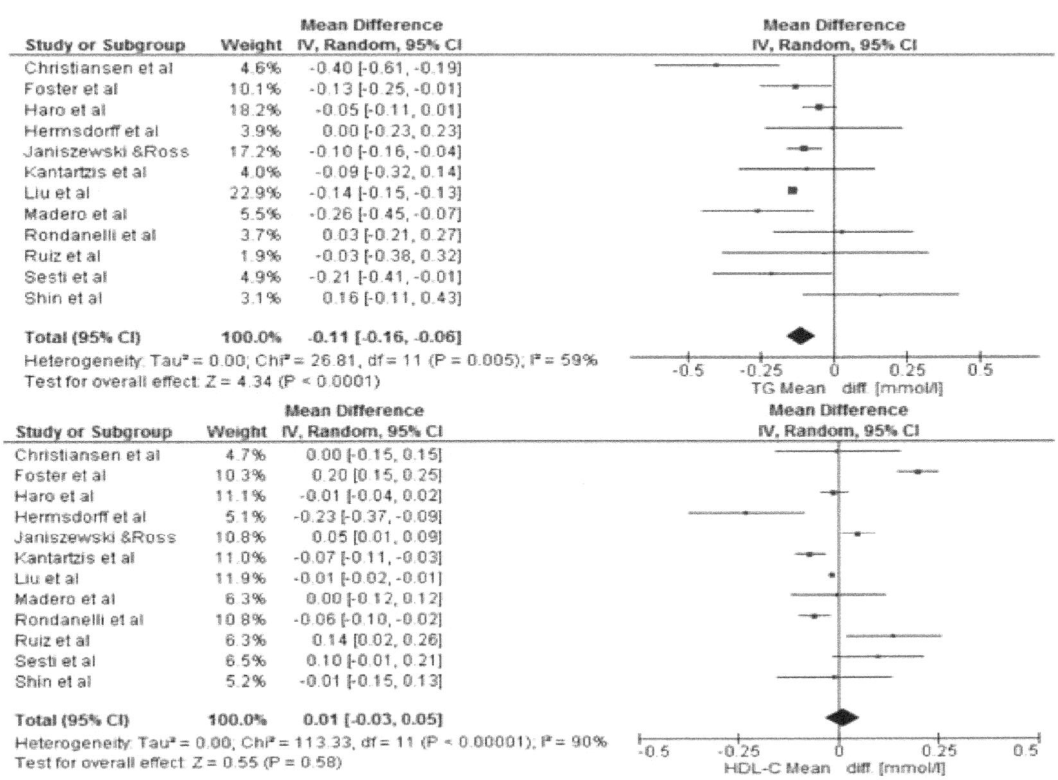

Figure 5. Forest plot of the random-effects meta-analysis of changes in Triglycerides and HDL-cholesterol according to reduction in energy intake shown as polled standard differences in the means with 95% Cis and in randomized and non-randomized trials. * For each study, the square represents the point estimate of the intervention effect. Horizontal lines join the lower and upper limits of the 95% CI of this effect. The area of shaded squares reflects the relative weight of the study in the meta-analysis. Diamonds represent the subgroup mean difference and pooled mean differences. CI indicates confidence interval.

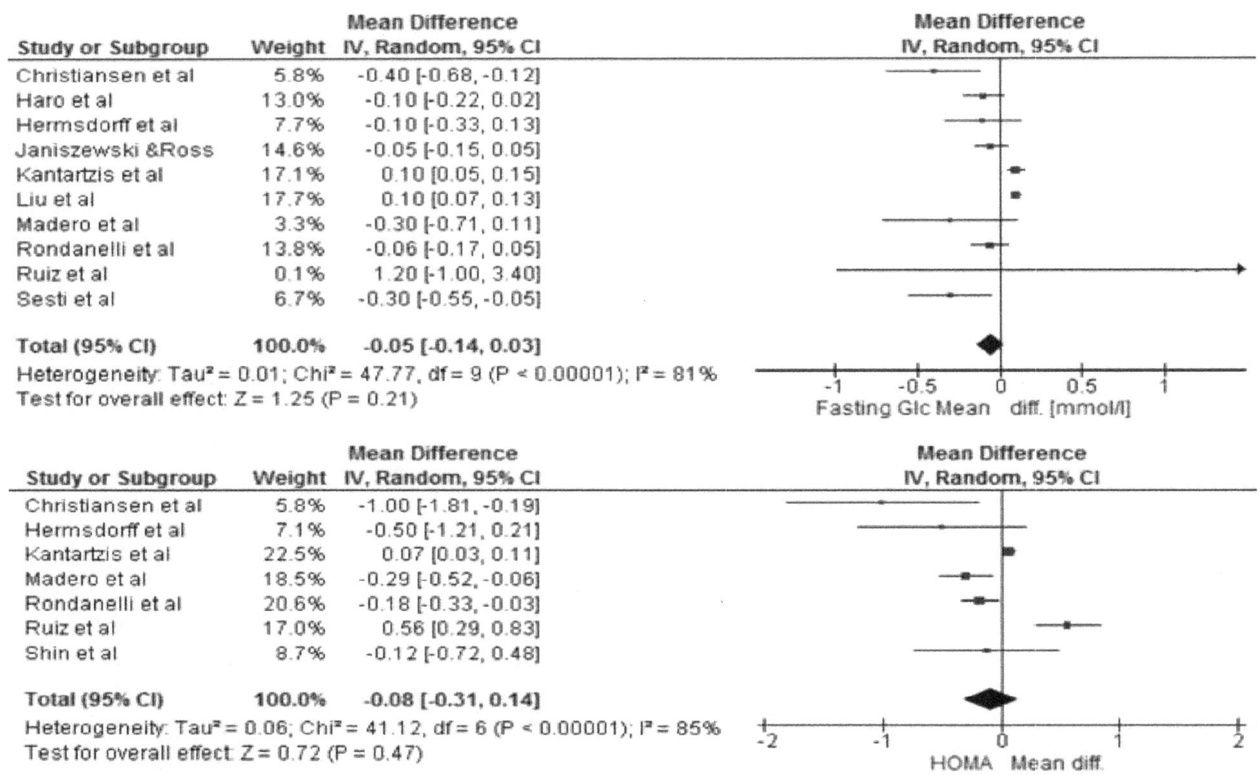

Figure 6. Forest plot of the random-effects meta-analysis of changes in Fasting Glucose and HOMA-IR according to reduction in energy intake shown as polled standard differences in the means with 95% Cis and in randomized and non-randomized trials. * For each study, the square represents the point estimate of the intervention effect. Horizontal lines join the lower and upper limits of the 95% CI of this effect. The area of shaded squares reflects the relative weight of the study in the meta-analysis. Diamonds represent the subgroup mean difference and pooled mean differences. CI indicates confidence interval.

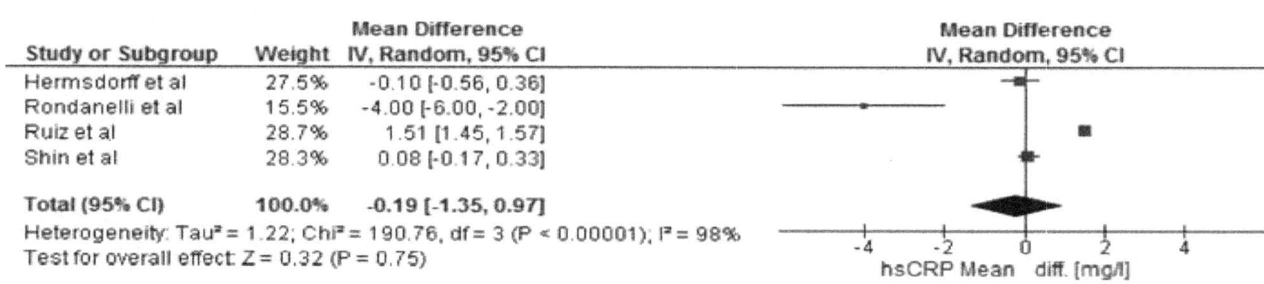

Figure 7. Forest plot of the random-effects meta-analysis of changes in high sensitivity C-Reactive Protein according to reduction in energy intake shown as polled standard differences in the means with 95% Cis and in randomized and non-randomized trials. * For each study, the square represents the point estimate of the intervention effect. Horizontal lines join the lower and upper limits of the 95% CI of this effect. The area of shaded squares reflects the relative weight of the study in the meta-analysis. Diamonds represent the subgroup mean difference and pooled mean differences. CI indicates confidence interval.

4. Discussion

Here, we present the first review summarizing the results from clinical studies performed in MHO with a primary interest in changes in BMI and selected cardio-metabolic outcomes. The findings of the conducted systematic review with meta-analysis did not find sufficient evidence to support the use of some specific diet in metabolically healthy obese subjects. However, it seems that effect of caloric restriction is related to reduction in BMI, blood pressure and triglycerides in the group of MHO patients.

It was imperative for the conducted review to show that the MHO subjects should be recognized as the core group with a primary interest in a changing lifestyle being the determinant of "metabolic health". Other longitudinal studies [29,30] with shorter follow-up (6–8.2 years) have indicated that only approximately half of MHO subjects maintained their "metabolic health" status. It was also suggested that initially MHO subjects undergo adverse metabolic changes associated with obesity over time [31]. Nevertheless, there is no clear data regarding the most beneficial dietary interventions, nor the effectiveness, of energy restricted diets in MHO patients taking into account clinical significance.

As previously demonstrated [32,33], obesity can be associated with a higher relative risk for CVD and cancer mortality compared to non-obese subjects. Therefore, the decrease in BMI can reflect the improvement in body composition, and consequently, reduce the mortality [34]. We have observed a significant association between the applications of energy restricted diets and BMI reduction in MHO individuals. Recently, Phillips and Perry [35] has also indicated that greater low density lipoprotein cholesterol (LDL-C) and HDL-C and less very low density lipoprotein cholesterol (VLDL-C) particles increase the likelihood of MHO. However, the results of our meta-analysis, through the applied dietary interventions, indicated only significantly beneficial association with the TG concentration within the MHO group. However, the inflammatory status in MHO can be reduced [36], partially stemming from more favorable fatty acid profiles [37] compared to MUHO, a significant decrease in hsCRP concentration was not observed in our analysis. As has been highlighted by Karelis et al. [38] health status may strongly influence the response to diet. For example, it was indicated in the MHO sedentary obese postmenopausal women without type 2 diabetes that the response to an energy-restricted diet may be different compared to at-risk individuals who achieve a similar weight loss, in that insulin sensitivity significantly improved in at-risk participants, but significantly deteriorated in MHO individuals in response to long-term diet. In our study, we did not find significant relation between energy restricted diets and biomarkers related to carbohydrates metabolism, i.e., fasting glucose and HOMA-IR within the MHO group of individuals. As shown in previously published studies [31,33], the baseline characteristic of metabolic profile can be more favorable in MHO compared to MUHO, which stay in line with some data selected for this systematic review [19,21]. As reported in Karelis et al. [39], MHO may have higher insulin sensitivity and a more favorable lipid profile. It has also been confirmed by Badoud et al. [40] that MHO individuals may show preserved insulin sensitivity and a greater ability to adapt to a caloric challenge compared to MUHO individuals. The postprandial response (i.e., area under the curve, AUC) for serum glucose and insulin were similar between MHO and lean healthy individuals and significantly lower than MUHO individuals ($p < 0.05$) [32]. However, a healthy metabolic profile and the absence of diabetic risk factors did not protect young adults from incident diabetes associated with overweight and obesity [40]. The intake of contraceptive pills by premenopausal women studied by Ruiz et al. [18] suggested that obtained results might be applied only for this sex and age group. Interestingly, the potential differences in body composition between MHO and MUHO were assessed in adults from the Pennington Center Longitudinal Study showing differences consistent between genders in both analyzed groups [34]. In clinical practice, as a goal for reducing CVD risk, the importance of body weight loss contributing to the maintenance of body weight loss is highlighted [4,41,42]. Camhi et al. [43] indicated that MHO young women demonstrate healthier lifestyle habits with less sedentary behavior, more time doing light physical activity, and healthier dietary quality for fat type and fiber in comparison to MUHO. Therefore, MUHO subjects are characterized by a higher risk of diabetes compared to MHO, which has been previously observed in Korean populations [44]. Indeed, metabolic health status, obesity and weight change were all independently associated with increased incidences of diabetes over five years of follow-up [44]. Nevertheless, we focused in our analysis on the MHO group of individuals only looking at the consequence of the applied dietary interventions. The data from the

International Population Study on Macro/Micronutrients and Blood Pressure (INTERMAP) cohort study did not support the hypothesis that diet composition accounts for the absence of cardio-metabolic abnormalities in MHO [45]. Furthermore, it has also been confirmed by Kimokoti et al. [46] in the cross-sectional analysis from the REasons for Geographic And Racial Differences in Stroke (REGARDS) study. Although HOMA-IR index can be slightly higher in MHO subjects than in subjects characterized by normal weight, it may also be lower compared to MUHO [21]. It has been also shown that a long-term intensive lifestyle program, including Mediterranean diet nutritional counselling and high-intensity interval training, may be an appropriate intervention in MHO and MUHO subjects with similar potential clinical health benefits including an improved body composition, blood pressure, fasting glucose levels, insulin sensitivity, peak oxygen uptake, and muscle endurance [47]. Therefore, it could be beneficial that the results obtained in intervention studies with regards to analyzed cardio-metabolic outcomes may have yielded stronger and more consistent support from the results of observational studies. More broadened interventional studies are needed to assess different dietary approaches in MHO subjects.

5. Limitations

The present findings are based on limited ethnicity (Caucasian, Asian), and, therefore, results could vary as a function of ethnic background. Although the duration of interventions in analyzed studies was relatively long, we could not analyze long-term follow-up changes of analyzed cardio-metabolic parameters (no data available in the literature). Although the applied dietary interventions were very different and heterogeneous in nature, all of them were based on energy restriction.

6. Conclusions

Based on the limited body of extracted data, we did not find sufficient evidence to support the use of some specific diet in metabolically healthy obese subjects. In general, it seems that the effect of caloric restriction is related to reduction in BMI, blood pressure and triglycerides in MHO individuals.

Acknowledgments: The authors are grateful to Robert J. Tower for English correction of the manuscript and Marcin Mardas for help in the updated search process.

Author Contributions: M.S.M. and J.W. designed the research and conducted the search. M.S.M. wrote the manuscript and analyzed data. J.W. critically reviewed manuscript content.

References

1. Kelly, T.; Yang, W.; Chen, C.S.; Reynolds, K.; He, J. Global burden of obesity in 2005 and projections to 2030. *Int. J. Obes.* **2008**, *32*, 1431–1437. [CrossRef] [PubMed]
2. Flegal, K.M.; Kit, B.K.; Orpana, H.; Graubard, B.I. Association of all-cause mortality with overweight and obesity using standard body mass index categories: A systematic review and meta-analysis. *JAMA* **2013**, *309*, 71–82. [CrossRef] [PubMed]
3. Ruderman, N.B.; Schneider, S.H.; Berchtold, P. The "metabolically obese", normal-weight individual. *Am. J. Clin. Nutr.* **1981**, *34*, 1617–1621. [CrossRef] [PubMed]
4. Wildman, R.P.; Muntner, P.; Reynolds, K.; McGinn, A.P.; Rajpathak, S.; Wylie-Rosett, J.; Sowers, M.R. The obese without cardiometabolic risk factor clustering and the normal weight with cardiometabolic risk factor clustering: Prevalence and correlates of 2 phenotypes among the US population (NHANES 1999–2004). *Arch. Intern. Med.* **2008**, *168*, 1617–1624. [CrossRef] [PubMed]

5. Meigs, J.B.; Wilson, P.W.; Fox, C.S.; Vasan, R.S.; Nathan, D.M.; Sullivan, L.M.; D'Agostino, R.B. Body mass index, metabolic syndrome, and risk of type 2 diabetes or cardiovascular disease. *J. Clin. Endocrinol. Metab.* **2006**, *91*, 2906–2912. [CrossRef] [PubMed]
6. Executive summary of the third report of the National Cholesterol Education Program (NCEP) expert panel on detection, evaluation, and treatment of high blood cholesterol in adults (adult treatment panel III). *JAMA* **2001**, *285*, 2486–2497.
7. Van Vliet-Ostaptchouk, J.V.; Nuotio, M.L.; Slagter, S.N.; Doiron, D.; Fischer, K.; Foco, L.; Gaye, A.; Gögele, M.; Heier, M.; Hiekkalinna, T.; et al. The prevalence of metabolic syndrome and metabolically healthy obesity in Europe: A collaborative analysis of ten large cohort studies. *BMC Endocr. Disord.* **2014**, *14*, 9. [CrossRef] [PubMed]
8. Soriguer, F.; Gutiérrez-Repiso, C.; Rubio-Martín, E.; García-Fuentes, E.; Almaraz, M.C.; Colomo, N.; de Antonio, I.E.; de Adana, M.S.R.; Chaves, F.J.; Morcillo, S.; et al. Metabolically healthy but obese, a matter of time? Findings from the prospective Pizarra study. *J. Clin. Endocrinol. Metab.* **2013**, *98*, 2318–2325. [CrossRef] [PubMed]
9. Schröder, H.; Ramos, R.; Baena-Díez, J.M.; Mendez, M.A.; Canal, D.J.; Fito, M.; Sala, J.; Elosua, R. Determinants of the transition from a cardiometabolic normal to abnormal overweight/obese phenotype in a Spanish population. *Eur. J. Nutr.* **2013**, *53*, 1345–1353. [CrossRef] [PubMed]
10. Moher, D.; Liberati, A.; Tetzlaff, J.; Altman, D.G.; PRISMA Group. Preferred reporting items for systematic reviews and meta-analyses: The PRISMA statement. *PLoS Med.* **2009**, *6*, e1000097. [CrossRef] [PubMed]
11. Stefan, N.; Häring, H.U.; Hu, F.B.; Schulze, M.B. Metabolically healthy obesity: Epidemiology, mechanisms, and clinical implications. *Lancet Diabetes Endocrinol.* **2013**, *1*, 152–162. [CrossRef]
12. Bo, S.; Musso, G.; Gambino, R.; Villois, P.; Gentile, L.; Durazzo, M.; Cavallo-Perin, P.; Cassader, M. Prognostic implications for insulin-sensitive and insulin-resistant normal-weight and obese individuals from a population-based cohort. *Am. J. Clin. Nutr.* **2012**, *96*, 962–969. [CrossRef] [PubMed]
13. Calori, G.; Lattuada, G.; Piemonti, L.; Garancini, M.P.; Ragogna, F.; Villa, M.; Mannino, S.; Crosignani, P.; Bosi, S.; Luzi, L.; et al. Prevalence, metabolic features, and prognosis of metabolically healthy obese Italian Individuals: The Cremona Study. *Diabetes Care* **2011**, *34*, 210–215. [CrossRef] [PubMed]
14. Hamer, M.; Stamatakis, E. Metabolically healthy obesity and risk of all-cause and cardiovascular disease mortality. *J. Clin. Endocrinol. Metab.* **2012**, *97*, 2482–2488. [CrossRef] [PubMed]
15. Wells, G.; Shea, B.; O'Connell, D.; Peterson, J.; Welch, V.; Losos, M.; Tugwell, P. The Newcastle-Ottawa Scale (NOS) for Assessing the Quality of Nonrandomized Studies in Meta–Analyses. Available online: http://www.ohri.ca/programs/clinical_epidemiology/oxford.htm (accessed on 17 June 2016).
16. Borenstein, M.; Hedges, L.V.; Higgins, J.P.T.; Rothstein, H.R. *Introduction to Meta-Analysis*; John Wiley & Sons Ltd.: Chichester, UK, 2009.
17. Rondanelli, M.; Klersy, C.; Perna, S.; Faliva, M.A.; Montorfano, G.; Roderi, P.; Colombo, I.; Corsetto, P.A.; Fioravanti, M.; Solerte, S.B.; et al. Effects of two-months balanced diet in metabolically healthy obesity: Lipid correlations with gender and BMI-related differences. *Lipids Health Dis.* **2015**, *14*, 139. [CrossRef] [PubMed]
18. Ruiz, J.R.; Ortega, F.B.; Labayen, I. A weight loss diet intervention has a similar beneficial effect on both metabolically abnormal obese and metabolically healthy but obese premenopausal women. *Ann. Nutr. Metab.* **2013**, *62*, 223–230. [CrossRef] [PubMed]
19. Kantartzis, K.; Machann, J.; Schick, F.; Rittig, K.; Machicao, F.; Fritsche, A.; Häring, H.-U.; Stefan, N. Effects of a lifestyle intervention in metabolically benign and malign obesity. *Diabetologia* **2011**, *54*, 864–868. [CrossRef] [PubMed]
20. Janiszewski, P.M.; Ross, R. Effects of weight loss among metabolically healthy obese men and women. *Diabetes Care* **2010**, *33*, 1957–1959. [CrossRef] [PubMed]
21. Shin, M.J.; Hyun, Y.J.; Kim, O.Y.; Kim, J.Y.; Jang, Y.; Lee, J.H. Weight loss effect on inflammation and LDL oxidation in metabolically healthy but obese (MHO) individuals: Low inflammation and LDL oxidation in MHO women. *Int. J. Obes.* **2006**, *30*, 1529–1534. [CrossRef] [PubMed]
22. Phillips, C.M. Metabolically healthy obesity: Definitions, determinants and clinical implications. *Rev. Endocr. Metab. Disord.* **2013**, *14*, 219–227. [CrossRef] [PubMed]
23. Liu, R.H.; Wharton, S.; Sharma, A.M.; Ardern, C.I.; Kuk, J.L. Influence of a clinical lifestyle-based weight loss program on the metabolic risk profile of metabolically normal and abnormal obese adults. *Obesity* **2013**, *21*, 1533–1539. [CrossRef] [PubMed]

24. Sesti, G.; Folli, F.; Perego, L.; Hribal, M.L.; Pontiroli, A.E. Effects of weight loss in metabolically healthy obese subjects after laparoscopic adjustable gastric banding and hypocaloric diet. *PLoS ONE* **2011**, *6*, e17737. [CrossRef] [PubMed]
25. Haro, C.; Montes-Borrego, M.; Rangel-Zúñiga, O.A.; Alcalá-Díaz, J.F.; Gómez-Delgado, F.; Pérez-Martínez, P.; Delgado-Lista, J.; Quintana-Navarro, G.M.; Tinahones, F.J.; Landa, B.B.; et al. Two Healthy Diets Modulate Gut Microbial Community Improving Insulin Sensitivity in a Human Obese Population. *J. Clin. Endocrinol. Metab.* **2016**, *101*, 233–242. [CrossRef] [PubMed]
26. Madero, M.; Arriaga, J.C.; Jalal, D.; Rivard, C.; McFann, K.; Pérez-Méndez, O.; Vázquez, A.; Ruiz, A.; Lanaspa, M.A.; Jimenez, C.R.; et al. The effect of two energy-restricted diets, a low-fructose diet versus a moderate natural fructose diet, on weight loss and metabolic syndrome parameters: A randomized controlled trial. *Metabolism* **2011**, *60*, 1551–1559. [CrossRef] [PubMed]
27. Foster, G.D.; Wyatt, H.R.; Hill, J.O.; Makris, A.P.; Rosenbaum, D.L.; Brill, C.; Stein, R.I.; Mohammed, B.S.; Miller, B.; Rader, D.J.; et al. Weight and metabolic outcomes after 2 years on a low-carbohydrate versus low-fat diet: A randomized trial. *Ann. Intern. Med.* **2010**, *153*, 147–157. [CrossRef] [PubMed]
28. Hermsdorff, H.H.M.; Zulet, M.Á.; Abete, I.; Martínez, J.A. A legume-based hypocaloric diet reduces proinflammatory status and improves metabolic features in overweight/obese subjects. *Eur. J. Nutr.* **2011**, *50*, 61–69. [CrossRef] [PubMed]
29. Christiansen, T.; Paulsen, S.K.; Bruun, J.M.; Pedersen, S.B.; Richelsen, B. Exercise training versus diet-induced weight-loss on metabolic risk factors and inflammatory markers in obese subjects: A 12-week randomized intervention study. *Am. J. Physiol. Endocrinol. Metab.* **2010**, *298*, E824–E831. [CrossRef] [PubMed]
30. Chang, Y.; Ryu, S.; Suh, B.S.; Yun, K.E.; Kim, C.-W.; Cho, S.-I. Impact of BMI on the incidence of metabolic abnormalities in metabolically healthy men. *Int. J. Obes.* **2012**, *36*, 1187–1194. [CrossRef] [PubMed]
31. Ortega, F.B.; Lee, D.C.; Katzmarzyk, P.T.; Ruiz, J.R.; Sui, X.; Church, T.S.; Blair, S.N. The intriguing metabolically healthy but obese phenotype: Cardiovascular prognosis and role of fitness. *Eur. Heart J.* **2013**, *34*, 389–397. [CrossRef] [PubMed]
32. Arnlov, J.; Ingelsson, E.; Sundstrom, J.; Lind, L. Impact of body mass index and the metabolic syndrome on the risk of cardiovascular disease and death in middle-aged men. *Circulation* **2010**, *121*, 230–236. [CrossRef] [PubMed]
33. Berentzen, T.L.; Jakobsen, M.U.; Halkjaer, J.; Tjønneland, A.; Overvad, K.; Sørensen, T.I.A. Changes in waist circumference and mortality in middle-aged men and women. *PLoS ONE* **2010**, *5*, e13097. [CrossRef] [PubMed]
34. Stelmach-Mardas, M.; Mardas, M.; Warchoł, W.; Jamka, M.; Walkowiak, J. Successful maintenance of body weight reduction after individualized dietary counseling in obese subjects. *Sci. Rep.* **2014**, *4*, 6620. [CrossRef] [PubMed]
35. Phillips, C.M.; Perry, I.J. Lipoprotein particle subclass profiles among metabolically healthy and unhealthy obese and non-obese adults: Does size matter? *Atherosclerosis* **2015**, *242*, 399–406. [CrossRef] [PubMed]
36. Perreault, M.; Zulyniak, M.A.; Badoud, F.; Stephenson, S.; Badawi, A.; Buchholz, A.; Mutch, D.M. A distinct fatty acid profile underlies the reduced inflammatory state of metabolically healthy obese individuals. *PLoS ONE* **2014**, *9*, e88539. [CrossRef] [PubMed]
37. Jung, H.S.; Chang, Y.; Eun Yun, K.; Kim, C.W.; Choi, E.S.; Kwon, M.J.; Cho, J.; Zhang, Y.; Rampal, S.; Zhao, D.; et al. Impact of body mass index, metabolic health and weight change on incident diabetes in a Korean population. *Obesity* **2014**, *22*, 1880–1887. [CrossRef] [PubMed]
38. Karelis, A.D.; Messier, V.; Brochu, M.; Rabasa-Lhoret, R. Metabolically healthy but obese women: Effect of an energy-restricted diet. *Diabetologia* **2008**, *51*, 1752–1754. [CrossRef] [PubMed]
39. Karelis, A.D.; St-Pierre, D.H.; Conus, F.; Rabasa-Lhoret, R.; Poehlman, E.T. Metabolic and body composition factors in subgroups of obesity: What do we know? *J. Clin. Endocrinol. Metab.* **2004**, *89*, 2569–2575. [CrossRef] [PubMed]
40. Badoud, F.; Lam, K.P.; Perreault, M.; Zulyniak, M.A.; Britz-McKibbin, P.; Mutch, D.M. Metabolomics Reveals Metabolically Healthy and Unhealthy Obese Individuals Differ in their Response to a Caloric Challenge. *PLoS ONE* **2015**, *10*, e0134613. [CrossRef] [PubMed]
41. Stelmach-Mardas, M.; Mardas, M.; Walkowiak, J.; Boeing, H. Long-term weight status in regainers after weight loss by lifestyle intervention: Status and challenges. *Proc. Nutr. Soc.* **2014**, *73*, 509–518. [CrossRef] [PubMed]

42. Phillips, C.M.; Dillon, C.; Harrington, J.M.; McCarthy, V.J.C.; Kearney, P.M.; Fitzgerald, A.P.; Perry, I.J. Defining metabolically healthy obesity: Role of dietary and lifestyle factors. *PLoS ONE* **2013**, *8*, e76188. [CrossRef] [PubMed]
43. Camhi, S.M.; Katzmarzyk, P.T. Differences in body composition between metabolically healthy obese and metabolically abnormal obese adults. *Int. J. Obes.* **2014**, *38*, 1142–1145. [CrossRef] [PubMed]
44. Camhi, S.M.; Crouter, S.E.; Hayman, L.L.; Must, A.; Lichtenstein, A.H. Lifestyle Behaviors in Metabolically Healthy and Unhealthy Overweight and Obese Women: A Preliminary Study. *PLoS ONE* **2015**, *10*, e0138548. [CrossRef] [PubMed]
45. Calanna, S.; Piro, S.; di Pino, A.; Zagami, R.M.; Urbano, F.; Purrello, F.; Rabuazzo, A.M. Beta and alpha cell function in metabolically healthy but obese subjects: Relationship with entero-insular axis. *Obesity* **2014**, *21*, 320–325. [CrossRef] [PubMed]
46. Hankinson, A.L.; Daviglus, M.L.; van Horn, L. Diet composition and activity level of at risk and metabolically healthy obese American adults. *Obesity* **2013**, *21*, 637–643. [CrossRef] [PubMed]
47. Kimokoti, R.W.; Judd, S.E.; Shikany, J.M.; Newby, P.K. Food intake does not differ between obese women who are metabolically healthy or abnormal. *J. Nutr.* **2014**, *144*, 2018–2026. [CrossRef] [PubMed]

5

Orthorexic Tendency in Polish Students: Exploring Association with Dietary Patterns, Body Satisfaction and Weight

Marta Plichta *, Marzena Jezewska-Zychowicz and Jerzy Gębski

Department of Organization and Consumption Economics, Faculty of Human Nutrition and Consumer Sciences, Warsaw University of Life Sciences (SGGW-WULS), 159C Nowoursynowska Street, 02-787 Warsaw, Poland; marzena_jezewska_zychowicz@sggw.pl (M.J.-Z.); jerzy_gebski@sggw.pl (J.G.)

* Correspondence: marta_plichta@sggw.pl

Abstract: Body dissatisfaction is central to clinically diagnosed eating disorders (ED) and seems to be important in causing other non-clinical disorders, including orthorexia nervosa (ON). It can also affect eating behaviors. The aim of this study was to assess the associations of ON tendency with dietary patterns (DPs) and body satisfaction. The data were collected in 2017 through questionnaire survey among 1120 students of health-oriented and other academic programs from seven universities in Poland. Principal components analysis (PCA) was conducted to derive DPs and body satisfaction factors. Six DPs, such as, 'High-sugar products & snacks', 'Fresh products & nuts', 'Fatty products & dressings', 'Oils & potatoes', 'Dairy products & whole-meal bread', 'Meat', and two body satisfaction factors, such as, 'Bottom body & weight', and 'Upper body' were identified. ON tendency was measured using ORTO-15 questionnaire with both cut-offs, i.e., 35 and 40. Logistic regression analysis was used to verify associations between ON tendency, body satisfaction factors, and DPs. More students of health related majors were characterized by ON tendency in comparison to students of other majors (35.9 vs. 37.2; $p < 0.001$). More women were dissatisfied with 'Bottom body & weight compared to men (<0.001). The higher the body mass index (BMI), the more people were dissatisfied with 'Bottom body & weight' ($p < 0.001$). More students with ON tendency were satisfied with their 'Upper body' than those without ON tendency, but there were no differences in ON tendency in regard to 'Bottom body & weight' satisfaction. ON tendency was associated with more frequent consumption of vegetables, fruits, nuts and seeds, and less frequent consumption of products high in sugar, snacks, fatty products and dressings. Using cut-off at 35 in ORTO-15 seems to be more appropriate than cut-off at 40 to identify external variables describing ON. Future research on orthorexia nervosa should use other research tools than ORTO-15 to better identify individuals with ON and to confirm our findings.

Keywords: dietary patterns; body satisfaction; orthorexia nervosa; students

---

1. Introduction

Dissatisfaction with one's body, distorted body image perception and obsession with thinness are central to clinically diagnosed eating disorders (ED) such as anorexia nervosa (AN), bulimia nervosa (BN), binge eating disorder (BED) and eating disorders not otherwise specified (EDNOS) [1]. It can be assumed, that these factors may also contribute to other non-clinical types of disorders including orthorexia nervosa (ON). ON expresses a pathological interest in healthy food. The healthy behavior and ON are placed as extreme poles on the continuum scale of states differing in the intensity of orthorexic symptoms [2].

ON was used to define an unhealthy obsession with healthy eating [3]. Individuals with ON eliminate certain food products that are perceived by them as unhealthy and impure. They avoid foods with high content of salt, sugar and fat, foods containing genetically-modified ingredients, herbicides, pesticides and artificial substances and also non-organic foods. Each meal is prepared with great concern and attention, often with repetitive activities which are to ensure the safety of food intake. This obsession is driven by a desire to optimize own health and well-being [4]. Individuals with ON may be on alternative diets (e.g., vegetarianism, veganism, raw foods, macrobiotics, fruitarianism) [5–7]. Recently, Dunn and Bratman [8] proposed the new criteria of classification of ON containing extreme preoccupation with healthy eating, restrictive eating behaviors, malnutrition, severe weight loss as a results of food choices as well as feeling guilt or self-loathing if diet is not followed correctly. However, no standardized tool for diagnosis currently exists [9–13].

To assess ON, ORTO-15 questionnaire [14] based on Bratman Orthorexia Test (BOT) [4] is widely used, despite criticism regarding this research tool [7]. Some researchers suggested that ORTO-15 questionnaire may not be able to distinguish pathological behaviors and is not clinically relevant [15]. However, the recent review of the studies using ORTO-15 showed that Cronbach's alpha coefficients were ranging from 0.83 to 0.91 [16]. The Italian version of ORTO-15 was translated into several languages, usually with the use of complicated multistep methods, and then administered to different samples. The results of confirmatory analysis and other methods allowed researchers to shorten original ORTO-15 [7]. In this way, the Turkish version of ORTO-11 [10] and ORTO-11-Hu, Hungarian adaptation of the ORTO-15 [12], were developed. In the original version of ORTO-15, to distinguish the orthorexic tendency it is recommended to use the cut-off point below 40 [17], and some researchers followed this recommendation [18,19]. Nevertheless, there are also suggestions to lower the cut-off point in this test to 35 [11,18]. Lowering the cut-off point would allow distinguishing a group of people in which the ON symptoms can be clearly identified. Thus, it enables a more effective search for the ON symptoms, its causes and consequences.

ON reveals several similarities with other eating disorders, such as avoidant/restrictive food intake disorder (AFRID) [20] and AN [21]. AFRID is characterized by the lack of interest in food, avoiding food products with specific shapes or colors, or anxiety about the aversive consequences of eating [22]. Nevertheless, the anxiety about eating results from a response to a preceding traumatic event (e.g., choking) or an aversive experience (e.g., repeated vomiting) [22,23] and not from excessive concerns for health as in ON. In contrast, AN and ON share traits of perfectionism, cognitive rigidity, high co-morbid anxiety, and need for control of life transferred to eating [5,21]. Both patients with AN and patients with ON perceive their behaviors as ego-syntonic [24]. Nonetheless, patients with ON are concerned about food quality rather than food quantity in contrast to patients with AN [25]. In addition to AN characteristics, individuals with ON may evince obsessive-compulsive disorders (OCD) [26] due to burdensome obsessions (e.g., intensive meal planning, intrusive thoughts of food) and compulsions (e.g., exact measuring and weighing of food). However, the obsessions in OCD are described as ego-dystonic [6].

ON may lead to severe physical and psychological complications such as, caloric deficit, lack of vitamins and minerals, gastrointestinal problems, stomach inflammation, anemia, osteopenia, hyponatremia, pancytopenia, heart failure, significant distress, and social isolation [2,5,27,28]. However, ON is still not diagnosed well and not recognized in the Diagnostic and Statistical Manual of Mental Disorders DSM-5 [1]. Thus, further research is needed to better understand the symptoms of ON [27,29].

Despite certain similarities between AN and ON, some researchers suppose that ON is not associated with weight control [24,30]. Nevertheless, young people are often dissatisfied with their bodies [31,32], and such negative body image may put them at severe health risk because it strongly predicts the development of disordered eating [33]. It has been showed that females with ON were characterized by striving for thinness, lower body satisfaction, and lower body acceptance [34]. Previous studies have shown that increased ON symptomatology was associated with calorie restriction and preoccupation with weight [10,13,18,35–39]. Nevertheless, the relationship of ON and body satisfaction requires further research.

Orthorexic individuals represented very specific eating habits, among others they avoid foods that may include genetically modified ingredients or pesticides, foods high in salt or sugar, and foods high in fat [24,40]. Previous research has shown that individuals eating whole wheat cereals, as well as fruits and vegetables more frequently were characterized by higher ON tendency compared to others [41]. However, despite the fact that ON is characterized by very specific eating behaviors, still little is known about food intake frequency in relation to this disorder [12,41]. To the best of our knowledge, the relationship between dietary patterns (DPs), body satisfaction and ON tendency was not examined. Therefore the aim of our study was first, to estimate the orthorexic tendency among students of different college majors, and second, to find the associations between ON tendency, body satisfaction, and dietary patterns in students taking into account gender, body mass index (BMI) and college majors, and third to recognize the usefulness of both cut-offs used to identify orthorexic tendency (at 35, and 40 points in ORTO-15) in the determination of external variables describing ON symptoms including dietary patterns and body satisfaction.

2. Materials and Methods

2.1. Ethical Approval

The study protocol was approved by the Ethics Committee of Faculty of Human Nutrition and Consumer Science, Warsaw University of Life Sciences (Resolution number 45/2017). Informed consent to participate in the study was collected from all participants.

2.2. Participants and Procedure

The study sample was selected in seven universities from Poland. The survey was conducted during lectures by a trained person. The teacher left the room after consenting to the survey among students. The persons participating in the study were informed about the purpose, course and duration of the study, as well as about the possibility of resigning from the study at any stage without bearing any legal liability. Participation in the study was voluntary. The questionnaire took approximately 15 min to complete. In total, 1300 students of health-oriented and other academic programs were invited to participate in the study. Male and female students at the age from 18 to 35 years old were included in the sample. As a result of incomplete questionnaires, 162 participants were excluded from the sample. Moreover, 18 students were excluded from the sample as they were older than 35 years old. Finally, the sample consisted of 1120 students who completed questionnaires correctly. The data were collected in 2017.

2.3. Questionnaire

The ORTO-15 questionnaire [19] was used to identify the ON tendency. The Polish version used in our study was adapted from the original Italian ORTO-15 [14], and has good repeatability and satisfactory reliability (Cronbach's alpha 0.70–0.90) [19]. The ORTO-15 is a validated measure consisting of 15 items that assesses beliefs about the perceived effects of eating healthy food, attitudes conditioning food selection, habits regarding food consumption, and the extent to which food concerns affect daily life [24]. Responses expressing the obsessive attitude of the individuals in choosing, buying, preparing and consuming food are scored on a 4-point scale (always, often, sometimes, never). Responses indicating ON symptoms were scored 1, while responses describing adequate eating behaviors were scored 4. The sum of scores was calculated for each participant with a minimum of 15 and a maximum of 60.

The Questionnaire of Body Particular Parts and Parameters Satisfaction [42] was used to measure body satisfaction. This tool was developed and then validated in the Polish population. The obtained reliability index for the entire scale was considered satisfactory (Cronbach's alpha

0.86) [42]. Respondents defined the satisfaction level with particular body parts on a nine-point scale, where: 1—totally dissatisfied; 5—neither dissatisfied nor satisfied; 9—totally satisfied. The following parts of the body were included in the questionnaire: face; shoulders; breast/chest; waist/midsection; abdomen; hips; thighs; legs; weight and height of body.

The Food Frequency Questionnaire (FFQ-6) was applied to determine respondents' dietary habits [43]. The FFQ-6 was validated in females aged 13–21 years old [43] and in both men and women aged 21–26 years old [44]. The FFQ-6 covered the diet thoroughly, including many of the most popular dishes consumed in Poland. The FFQ contained a list of 165 products and dishes which represented such food groups as: sweets and snacks; dairy products and eggs; cereal products; fats; fruits; vegetables and grains; meat and fish products; beverages. The frequency of food consumption throughout the year preceding the study was assessed. For this analysis, 26 products and dishes were chosen, including: sugar; chocolate, chocolate candies and chocolate bars; non-chocolate candies; biscuits and cookies; salty snacks; milk and natural milk drinks; sweetened milk drinks; cheese; whole-meal bread; refined bread; oils; butter; margarine; sour cream and sweet cream; other animal fats; mayonnaise and dressings; fresh fruits; processed fruit products; fresh vegetables; potatoes; nuts; grains and wheat germ; red meat; poultry meat and rabbit meat; fatty fish; sweetened fizzy drinks. When selecting 26 products, the results of other studies on the relationship between body dissatisfaction and consumed foods were taken into account [45,46]. In addition, the choice of items resulted from their importance in diet of individuals with ON tendency. FFQ-6 included six categories of food intake frequency: never or almost never (1 points); once a month or less frequently (2 points); several times per month (3 points); several times per week (4 points); every day (5 points); and several times per day (6 points).

Socioeconomic profile of participants was assessed based on questions regarding gender, age (in years), place of residence, and college major. Body Mass Index (BMI) was calculated using self-reported weight and height and categorized accordingly World Health Organization [47] into four groups: underweight ($BMI < 18.5\ kg/m^2$), normal weight ($18.5 \leq BMI \leq 24.9\ kg/m^2$), overweight ($25.0 \leq BMI \leq 29.9\ kg/m^2$) and obesity ($BMI \geq 30.0\ kg/m^2$).

2.4. The Sample Characteristics

The characteristics of the sample are presented in Table 1. The sample included 1120 college students, of which 70.4% were female and 29.6% were male. The highest number of participants were younger than 20 years old (36.1%). Majority of the students lived in cities (71.6%). More participants were enrolled in bachelor or engineering studies (88.7%) than in master studies (11.3%). Almost a half of the sample (48.8%) represented health related majors (Food Technology and Human Nutrition, Dietetics, Physiotherapy, Physical Education and Wellness) and 51.2% were students of other majors. The majority of participants had normal weight (72.9%).

Table 1. Sociodemographic characteristics of the study sample.

Variables		*N* = 1120	%
Gender	Female	789	70.4
	Male	331	29.6
Age	18–19	404	36.1
	20–22	388	34.6
	23–25	253	22.6
	26–35	75	6.7
Place of residence	Village	318	28.4
	City ≤ 100.000 citizens	319	28.5
	City > 100.000 citizens	483	43.1
Level of studies	Bachelor or engineering studies	994	88.7
	Master studies	126	11.3

Table 1. *Cont.*

Variables		*N* = 1120	%
College major	Health related	547	48.8
	Non health related	573	51.2
BMI categories	Underweight	123	11.0
	Normal weight	817	72.9
	Overweight	154	13.8
	Obesity	26	2.3

N—number of participants, BMI—body mass index.

2.5. Data Analysis

Descriptive statistics including frequency distributions and cross-tabulations were carried out. The Principal Component Analysis (PCA) was applied to identify body satisfaction factors and dietary patterns (DPs), separately. The factors were orthogonally rotated (the varimax option) to maintain uncorrelated factor variables. The number of factors was based on the following criteria: components with an eigenvalue of 0.1, scree plot test and the interpretability of the factors. The factorability of data was confirmed with Kaiser–Meyer–Olkin (KMO) measure of sampling adequacy and Bartlett's test of sphericity achieving statistical significance. Bartlett's tests have a significance of $p < 0.001$ for both data. KMO value for body satisfaction data was 0.862 and for dietary data was 0.842. Factor loadings higher than 0.4 assure that the variables extracted are shown through a specific factor, therefore both food items and body parts with factor-loadings of at least 0.50 have been taken into consideration and used to label the dietary patterns and body satisfaction factors, respectively [48].

Two body satisfaction factors were identified: 'Bottom body & weight' and 'Upper body'. Total variance explained was 57.6%. The factor-loading matrix for the body satisfaction identified by principal component analysis (PCA) is presented in detail in Table 2.

Table 2. Factor-loading matrix for the body satisfaction factors identified by principal component analysis (PCA).

Variables	Bottom Body & Weight	Upper Body
Waist/midsection	**0.617**	0.438
Abdomen	**0.692**	0.321
Hips	**0.800**	0.261
Thighs	**0.853**	0.137
Legs	**0.795**	0.141
Weight	**0.758**	0.436
Face	0.186	**0.715**
Shoulders	0.282	**0.666**
Breasts/chest	0.064	**0.750**
Variance Explained (%)	46.0	11.6
Total Variance Explained (%)	57.6	
Kaiser's Measure of Sampling Adequacy	0.862	

Bolded values are marked for the main components of PCA-derived body satisfaction factors with absolute loadings ≥ 0.5.

Six dietary patterns were identified: 'High-sugar products & snacks', 'Fresh products & nuts', 'Fatty products & dressings', 'Oils & potatoes', 'Dairy products & whole-meal bread', and 'Meat'. Total variance explained was 51.3%. For each factor the explained variance was: 19.1%, 10.9%, 6.7%, 5.4%, 4.8%, and 4.4%, respectively. The factor-loading matrix for the DPs identified by principal component analysis (PCA) is presented in detail in Table 3.

Table 3. Factor-loading matrix for the DPs identified by principal component analysis (PCA).

Variables	High-Sugar Products & Snacks	Fresh Products & Nuts	Fatty Products & Dressings	Oils & Potatoes	Dairy Products & Whole-Meal Bread	Meat
Chocolate, chocolate candies and chocolate bars	**0.722**	−0.094	−0.020	0.090	0.084	0.016
Biscuits and cookies	**0.709**	−0.023	0.028	0.115	0.195	0.032
Non chocolate candies	**0.757**	0.024	0.103	−0.046	0.006	0.125
Salty snacks	**0.580**	−0.093	0.251	0.121	−0.075	0.045
Sweetened milk drinks	**0.506**	−0.083	0.243	−0.017	0.461	0.022
Milk and natural milk drinks	0.095	0.073	−0.001	0.007	**0.785**	0.034
Cheese, blue cheese, melted cheese, spread cheese	0.111	−0.075	0.250	0.159	**0.616**	0.034
Whole-meal bread	−0.085	0.249	−0.225	0.054	**0.525**	−0.058
Margarine	0.190	−0.028	**0.561**	0.064	0.012	−0.187
Sour cream and sweet cream	0.178	−0.001	**0.537**	0.312	0.312	0.073
Other animal fats	0.048	0.139	**0.640**	0.047	−0.051	0.381
Mayonnaise and dressings	0.229	−0.066	**0.502**	0.298	0.166	0.141
Fresh fruits	−0.006	**0.640**	−0.372	0.304	0.134	−0.088
Fresh vegetables	−0.207	**0.594**	−0.328	0.311	0.106	0.013
Nuts	−0.099	**0.728**	0.084	−0.058	−0.037	0.093
Seeds (e.g., pumpkin, sesame, sunflower, wheat germ)	−0.068	**0.738**	0.104	−0.111	0.018	−0.047
Red meat (e.g., pork, beef, veal)	0.065	−0.010	0.233	0.139	−0.018	**0.770**
Poultry meat and rabbit meat	0.115	−0.039	−0.095	0.123	0.030	**0.764**
Oils	−0.008	0.172	−0.008	0.658	0.082	0.068
Potatoes	0.258	−0.017	0.159	0.631	−0.053	0.129
Variance Explained (%)	19.1	10.9	6.7	5.4	4.8	4.4
Total Variance Explained (%)	51.3					
Kaiser's Measure of Sampling Adequacy			0.842			

Bolded values are marked for the main components of PCA-derived dietary patterns factors with absolute loadings ≥ 0.5.

Respondents allocated to each of the dietary patterns were divided into three groups based on tertile distribution: bottom, middle and upper tertile. Participants in the upper tertile had the strongest adherence to the pattern.

Two categories within each body satisfaction factors, such as, satisfaction and dissatisfaction, were created using factor scores obtained with regression approach. The factor scores of 0 and below is interpreted as 'dissatisfaction', whereas the value above 0 as 'satisfaction' with body.

According to Donini et al. [14], a score lower than or equal to 40 indicates ON tendency, while higher scores inform about adequate eating behaviors. Whereas according to Ramacciotti et al. [11], a cut-off at 35 provides a lower and more accurate estimate of ON tendency, than the cut-off at 40. Both cut-offs were included in our study. Cronbach's alpha for ORTO-15 was 0.7.

The differences between groups were verified by Chi-square test (the ON tendency groups versus sociodemographic characteristics, including gender, age bracket, place of residence, level of studies, college major and BMI categories); student's t-test (mean score of ORTO-15 versus gender and college majors); the one-way analysis of variance ANOVA (mean score of ORTO-15 versus BMI categories).

A simple logistic regression analysis was applied to the models verifying associations between ON tendency, body satisfaction, and DPs. The odds ratio (OR) and 95% confidence interval (95% CI) were calculated. Such dichotomous variables as ON tendency, 'Bottom body & weight' and 'Upper body' have been introduced into models as dependent variables. The independent variables in the models were dietary patterns. The OR calculated for each independent variable represents the odds ratio between a given variable level (the upper tertile of each dietary pattern), and the adopted level of reference (the bottom tertile—OR = 1.00) while the remaining explanatory (independent) variables remain constant. The adjusted models were developed for the potential confounders, such as, gender (categorical, female/men), age (continuous, years), place of residence (categorical, village/city $\leq$ 100.000 citizens/city > 100.000 citizens), level of studies (categorical, bachelor or engineering studies/master studies), college major (categorical, health related/non health related), and BMI (continuous, kg/m^2). The level of significance of the odds ratio was assessed with a Wald test. A p-value ≤ 0.05 was considered statistically significant for all tests. All analyses were carried out applying sample weights to adjust for non-response and missing data. All analyses were performed using SAS 9.4. software (SAS Institute, Cary, NC, USA).

3. Results

3.1. Orthorexia Nervosa Tendency and Body Satisfaction across Gender, BMI and College Major

The ON tendency was observed among 75.0% of the sample when the cut-off at 40 was used. However, only 28.3% of students showed ON tendency when the cut-off at 35 was implemented. Mean value of ORTO-15 was 36.6 (standard deviation 4.2). More than a half of participants were satisfied with both 'Bottom body & weight' (52.9%) and 'Upper body' (51.4%). Twice more females than males were dissatisfied with 'Bottom body & weight' ($p < 0.001$). There were no significant differences in ON tendency and 'Upper body' satisfaction between gender groups (Table 4).

The differences between BMI categories regarding 'Bottom body & weight' satisfaction were observed (<0.001). The higher the BMI, the more people were dissatisfied with 'Bottom body & weight'. No significant differences were observed between BMI categories in regard to the ON tendency (regardless of the cut-off point) and 'Upper body' satisfaction (Table 5).

Students of health related majors (35.9 $\pm$ 4.1) scored significantly lower in ORTO-15 than students of other majors (37.2 $\pm$ 4.2). More students of health related majors (79.3%) than students of other majors (70.9%) displayed ON tendency (cut-off at 40). Similarly, such difference was observed with the cut-off at 30 (32.9 and 23.9%, respectively). There were no significant differences both in 'Bottom body & weight' and 'Upper body' satisfaction across the college majors (Table 6).

Table 4. Orthorexia nervosa tendency and body satisfaction in the total sample and gender groups.

Variables	Total Sample	Female	Male	Chi-Squared Test/Student's *t*-Test	*p*-Value
	N = 1120	*N* = 789	*N* = 331		
Orthorexia nervosa *n* (%)					
ON tendency (<40)	840 (75.0)	595 (75.4)	245 (74.0)	0.24 *	0.623
Without ON tendency (<40)	280 (25.0)	194 (24.6)	86 (26.0)		
ON tendency (<35)	317 (28.3)	219 (27.8)	98 (29.6)	0.39 *	0.530
Without ON tendency (<35)	803 (71.7)	570 (72.2)	233 (70.4)		
ORTO-15 score (M ± SD)	36.6 ± 4.2	36.6 ± 4.1	36.6 ± 4.4	0.03 **	0.973
'Bottom body & weight' *n* (%)					
Dissatisfaction	527 (47.1)	437 (55.4)	90 (27.2)	74.41 *	<0.001
Satisfaction	593 (52.9)	352 (44.6)	241 (72.8)		
'Upper body' *n* (%)					
Dissatisfaction	544 (48.6)	372 (47.2)	172 (52.0)	2.16 *	0.141
Satisfaction	576 (51.4)	417 (52.8	159 (58.0)		

* Chi-squared test; ** Student's *t*-test (t); ON—orthorexia nervosa; M—mean; SD—standard deviation.

Table 5. Orthorexia nervosa tendency and body satisfaction according to BMI categories.

Variables	Underweight	Normal Weight	Overweight	Obesity	Chi-Squared Test/ANOVA	*p*-Value
	N = 123	*N* = 817	*N* = 154	*N* = 26		
Orthorexia nervosa *n* (%)						
ON tendency (<40)	91 (74.0)	620 (75.9)	111 (72.1)	18 (69.2)	1.57 *	0.665
Without ON tendency (<40)	32 (26.0)	197 (24.1)	43 (27.9)	8 (30.8)		
ON tendency (<35)	38 (30.9)	230 (28.2)	43 (27.9)	6 (23.1)	0.78 *	0.855
Without ON tendency (<35)	85 (69.1)	587 (71.9)	111 (72.1)	20 (76.9)		
ORTO-15 score (M ± SD)	36.5 ± 4.4	36.6 ± 4.1	36.6 ± 4.6	37.7 ± 3.6	1.23 **	0.197
'Bottom body & weight' *n* (%)						
Dissatisfaction	32 (26.0)	382 (46.8)	93 (60.4)	20 (76.9)	42.18 *	<0.001
Satisfaction	91 (74.0)	435 (53.2)	61 (39.6)	6 (23.1)		
'Upper body' *n* (%)						
Dissatisfaction	70 (56.9)	389 (47.6)	69 (44.8)	16 (61.5)	6.35 *	0.096
Satisfaction	53 (43.1)	428 (52.4)	85 (55.2)	10 (38.5)		

* Chi squared test; ** one-way analysis of variance ANOVA (F).

Table 6. Orthorexia nervosa tendency and body satisfaction according to majors of the study.

Variables	Health Related Majors	Non Health Related Majors	Chi-Squared Test/Student's *t*-Test	*p*-Value
	N = 547	*N* = 573		
Orthorexia nervosa *n* (%)				
ON tendency (<40)	434 (79.3)	406 (70.9)	10.75 *	0.001
Without ON tendency (<40)	113 (20.7)	167 (29.1)		
ON tendency (<35)	180 (32.9)	137 (23.9)	11.16 *	<0.001
Without ON tendency (<35)	367 (67.1)	436 (76.1)		
ORTO-15 score (M ± SD)	35.9 ± 4.1	37.2 ± 4.2	4.95 **	<0.001
'Bottom body & weight' *n* (%)				
Dissatisfaction	270 (49.4)	257 (44.9)	2.28 *	0.131
Satisfaction	277 (50.6)	316 (55.2)		
'Upper body' *n* (%)				
Dissatisfaction	269 (49.2)	275 (48.0)	0.16 *	0.692
Satisfaction	278 (50.8)	298 (52.0)		

* Chi squared test; ** Student's *t*-test (t).

3.2. *Orthorexia Nervosa Tendency and Body Satisfaction*

More students with ON tendency were satisfied with their 'Upper body' in comparison with students without ON tendency. There was not a significant difference in 'Bottom body & weight' satisfaction in respect to ON tendency. Such relationships were demonstrated for categories identified using both cut-offs ($p = 0.027$ and $p = 0.005$, respectively at 40 and 35) (Table 7).

3.3. *Associations between Orthorexia Nervosa Tendency, Body Satisfaction and Dietary Patterns*

The results from the adjusted model have demonstrated that students who consumed high-sugar products and snacks most often (the upper tertile of DP) were less likely to display ON tendency, regardless of the cut-off point. Odds Ratio (OR) was higher at the cut-off at 35 points compared to the cut-off at 40 points (0.32 and 0.34, respectively). In addition, students in the upper tertile of 'Fatty products & dressings' pattern were less likely to display ON tendency compared to those in the bottom tertile of this DP. However, Odds Ratio (OR) was lower at the cut-off at 35 compared to the cut-off at 40 (0.52 and 0.59, respectively). In contrast, students in the upper tertile of 'Fresh products & nuts' were more than twice as likely to have ON tendency compared to those in the bottom tertile of this DP. Odds Ratio (OR) was higher at the cut-off at 35 compared to the cut-off at 40 (2.49 and 2.30, respectively) (Table 8).

Table 7. Orthorexia nervosa tendency and body satisfaction in the total sample.

Variables	ON Tendency (<40)	Without ON Tendency (<40)	Chi-Squared Test	*p*-Value	ON Tendency (<35)	Without ON Tendency (<35)	Chi-Squared Test	*p*-Value
	N = 840	*N* = 280			*N* = 317	*N* = 803		
'Bottom body & weight' *n* (%)								
Dissatisfaction	392 (46.7)	135 (48.2)	0.20	0.653	139 (43.9)	388 (48.3)	1.82	0.177
Satisfaction	448 (53.3)	145 (51.8)			171 (56.1)	415 (51.7)		
'Upper body' *n* (%)								
Dissatisfaction	392 (46.7)	152 (54.3)	4.88	0.027	133 (42.0)	411 (51.2)	7.75	0.005
Satisfaction	448 (53.3)	128 (45.7)			184 (58.0)	392 (48.8)		

Table 8. Dietary patterns by orthorexia nervosa tendency and body satisfaction: adjusted logistic regression model (odds ratios with 95% confidence interval).

ON Tendency/Body Satisfaction	Dietary Patterns											
	High-Sugar Products & Snacks [c] (Ref. Bottom Tertile)		Fresh Products & Nuts [c] (Ref. Bottom Tertile)		Fatty Products & Dressings [c] (Ref. Bottom Tertile)		Oils & Potatoes [c] (Ref. Bottom Tertile)		Dairy Products & Whole-Meal Bread [c] (Ref. Bottom Tertile)		Meat [c] (Ref. Bottom Tertile)	
	Upper Tertile	*p*	Upper Tertile	*p*	Upper Tertile	*p*	Upper Tertile	*p*	Upper Tertile	*p*	Upper Tertile	*p*
Orthorexia nervosa [a] (ON tendency <40) [b]	0.32 [d] (0.22; 0.46) [e]	<0.001	2.30 (1.59; 3.32)	<0.001	0.59 (0.41; 0.85)	0.004	0.93 (0.65; 1.32)	0.690	1.06 (0.74; 1.51)	0.771	1.15 (0.79; 1.68)	0.471
Orthorexia nervosa [a] (ON tendency <35) [b]	0.33 (0.24; 0.48)	<0.001	2.46 (1.72; 3.52)	<0.001	0.52 (0.36; 0.75)	<0.001	0.75 (0.53; 1.05)	0.094	0.93 (0.66; 1.32)	0.687	1.00 (0.70; 1.43)	0.994
'Bottom body & weight' [a] (dissatisfaction) [b]	0.92 (0.66; 1.28)	0.606	0.82 (0.59; 1.15)	0.248	0.94 (0.66; 1.32)	0.714	0.81 (0.59; 1.13)	0.217	1.00 (0.72; 1.39)	0.992	0.78 (0.55; 1.11)	0.163
'Upper body' [a] (dissatisfaction) [b]	1.75 (1.29; 2.37)	<0.001	0.65 (0.48; 0.88)	0.005	1.03 (0.76; 1.41)	0.832	0.76 (0.57; 1.03)	0.073	1.02 (0.75; 1.37)	0.922	1.07 (0.78; 1.47)	0.669

[a] dependent variable; [b] predicted level of dependent variable; [c] independent variables; [d] OR point estimate (e^{β}) upper tertile vs. lower tertile; [e] 95% Wald Confidence Intervals. All data adjusted for sample weights. ORs were adjusted for: gender (categorical, female/men), age (continuous, years), place of residence (categorical, village/city $\leq$ 100.000 citizens/city > 100.000 citizens), level of studies (categorical, bachelor or engineering studies/master studies), college major (categorical, health related/non health related), BMI (continuous, kg/m^2); $p < 0.05$ (Wald's test).

Students in the upper tertile of 'High-sugar products & snacks' were more likely to be dissatisfied with their 'Upper body' ((OR) 1.75, 95% CI: 1.29–2.37) compared to those in the bottom tertile. Students who consumed fresh products and nuts most often (the upper tertile of 'Fresh products & nuts') were less likely to be dissatisfied with their 'Upper body' ((OR) 0.65, 95% CI: 0.48–0.88) than those in the bottom tertile. No significant associations between 'Bottom body & weight' satisfaction and DPs were revealed (Table 8).

4. Discussion

In our study we attempted to assess the occurrence of the ON tendency amongst students, who, due to their young age, are prone to developing incorrect eating behaviors [49]. Our results obtained in the ORTO-15 test for the cut-off of 40 are in accordance with other studies [12,38,50,51]. After reducing the cut-off limit to 35 points, there was almost a three-fold decrease in the number of people with ON tendency (from 75.0% to 28.3%). Other researchers also pointed out the validity of lowering the cut-off below 35 points in the ORTO-15 test [11,18].

Previous research indicate that the occurrence of ON is more common among students of medicine [10], exercise science [52], dietetics [53] and majors related to nutrition [9]. Our results also confirm these observations in relation to health-related majors. Both the percentage of people with ON symptoms and the mean value of ORTO-15 indicate differences between students of majors related to health and the rest of participants, but these differences were not of clinical significance. However, they can be used in the development of education programs. Students of health-related majors acquire knowledge about the principles of adequate nutrition and health consequences resulting from their non-observance. In addition, they use other sources of information (e.g., Internet sources) about food and its impact on health [54]. This may result in the application of strict nutritional rules aimed at maintaining health or normal body weight, however this can also lead to the development of eating disorders [55,56].

Our study did not reveal differences in the occurrence of ON tendency between the categories identified due to BMI, both for the cut-off limit at 35, and at 40 points in the ORTO-15 test. Previous research did not confirm the association between ON and BMI as well [36,57,58], which indicates the distinctiveness of ON from AN in terms of this index [21,24,59,60]. Excessive concentration of people with the ON tendency on the quality of food [24] does not have to be combined with control of the amount of food consumed. In studies on stereotypical thinking about healthy food, it was shown that when people assessed its impact on weight gain mainly the health-related properties of the food consumed were taken into account and not its quantity [61,62]. The lack of association between orthorexic symptoms and BMI, but also stereotypical thinking of healthy food as good for body could therefore suggest that encouraging the choice of healthy food is not sufficient to limit overweight and obesity. The recommendation to choose healthy food has to be supplemented with the recommendation to control the amount in which healthy food is consumed.

The results of our study revealed the relationship of BMI with the student's satisfaction with 'Bottom body & weight', with the highest number of underweight individuals being satisfied with 'Bottom body & weight'. Likewise Goswami et al. [63] we observed a higher level of body satisfaction among the respondents with BMI < 18.5 kg/m^2 in comparison to people with higher BMI (>25 kg/m^2). The majority of obese people were dissatisfied with their 'Bottom body & weight', which may result from excess of body fat deposited especially in the lower body parts, as well as excessive body weight. The overweight or obese individuals may experience strong stigma and discrimination due to weight and size of their body, leading them to focus increasingly and obsessively on dieting for weight loss and body dissatisfaction [64]. Low body satisfaction may lead to development of an ED, as well as to sadness, low self-esteem and depression [49]. However, it is alarming that among people with a normal body weight, almost half were dissatisfied with 'Bottom body & weight', which may lead them to implementing dietary restrictions. An important factor causing the lack of satisfaction with one's own body is the internalization of information provided by parents, peers and mass media [65]. Interestingly, the messages addressed to men and women significantly differ from each other [66]. In the case of women, the information transmit the pressure of having a slim figure. For men, the pressure concentrates on having an athletic and muscular body. Dissatisfaction with one's own body may stem from the inability to meet the imposed ideals [67]. Women internalize messages regarding the body image more often and they tend to be more severe judges of their looks in comparison to men [68–70]. This tendency occurs alike among children [71], adolescents [72], and grown-ups [73]. The lack of associations between body satisfaction and BMI demonstrated in our study can be used in the development of messages aimed at reducing obesity. In order to encourage people to maintain or reduce weight, both health and body satisfaction should be emphasized as resulting from controlling one's diet. Body satisfaction would be presented as a result of the action undertaken, and at the same time a reward for the effort made, which may increase the effectiveness of the process of behaviors' change.

Although more women than men experience ED [74–77], our results did not confirm the relationship between gender and ON tendency regardless of the cut-off point used in the ORTO-15 test. Previous studies also did not show any definite relationship between gender and ON. Some research papers have pointed to a higher incidence of ON among men [10,14,78], whereas others observed it more often in women [26,36,79]. Considerable number of publications, like our study, did not indicate any significant relationship between gender and ON [80,81]. The discrepancies in results may be related to the specificity of ON. An unhealthy obsession with proper nutrition resulting from the preoccupation with one's health is the main characteristic of ON [3,4]. The increasing awareness of the relationship between nutrition and health induces growing interest in this issue [82], which may favor the application of strict nutrition rules regardless of gender. Their use can reach the pathological level and turn into ON, also regardless of gender. In the case of ED, such as AN or BN, dissatisfaction with body image, fear of obesity and distorted assessment of body dimensions are the main factors affecting the formation of these disorders [1]. Thus, women who are generally less satisfied with the image of their own body constitute a group that is particularly vulnerable to this type of disorders.

Previous studies did not indicate a connection between the negative image of one's body and ON [30,83], but the fact that the perception of one's own body is a frequent cause of changing one's eating behaviors has prompted us to include this variable in our study. The obtained results indicate the lack of relationship between ON tendency (both cut-offs in ORTO-15 test) and satisfaction with own body, but only in regard to 'Bottom body & weight'. In ED, concerns about the body image refer primarily to those parts of the body (i.e., abdomen, hip, thighs and buttocks) in which fatty tissue accumulates [42]. The lack of this relationship could confirm the differences between ON and BN, due to the lack of a characteristic symptom of AN and BN (i.e., body dissatisfaction). Nevertheless, our results indicate a relationship of satisfaction with the upper body with ON tendency. Higher satisfaction with the upper body of people with ON tendency may result from the fact that they eliminate products with a high sugar content and processed food from their diet [3,4], which may affect skin condition adversely [84]. Our results confirm that the respondents from the upper tertile of 'High-sugar products & snacks' pattern were more likely to be dissatisfied with upper body and those in the upper tertile of 'Fresh products & nuts' pattern were less likely to be dissatisfied with upper body. Thus, the restrictions introduced by people with ON tendency can positively affect the skin condition of these parts of the body, and thus increase the satisfaction with their body.

Our research has pointed to the lower risk of ON tendency (regardless of the cut-off limit in ORTO-15) among the respondents in the upper tertile of 'High-sugar products & snacks' and 'Fatty products & dressings' patterns. People with ON avoid foods rich in sugar, fat and salt [13,24,41], which is confirmed by our results. In addition, in our study greater ON tendency (for both cut-offs in ORTO-15 test) in people from the upper tertile of 'Fresh products & nuts' pattern was observed. An earlier study also showed higher intake of vegetables and fruits among people with ON [12]. Our results did not confirm the relationship between 'Meat' DP and ON tendency, regardless of the cut-offs used in ORTO-15. Some researchers suggest that vegetarian diet does not lead directly to ED, however, the prevalence of ON among vegans and vegetarians is higher than among people who eat meat [85–88]. It seems that only the complete elimination of meat from the diet, and not the varied frequency of its consumption may be the reason for the more frequent occurrence of ON tendency among vegans and vegetarians. However, further research into ON should be carried out in the context of the use of alternative diets.

The use of both cut-off points in our analysis (at 35 and at 40 points in ORTO-15) in the determination of ON tendency has not provided us with findings which we expected. There were no major differences in the results after applying both cut-offs, except for the estimation of the occurrence of ON tendency. The differences shown in the dietary patterns after taking into account both cut-off points in ORTO-15 were only minimal. However, slightly higher chances of representing the upper tertile of 'Fresh products & nuts' and lower chances of representing the upper tertile of 'Fatty products & dressing' were observed in people with higher symptoms of ON when the cut-off at 35 was used, which is also confirmed in other studies [12,13,24,41]. Although the use of cut-off at 35 in ORTO-15 seems more appropriate to diagnose external variables describing ON, further studies are needed to confirm our results.

Strengths and Limitations

The strength of our results is a relatively large sample of Polish students. Although our findings are specific to Polish cultural background and should not be generalized to populations of students of various nationalities, the findings could be of potential use in further research on ON tendency and its symptoms, especially when methodological issues are concerned. We believe that including body satisfaction and dietary patterns in the study brought a wider perspective on symptoms of ON tendency.

Nevertheless, there are several limitations within the study. The first limitation of the current study is carrying out the survey in lectures, which limited the anonymity of the respondents. The literature suggests that anonymity may enhance the accuracy of disclosure among college students for questions of a sensitive nature [89]. Secondly, the self-reported weight and height could have led to an inaccurate body mass index classification. The ability to self-report weight and height data may be influenced by sociodemographic features such as age, gender and economic status [90]. Next, the three identified dietary patterns explained only 5.4% or less of the total variance in the dietary intake data, which is lower compared to another studies undertaking similar type of analyses [91,92]. This value may be a results of the inclusion of a high numbers of variables in the PCA [93]. Finally, the cross-sectional design of the present study and data collection at a single point in time did not allow conclusions to be drawn about causality, but only on the associations of ON tendency with both dietary patterns and body satisfaction. Moreover, using the ORTO-15 for examining ON tendencies can be questioned due to its limitations [94,95].

5. Conclusions

The results of our study indicate that there was no body dissatisfaction among people with ON tendency. What's more, people with ON tendency were more satisfied with their upper body in comparison to people with no orthorexic characteristics. In addition, there was no relationship between ON tendency and BMI. The obtained results do not confirm the suggested relationship between ON and AN due to the lack of ON relationship with dissatisfaction with one's body and BMI. However, further research in this area is needed in order to confirm the relationship between the one's body satisfaction and ON in different populations, including youth that does not attend college, adults and people with ED. Moreover, the assessment of the relationship of ON tendency with dietary patterns allowed characterizing dietary behaviors of people with ON tendency, which may be important in the development of educational programs and nutritional interventions directed to people with ON.

The use of both cut-off points for results obtained in ORTO-15, and then their inclusion in the analyses suggests the legitimacy of using the cut-off point 35, because it results in a decrease in the number of people with ON tendency. However, in the diagnosis of ON symptoms such as body satisfaction and dietary patterns, there were no major differences from the cut-off point at 40. This can confirm the limitations of the ORTO-15 demonstrated by other researchers. Future research on ON should use other research tools than ORTO-15 to identify individuals with ON and to confirm our findings. Simultaneously, research should be intensified in order to create a new tool for better identification of ON and its symptoms, both behavioral and related to psychological characteristics.

Author Contributions: M.P. made substantial contributions to the study conception, design, and data acquisition; J.G. and M.P. analyzed the data; M.P. and M.J.-Z. interpreted the data and wrote the manuscript; M.J.-Z., and J.G. were involved in critically revising the manuscript, and have given their approval to the manuscript submitted.

Acknowledgments: Thanks are expressed to the participants for their contributions to the study.

References

1. American Psychiatric Associaton. *Diagnostic and Statistical Manual of Mental Disorders DSM-5*; American Psychiatric Publishing: Arlington, VA, USA, 2013.
2. Varga, M.; Dukay-Szabó, S.; Túry, F.; Van Furth, E.F. Evidence and gaps in the literature on orthorexia nervosa. *Eat. Weight Disord.* **2013**, *18*, 103–111. [CrossRef]
3. Bratman, S. Health Food Junkie. *Yoga J.* **1997**, 42–50.
4. Bratman, S.; Knight, D. *Healthy Food Junkies: Overcoming the Obsession with Healthful Eating*; Broadway Books: New York, NY, USA, 2000.
5. Catalina Zamora, M.L.; Bonaechea, B.; Sánchez, G.; Rial, R. Orthorexia nervosa. A new eating behavior disorder? *Actas Esp. Psiquiatr.* **2005**, *33*, 66–68. [PubMed]
6. Dell'Osso, L.; Abelli, M.; Carpita, B.; Massimetti, G.; Pini, S.; Rivetti, L.; Gorrasi, F.; Tognetti, R.; Ricca, V.; Carmassi, C. Orthorexia nervosa in a sample of Italian university population. *Riv. Psichiatr.* **2016**, *51*, 190–196. [CrossRef] [PubMed]
7. Missbach, B.; Dunn, T.M.; König, J.S. We need new tools to assess Orthorexia Nervosa. A commentary on "Prevalence of Orthorexia Nervosa among College Students Based on Bratman's Test and Associated Tendencies". *Appetite* **2017**, *108*, 521–524. [CrossRef]
8. Dunn, T.M.; Bratman, S. On orthorexia nervosa: A review of the literature and proposed diagnostic criteria. *Eat. Behav.* **2016**, *21*, 11–17. [CrossRef] [PubMed]
9. Bo, S.; Zoccali, R.; Ponzo, V.; Soldati, L.; De Carli, L.; Benso, A.; Fea, E.; Rainoldi, A.; Durazzo, M.; Fassino, S.; et al. University courses, eating problems and muscle dysmorphia: Are there any associations? *J. Transl. Med.* **2014**, *12*, 221. [CrossRef]
10. Fidan, T.; Ertekin, V.; Işikay, S.; Kirpinar, I. Prevalence of orthorexia among medical students in Erzurum, Turkey. *Compr. Psychiatry* **2010**, *51*, 49–54. [CrossRef]
11. Ramacciotti, C.E.; Perrone, P.; Coli, E.; Burgalassi, A.; Conversano, C.; Massimetti, G.; Dell'Osso, L. Orthorexia nervosa in the general population: A preliminary screening using a self-administered questionnaire (ORTO-15). *Eat. Weight Disord.* **2011**, *16*, e127–e130. [CrossRef]
12. Varga, M.; Thege, B.K.; Dukay-Szabó, S.; Túry, F.; van Furth, E.F. When eating healthy is not healthy: Orthorexia nervosa and its measurement with the ORTO-15 in Hungary. *BMC Psychiatry* **2014**, *14*, 59. [CrossRef]
13. Bundros, J.; Clifford, D.; Silliman, K.; Neyman Morris, M. Prevalence of Orthorexia nervosa among college students based on Bratman's test and associated tendencies. *Appetite* **2016**, *101*, 86–94. [CrossRef] [PubMed]
14. Donini, L.M.; Marsili, D.; Graziani, M.P.; Imbriale, M.; Cannella, C. Orthorexia nervosa: Validation of a diagnosis questionnaire. *Eat. Weight Disord.* **2005**, *10*, e28–e32. [CrossRef] [PubMed]
15. Dunn, T.M.; Gibbs, J.; Whitney, N.; Starosta, A. Prevalence of orthorexia nervosa is less than 1%: Data from a US sample. *Eat. Weight Disord.* **2017**, *22*, 185–192. [CrossRef] [PubMed]

16. Costa, C.B.; Hardan-Khalil, K.; Gibbs, K. Orthorexia Nervosa: A Review of the Literature. *Issues Ment. Health Nurs.* **2017**, *38*, 980–988. [CrossRef] [PubMed]
17. Clifford, T.; Blyth, C. A pilot study comparing the prevalence of orthorexia nervosa in regular students and those in University sports teams. *Eat. Weight Disord.* **2018**. [CrossRef] [PubMed]
18. Segura-García, C.; Papaianni, M.C.; Caglioti, F.; Procopio, L.; Nisticò, C.G.; Bombardiere, L.; Ammendolia, A.; Rizza, P.; De Fazio, P.; Capranica, L. Orthorexia nervosa: A frequent eating disordered behavior in athletes. *Eat. Weight Disord.* **2012**, *17*, 226–233. [CrossRef]
19. Stochel, M.; Janas-Kozik, M.; Zejda, J.E.; Hyrnik, J.; Jelonek, I.; Siwiec, A. Validation of ORTO-15 Questionnaire in the group of urban youth aged 15–21. *Psychiatr. Pol.* **2015**, *49*, 119–134. [CrossRef] [PubMed]
20. Brytek-Matera, A.; Rogoza, R.; Gramaglia, C.; Zeppegno, P. Predictors of orthorexic behaviours in patients with eating disorders: A preliminary study. *BMC Psychiatry* **2015**, *15*, 252. [CrossRef]
21. Koven, N.S.; Abry, A. The clinical basis of orthorexia nervosa: Emerging perspectives. *Neuropsychiatr. Dis. Treat.* **2015**, *11*, 385–394. [CrossRef]
22. Kreipe, R.E.; Palomaki, A. Beyond picky eating: Avoidant/restrictive food intake disorder. *Curr. Psychiatry Rep.* **2012**, *14*, 421–431. [CrossRef]
23. Bryant-Waugh, R.; Kreipe, R.E. Avoidant/Restrictive Food Intake Disorder in *DSM-5*. *Psychiatr. Ann.* **2012**, *42*, 402–405. [CrossRef]
24. Brytek-Matera, A. Orthorexia nervosa—An eating disorder, obsessive-compulsive disorder or disturbed eating habit? *Arch. Psychiatry Psychother.* **2012**, *14*, 55–60. [CrossRef]
25. Turner, P.G.; Lefevre, C.E. Instagram use is linked to increased symptoms of orthorexia nervosa. *Eat. Weight Disord.* **2017**, *22*, 277–284. [CrossRef] [PubMed]
26. Koven, N.S.; Senbonmatsu, R. A neuropsychological evaluation of orthorexia nervosa. *Open J. Psychiatry* **2013**, *3*, 214–222. [CrossRef]
27. Moroze, R.M.; Dunn, T.M.; Craig Holland, J.; Yager, J.; Weintraub, P. Microthinking About Micronutrients: A Case of Transition From Obsessions About Healthy Eating to Near-Fatal "Orthorexia Nervosa" and Proposed Diagnostic Criteria. *Psychosomatics* **2015**, *56*, 397–403. [CrossRef]
28. Park, S.W.; Kim, J.Y.; Go, G.J.; Jeon, E.S.; Pyo, H.J.; Kwon, Y.J. Orthorexia nervosa with hyponatremia, subcutaneous emphysema, pneumomediastinum, pneumothorax, and pancytopenia. *Electrolyte Blood Press.* **2011**, *9*, 32–37. [CrossRef]
29. Frances, A. *Saving Normal: An Insider's Revolt Against Out-Of-Control Psychiatric Diagnosis, DSM-5, Big Pharma, and the Medicalization of Ordinary Life*, 3rd ed.; Sage Publications: New York, NY, USA, 2013.
30. Brytek-Matera, A.; Fonte, M.L.; Poggiogalle, E.; Donini, L.M.; Cena, H. Orthorexia nervosa: Relationship with obsessive-compulsive symptoms, disordered eating patterns and body uneasiness among Italian university students. *Eat. Weight Disord.* **2017**, *22*, 609–617. [CrossRef]
31. Grabe, S.; Hyde, J.S. Ethnicity and body dissatisfaction among women in the United States: A meta-analysis. *Psychol. Bull.* **2006**, *132*, 622–640. [CrossRef]
32. Olivardia, R.; Pope, H.G.; Borowiecki, J.J.; Cohane, G.H. Biceps and body image: The relationship between muscularity and self-esteem, depression, and eating disorder symptoms. *Psychol. Men Masc.* **2004**, *5*, 112–120. [CrossRef]
33. Harrison, K.; Cantor, J. The Relationship Between Media Consumption and Eating Disorders. *J. Commun.* **1997**, *47*, 40–67. [CrossRef]
34. Barthels, F.; Meyer, F.; Pietrowsky, R. Orthorektisches Ernährungsverhalten. *Ernahrungs Umschau* **2015**, *62*, 156–161. [CrossRef]
35. Segura-Garcia, C.; Ramacciotti, C.; Rania, M.; Aloi, M.; Caroleo, M.; Bruni, A.; Gazzarrini, D.; Sinopoli, F.; De Fazio, P. The prevalence of orthorexia nervosa among eating disorder patients after treatment. *Eat. Weight Disord.* **2015**, *20*, 161–166. [CrossRef] [PubMed]
36. Arusoğlu, G.; Kabakçi, E.; Köksal, G.; Merdol, T.K. Orthorexia Nervosa and Adapta on of ORTO-11 into Turkish. *Türk Psikiyatr. Derg. Turkish J. Psychiatry* **2008**, *19*, 283–291.
37. Brytek-Matera, A.; Krupa, M.; Poggiogalle, E.; Donini, L.M. Adaptation of the ORTHO-15 test to Polish women and men. *Eat. Weight Disord.* **2014**, *19*, 69–76. [CrossRef] [PubMed]

38. Sanlier, N.; Yassibas, E.; Bilici, S.; Sahin, G.; Celik, B. Does the rise in eating disorders lead to increasing risk of orthorexia nervosa? Correlations with gender, education, and body mass index. *Ecol. Food Nutr.* **2016**, *55*, 266–278. [CrossRef] [PubMed]
39. Asil, E.; Sürücüoğlu, M.S. Orthorexia Nervosa in Turkish Dietitians. *Ecol. Food Nutr.* **2015**, *54*, 303–313. [CrossRef]
40. Sellin, J. Dietary Dilemmas, Delusions, and Decisions. *Clin. Gastroenterol. Hepatol.* **2014**, *12*, 1601–1604. [CrossRef]
41. Kaźmierczak, N.; Łukasiewicz, K.; Niedzielski, A. The outlook, behavior and eating habits occurring in the course of orthorexia nervosa. *Nurs. Public Heal.* **2017**, *7*, 125–133. [CrossRef]
42. Głębocka, A. *Niezadowolenie z Wyglądu a Rozpaczliwa Kontrola Wagi*; Oficyna Wydawnicza "Impuls": Kraków, Poland, 2009.
43. Wadolowska, L.; Niedzwiedzka, E.; Kowalkowska, J. Kwestionariusz Częstotliwości Spożycia Żywności FFQ-6 [Food Frequency Questionnaire FFQ-6]. Available online: http://www.uwm.edu.pl/edu/lidiawadolowska/ (accessed on 15 October 2018).
44. Wądołowska, L. Validation of food frequency questionaire–FFQ. Rreproducibility assessment. *Bromatol. Chem. Toksykol.* **2005**, *38*, 27–33.
45. Ribeiro-Silva, R.C.; Fiaccone, R.L.; Conceição-Machado, M.E.P.D.; Ruiz, A.S.; Barreto, M.L.; Santana, M.L.P. Body image dissatisfaction and dietary patterns according to nutritional status in adolescents. *J. Pediatr.* **2018**, *94*, 155–161. [CrossRef]
46. Bibiloni, M.D.M.; Pich, J.; Pons, A.; Tur, J.A. Body image and eating patterns among adolescents. *BMC Public Health* **2013**, *13*, 1104. [CrossRef] [PubMed]
47. World Health Organization. Body Mass Index—BMI. Available online: http://www.euro.who.int/en/health-topics/disease-prevention/nutrition/a-healthy-lifestyle/body-mass-index-bmi (accessed on 15 September 2018).
48. Field, A. *Discovering Statistics Using SPSS*, 3rd ed.; Sage Publications: London, UK, 2009.
49. Wong, Y.; Lin, J.S.; Chang, Y.J. Body satisfaction, emotional intelligence, and the development of disturbed eating: A survey of Taiwanese students. *Asia Pac. J. Clin. Nutr.* **2014**, *23*, 651–659. [CrossRef] [PubMed]
50. Ab Hamid, M.R.; Azman, N.N.; Said, N.; Rahman, A.N.A. Orthorexia Nervosa and the Quality of Life among Health Sciences Students in Universiti Teknologi MARA, Selangor. *Environ. Proc. J.* **2018**, *3*, 121. [CrossRef]
51. De Souza, Q.J.O.V.; Rodrigues, A.M. Comportamento de risco para ortorexia nervosa em estudantes de nutrição. *J. Bras. Psiquiatr.* **2014**, *63*, 201–204. [CrossRef]
52. Malmborg, J.; Bremander, A.; Olsson, M.C.; Bergman, S. Health status, physical activity, and orthorexia nervosa: A comparison between exercise science students and business students. *Appetite* **2017**, *109*, 137–143. [CrossRef] [PubMed]
53. Grammatikopoulou, M.G.; Gkiouras, K.; Markaki, A.; Theodoridis, X.; Tsakiri, V.; Mavridis, P.; Dardavessis, T.; Chourdakis, M. Food addiction, orthorexia, and food-related stress among dietetics students. *Eat. Weight Disord.* **2018**, *23*, 459–467. [CrossRef] [PubMed]
54. Gubiec, E.; Stetkiewicz-Lewandowicz, A.; Rasmus, P.; Sobów, T. Orthorexia in a group of dietetics students. *Medycyna Ogólna i Nauki o Zdrowiu* **2015**, *21*, 95–100. [CrossRef]
55. Borzekowski, D.L.G.; Schenk, S.; Wilson, J.L.; Peebles, R. E-Ana and e-Mia: A content analysis of pro-eating disorder web sites. *Am. J. Public Health* **2010**, *100*, 1526–1534. [CrossRef]
56. Norris, M.L.; Boydell, K.M.; Pinhas, L.; Katzman, D.K. Ana and the Internet: A review of pro-anorexia websites. *Int. J. Eat. Disord.* **2006**, *39*, 443–447. [CrossRef]
57. Aksoydan, E.; Camci, N. Prevalence of orthorexia nervosa among Turkish performance artists. *Eat. Weight Disord.* **2009**, *14*, 33–37. [CrossRef]
58. Kinzl, J.F.; Hauer, K.; Traweger, C.; Kiefer, I. Orthorexia nervosa in dieticians. *Psychother. Psychosom.* **2006**, *75*, 395–396. [CrossRef] [PubMed]
59. Dell'Osso, L.; Abelli, M.; Carpita, B.; Pini, S.; Castellini, G.; Carmassi, C.; Ricca, V. Historical evolution of the concept of anorexia nervosa and relationships with orthorexia nervosa, autism, and obsessive-compulsive spectrum. *Neuropsychiatr. Dis. Treat.* **2016**, *12*, 1651–1660. [CrossRef] [PubMed]
60. Zipfel, S.; Giel, K.E.; Bulik, C.M.; Hay, P.; Schmidt, U. Anorexia nervosa: Aetiology, assessment, and treatment. *Lancet Psychiatry* **2015**, *2*, 1099–1111. [CrossRef]

61. Oakes, M.E. Differences in judgments of food healthfulness by young and elderly women. *Food Qual. Prefer.* **2003**, *14*, 227–236. [CrossRef]
62. Jeżewska-Zychowicz, M. Stereotypical thinking about food in the context of promoting weight gain. *Ann. Natl. Inst. Hyg.* **2007**, *58*, 437–444.
63. Goswami, S.; Sachdeva, S.; Sachdeva, R. Body image satisfaction among female college students. *Ind. Psychiatry J.* **2012**, *21*, 168–172.
64. Szyszkowska, B.; Łepecka-Klusek, C.; Kozłowicz, K. The change of the image of women in the modern world and eating disorders. *Arch. Physiother. Glob. Res.* **2014**, *18*, 11–16. [CrossRef]
65. Goncalves, J.D.A.; Moreira, E.A.M.; Trindade, E.B.S.D.M.; Fiates, G.M.R. Eating disorders in childhood and adolescence. *Rev. Paul. Pediatr.* **2013**, *31*, 96–103. [CrossRef]
66. Tiggemann, M. Sociocultural perspectives on human appearance and body image. In *Body Image: A Handbook od Science, Practice and Prevention*; Cash, T.F., Smolak, L., Eds.; Guilford Press: New York, NY, USA, 2011.
67. Czepczor, K.; Kościcka, K.; Brytek-Matera, A. The sociocultural attitudes towards appearance and body dissatisfaction among late adolescence: A pilot study. *Pol. Forum Psychol.* **2016**, *21*, 364–377.
68. Brechan, I.; Kvalem, I.L. Relationship between body dissatisfaction and disordered eating: Mediating role of self-esteem and depression. *Eat. Behav.* **2015**, *17*, 49–58. [CrossRef]
69. Ferguson, C.J. In the eye of the beholder: Thin-ideal media affects some, but not most, viewers in a meta-analytic review of body dissatisfaction in women and men. *Psychol. Pop. Media Cult.* **2013**, *2*, 20–37. [CrossRef]
70. Mitchell, S.H.; Petrie, T.A.; Greenleaf, C.A.; Martin, S.B. Moderators of the internalization-body dissatisfaction relationship in middle school girls. *Body Image* **2012**, *9*, 431–440. [CrossRef] [PubMed]
71. Heron, K.E.; Smyth, J.M.; Akano, E.; Wonderlich, S.A. Assessing body image in young children: A preliminary study of racial and developmental differences. *SAGE Open* **2013**, *3*, 1–7. [CrossRef]
72. Bucchianeri, M.; Arikian, A.; Hannan, P.; Eisenberg, M. Body Dissatisfaction from Adolescence to Young Adulthood: Findings from a 10-Year Longitudinal Study. *Body Image* **2013**, *10*, 1–15. [CrossRef] [PubMed]
73. Blake, C.E.; Hébert, J.R.; Lee, D.C.; Adams, S.A.; Steck, S.E.; Sui, X.; Kuk, J.L.; Baruth, M.; Blair, S.N. Adults with greater weight satisfaction report more positive health behaviors and have better health status regardless of BMI. *J. Obes.* **2013**, *2013*, 291371. [CrossRef] [PubMed]
74. Afifi, T.O.; Sareen, J.; Fortier, J.; Taillieu, T.; Turner, S.; Cheung, K.; Henriksen, C.A. Child maltreatment and eating disorders among men and women in adulthood: Results from a nationally representative United States sample. *Int. J. Eat. Disord.* **2017**, *50*, 1281–1296. [CrossRef] [PubMed]
75. Brown, K.L.; LaRose, J.G.; Mezuk, B. The relationship between body mass index, binge eating disorder and suicidality. *BMC Psychiatry* **2018**, *18*, 196. [CrossRef]
76. Fisher, M.M.; Rosen, D.S.; Ornstein, R.M.; Mammel, K.A.; Katzman, D.K.; Rome, E.S.; Callahan, S.T.; Malizio, J.; Kearney, S.; Walsh, B.T. Characteristics of Avoidant/Restrictive Food Intake Disorder in Children and Adolescents: A "new disorder" in DSM-5. *J. Adolesc. Health* **2014**, *55*, 49–52. [CrossRef]
77. Norris, M.L.; Robinson, A.; Obeid, N.; Harrison, M.; Spettigue, W.; Henderson, K. Exploring avoidant/restrictive food intake disorder in eating disordered patients: A descriptive study. *Int. J. Eat. Disord.* **2014**, *47*, 495–499. [CrossRef]
78. Donini, L.M.; Marsili, D.; Graziani, M.P.; Imbriale, M.; Cannella, C. Orthorexia nervosa: A preliminary study with a proposal for diagnosis and an attempt to measure the dimension of the phenomenon. *Eat. Weight Disord.* **2004**, *9*, 151–157. [CrossRef]
79. Eriksson, L.; Baigi, A.; Marklund, B.; Lindgren, E.C. Social physique anxiety and sociocultural attitudes toward appearance impact on orthorexia test in fitness participants. *Scand. J. Med. Sci. Sport.* **2008**, *18*, 389–394. [CrossRef] [PubMed]
80. Bağci Bosi, A.T.; Çamur, D.; Güler, Ç. Prevalence of orthorexia nervosa in resident medical doctors in the faculty of medicine (Ankara, Turkey). *Appetite* **2007**, *49*, 661–666. [CrossRef] [PubMed]
81. Korinth, A.; Schiess, S.; Westenhoefer, J. Eating behaviour and eating disorders in students of nutrition sciences. *Public Health Nutr.* **2010**, *13*, 32–37. [CrossRef] [PubMed]
82. Kiss-Leizer, M.; Rigó, A. People behind unhealthy obsession to healthy food: The personality profile of tendency to orthorexia nervosa. *Eat. Weight Disord.* **2018**. [CrossRef] [PubMed]
83. Brytek-Matera, A.; Donini, L.M.; Krupa, M.; Poggiogalle, E.; Hay, P. Orthorexia nervosa and self-attitudinal aspects of body image in female and male university students. *J. Eat. Disord.* **2015**, *3*, 2. [CrossRef] [PubMed]

84. Katta, R.; Desai, S.P. Diet and Dermatology. *Clin. Aesthet. Dermatol.* **2014**, *7*, 46–51. [CrossRef]
85. Barnett, M.J.; Dripps, W.R.; Blomquist, K.K. Organivore or organorexic? Examining the relationship between alternative food network engagement, disordered eating, and special diets. *Appetite* **2016**, *105*, 713–720. [CrossRef] [PubMed]
86. Barthels, F.; Meyer, F.; Pietrowsky, R. Orthorexic and restrained eating behaviour in vegans, vegetarians, and individuals on a diet. *Eat. Weight Disord.* **2018**, *23*, 159–166. [CrossRef] [PubMed]
87. Brytek-Matera, A.; Czepczor-Bernat, K.; Jurzak, H.; Kornacka, M.; Kołodziejczyk, N. Strict health-oriented eating patterns (orthorexic eating behaviours) and their connection with a vegetarian and vegan diet. *Eat. Weight Disord.* **2018**. [CrossRef]
88. Luck-Sikorski, C.; Jung, F.; Schlosser, K.; Riedel-Heller, S.G. Is orthorexic behavior common in the general public? A large representative study in Germany. *Eat. Weight Disord.* **2018**. [CrossRef]
89. Kays, K.; Gathercoal, K.; Buhrow, W. Does survey format influence self-disclosure on sensitive question items? *Comput. Hum. Behav.* **2012**, *28*, 251–256. [CrossRef]
90. Johansson, G.; Wikman, Å.; Åhrén, A.-M.; Hallmans, G.; Johansson, I. Underreporting of energy intake in repeated 24-hour recalls related to gender, age, weight status, day of interview, educational level, reported food intake, smoking habits and area of living. *Public Health Nutr.* **2001**, *4*, 919–927. [CrossRef] [PubMed]
91. Hamer, M.; Mishra, G.D. Dietary patterns and cardiovascular risk markers in the UK Low Income Diet and Nutrition Survey. *Nutr. Metab. Cardiovasc. Dis.* **2010**, *20*, 491–497. [CrossRef] [PubMed]
92. McCourt, H.J.; Draffin, C.R.; Woodside, J.V.; Cardwell, C.R.; Young, I.S.; Hunter, S.J.; Murray, L.J.; Boreham, C.A.; Gallagher, A.M.; Neville, C.E.; et al. Dietary patterns and cardiovascular risk factors in adolescents and young adults: The Northern Ireland Young Hearts Project. *Br. J. Nutr.* **2014**, *112*, 1685–1698. [CrossRef] [PubMed]
93. Roberts, K.; Cade, J.; Dawson, J.; Holdsworth, M. Empirically derived dietary patterns in uk adults are associated with sociodemographic characteristics, lifestyle, and diet quality. *Nutrients* **2018**, *10*, 177. [CrossRef] [PubMed]
94. Roncero, M.; Barrada, J.R.; Perpiñá, C. Measuring Orthorexia Nervosa: Psychometric Limitations of the ORTO-15. *Span. J. Psychol.* **2017**, *20*, E41. [CrossRef] [PubMed]
95. Missbach, B.; Hinterbuchinger, B.; Dreiseitl, V.; Zellhofer, S.; Kurz, C.; König, J. When eating right, is measured wrong! A validation and critical examination of the ORTO-15 questionnaire in German. *PLoS ONE* **2015**, *10*, e0235772. [CrossRef]

6

Individuals with Metabolically Healthy Overweight/Obesity have Higher Fat Utilization than Metabolically Unhealthy Individuals

Arturo Pujia [1], Carmine Gazzaruso [2], Yvelise Ferro [1], Elisa Mazza [1], Samantha Maurotti [1], Cristina Russo [1], Veronica Lazzaro [3], Stefano Romeo [1,4] and Tiziana Montalcini [1,*]

1 Department of Medical and Surgical Science, University Magna Grecia, Catanzaro 88100, Italy; pujia@unicz.it (A.P.); yferro@unicz.it (Y.F.); elisamazza@inwind.it (E.M.); samabiotec@yahoo.it (S.M.); cristina_russo_cr@libero.it (C.R.); romeo@unicz.it (S.R.)

2 Clinical Institute "Beato Matteo", Vigevano 27029, Italy; c.gazzaruso@gmail.com

3 Department of Health Science, University Magna Grecia, Catanzaro 88100, Italy; veronicalazzaro09@gmail.com

4 Department of Molecular and Clinical Medicine, University of Gothenburg, Gothenburg 40530, Sweden

* Correspondence: tmontalcini@unicz.it

Abstract: The mechanisms underlying the change in phenotype from metabolically healthy to metabolically unhealthy obesity are still unclear. The aim of this study is to investigate whether a difference in fasting fat utilization exists between overweight/obese individuals with a favorable cardiovascular risk profile and those with Metabolic Syndrome and Type 2 diabetes. Furthermore, we sought to explore whether there is an association between fasting fat utilization and insulin resistance. In this cross-sectional study, 172 overweight/obese individuals underwent a nutritional assessment. Those with fasting glucose ⩾126 mg/dL or antidiabetic treatment were considered to be diabetics. If at least three of the NCEP criteria were present, they had Metabolic Syndrome, while those with less criteria were considered to be healthy overweight/obese. An indirect calorimetry was performed to estimate Respiratory Quotient, an index of nutrient utilization. A lower Respiratory Quotient (*i.e.*, higher fat utilization) was found in healthy overweight/obese individuals than in those with Metabolic Syndrome and Type 2 diabetes (0.85 ± 0.05; 0.87 ± 0.06; 0.88 ± 0.05 respectively, p = 0.04). The univariate and multivariable analysis showed a positive association between the Respiratory Quotient and HOMA-IR (slope in statistic (B) = 0.004; β = 0.42; p = 0.005; 95% Confidence interval = 0.001–0.006). In this study, we find, for the first time, that the fasting Respiratory Quotient is significantly lower (fat utilization is higher) in individuals who are metabolically healthy overweight/obese than in those with metabolically unhealthy obesity. In addition, we demonstrated the association between fat utilization and HOMA-IR, an insulin resistance index.

Keywords: obesity; nutrition assessment; fat utilization; Metabolic Syndrome; metabolically unhealthy Obesity; diabetes

1. Introduction

Epidemiological research established that overweight and obese individuals do not always show high rates of cardiovascular diseases (CVD) and mortality [1,2]. Those without dyslipidemia, insulin resistance, and hypertension are characterized by a low risk, despite the presence of an elevated body mass index (BMI) [3]. However, this phenotype seems to be a transient state [4,5] since a high risk of developing Type 2 diabetes mellitus (T2DM) has been demonstrated in those who maintain an unhealthy lifestyle over time [5]. The mechanism underlying the switch in phenotype from the metabolically healthy status to T2DM is still unclear. Obesity, inflammation, and worsening of insulin resistance are recognized as important risk factor in the pathogenesis of diabetes [6,7] but other mechanisms could play a role. A high fat (HF) diet results in an increase in β-oxidation [8]. However, other investigations demonstrated a reduction in β-oxidation [9–16]. These studies are not conflicting because the mechanisms described above could be sequential (first it increases and then, it decreases), leading to the switch from a metabolically healthy but overweight/obesity status to T2DM. In this regard, it is well known that nutrient utilization can be assessed with Indirect Calorimetry by measuring the ratio between carbon dioxide production and oxygen consumption (Respiratory Quotient (RQ)) [17]. Some investigations have demonstrated that subjects who tend to burn less fat have an increased RQ value [18,19]. High RQ is associated with a high rate of subsequent weight gain [20]. Recently, a high post-absorptive RQ was associated with hypertension [21] and increased Carotid Intima-Media Thickness (CIMT), a well-known predictor of cardiovascular events [22,23] in individuals with obesity [24]. Furthermore, fasting RQ is higher in individuals with obesity and hypertriglyceridemia [25] and in overweight/obese individuals with cardiac remodelling than in those who are just obese [26]. In this study, we sought to investigate whether a difference in RQ (and thus, in fat utilization) exists between overweight/obese individuals with a favorable cardiovascular risk profile and those with Metabolic Syndrome (MS) and T2DM, and whether RQ is associated with insulin resistance. This investigation could be useful to hypothesize the mechanisms underlying the progression from a metabolically healthy but overweight/obese phenotype towards metabolically unhealthy obesity and T2DM, and probably to distinguish subjects who will be at a high risk for T2DM and cardiovascular diseases.

2. Methods

In this cross-sectional study, the population consisted of white overweight/obese subjects who were undergoing health-screening tests at our outpatient nutrition clinic. All the participants were over 45 years old with a BMI of more than 24.9. Participants underwent a medical interview and the nutritional assessment to verify if there had been any changes in their food habits or if they followed a special diet or used any dietary supplements in the three months prior to our tests. We enrolled consecutively only those who had not performed these actions. All enrolled individuals had the same diet, determined by nutritional intake assessment, *i.e.*, a solid-food diet that supplied 50%–55% of the calories as carbohydrate, 18%–20% as protein, and no more than 30% as fat.

All patients included in the study were not suffering from any diseases (like chronic obstructive pulmonary disease, thyroid dysfunction, cancer, congestive heart failure, myocardial infarction, stroke) and did not take any drug (anti-obesity medications, psychotropic drugs and chronotropic agents)which could affect respiratory gas exchange or had debilitating diseases known to affect blood pressure or plasma glucose or lipid concentrations (like stage 2–5 chronic kidney disease and end stage liver failure) as determined by medical history, a physical examination, and laboratory tests.

Furthermore, we assessed the presence of the known classical cardiovascular (CV) risk factors, MS presence and anthropometric characteristics. The following criteria were used to define the distinct CV risk factors: diabetes: fasting blood glucose ⩾126 mg/dL or antidiabetic treatment; hyperlipidemia: total cholesterol >200 mg/dL and/or triglycerides >200 mg/dL or lipid lowering drugs use; hypertension: systolic blood pressure ⩾130 mmHg and/or diastolic blood pressure ⩾85 mmHg or antihypertensive treatment; overweight: 25 $kg/m^2 \leqslant$ BMI < 30 kg/m^2; obesity: body mass index (BMI) ⩾30 kg/m^2; smoking: a current smoker who has smoked more than 100 cigarettes in their lifetime and smokes cigarettes every day or some days [27,28].

The selection criteria for MS individuals were based on the National Cholesterol Education Program's (NCEP) Adult Treatment Panel III report (ATP III). Individuals with 0–2 cardiometabolic abnormalities were identified as having a metabolically healthy but overweight/obese phenotype, while those with at least three or more abnormalies were identified as having MS [29]. Furthermore, all participants underwent the instrumental evaluation of the carotid intima-media thickness (CIMT).

Therefore, in this study we enrolled 172 overweight/obese subjects, categorized into the following three groups: healthy overweight/obese (with maximum two NCEP abnormalities and without T2DM); MS (with three or more NCEP abnormality and without T2DM) and T2DM (only those with fasting glucose ⩾126 mg/dL or antidiabetic treatment). Written informed consent was obtained. The protocol was approved by local ethic committee at the University Hospital (projects codes 2013-1/CE). The investigation conforms to the principles outlined in the Declaration of Helsinki.

2.1. Blood Pressure Measurement

The measurement of the systemic blood pressure (systolic blood pressure (SBP) and diastolic blood pressure (DBP)) of both arms was obtained by an auscultatory blood pressure technique with aneroid sphygmomanometer. Clinic BP was obtained in supine patients, after 5 min of quiet rest. A minimum of three BP readings were taken using an appropriate BP cuff size (the inflatable part of the BP cuff covered about 80 percent of the circumference of upper arm) as previously described [30].

2.2. Biochemical Evaluation

Venous blood was collected after fasting overnight into vacutainer tubes (Becton & Dickinson, Plymouth, UK) and centrifuged within 4 h. Serum glucose, total cholesterol, high density lipoprotein (HDL)-cholesterol, and triglycerides were measured with enzymatic colorimetric test. Low-density lipoprotein (LDL) cholesterol level was calculated by the Friedewald formula: total cholesterol—HDL cholesterol—(triglycerides/5). Plasma insulin concentration was determined by radioimmunoassay. We calculated Homeostasis Model Assessment of Insulin Resistance (HOMA-IR) by the following formula:

$$\text{HOMA-IR} = \text{Fasting blood glucose (mg/dL)} \times \text{insulin (U/mL)}/405$$

Quality control was assessed daily for all determinations.

2.3. Anthropometric Measurements

All tests were performed after a 12 h overnight fast. Body weight was measured with a calibrated scale with the subjects lightly dressed, subtracting the weight of clothes. Height was measured with a wall-mounted stadiometer (TANITA, Middlesex, UK). BMI was calculated with the following formula: weight (kg)/height (m)^2. Waist circumferences and hip circumferences (WC and HC) were measured with a nonstretchable tape over the unclothed abdomen at the narrowest point between costal margin and iliac crest at the level of the widest diameter around the buttocks, respectively [31]. Bioelectrical impedance analysis (BIA) (BIA-101, Akernsrl, Florence, Italy) was performed to estimate the percentage of Total Body Water (TBW), Fat Mass (FM), Muscle Mass (MM), total Fat-Free Mass (FFM) [32].

2.4. Dietary Intake Assessment

The participant's nutritional intake was calculated using nutritional software MetaDieta 3.0.1 (Metedasrl, San Benedetto del Tronto, Italy). Dietary intake data comprised a 24-h recall and a seven-day diet record. The 24-h recall was collected via an interview by a dietitian who used images associated with a comprehensive food list in the program. All participants were also given a food diary, measuring sheet with life-size images of a spoon, cup and bottle sizes for food diaries. The INRAN (National Institute of Food Research) 2000 and IEO (European Institute of Oncology) 2008 database serves as the source of food composition information in the program. The data was entered by dietitians into the program. All foods are assigned a unique code which allows categorization of foods into food groups. The resulting database was exported into SPSS (IBM Corporation, New York, NY, USA) for analysis.

2.5. RQ Assessment—Indirect Calorimetry

RQ and the Resting Energy Expenditure (REE) were measured by Indirect Calorimetry using the open circuit technique (Viasys Healthcare, Hoechberg, Germany). All tests were performed after fasting overnigh, between hours of 7 a.m. and 8:30 a.m. after 48 h abstention from exercise, in a sedentary position. The participant rested quietly for 30 min in an isolated room at a controlled temperature (21–24 °C). Respiratory gas exchange was measured within a canopy circuit for at least 30 min, until steady state was achieved. The calorimeter quantifies the volume of O2 inspired and CO2 expired by the subject. Resting Energy Expenditure is calculated by the Weir formula. RQ was calculated as CO2 production/O2 consumption. Criteria for a valid measurement was at least 15 min of steady state, with less than 10% fluctuation in minute ventilation and oxygen consumption and less than 5% fluctuation in RQ [26,33].

2.6. Carotid Arteries Assessment

The participants underwent B-mode ultrasonography of the extracranial carotid arteries by use of a high-resolution ultrasound instrument (Toshiba Medical Systems Corporation, model TUS-A500, 1385, Shimoishigami, Otawara-Shi, Tochigi, Japan). We used a 5- to 12-MHz linear array multifrequency transducer. All the examinations were performed by the same ultrasonographer blinded to clinical information with patients in the supine position. ECG leads were attached to the ultrasound recorder for on-line continuous heart rate monitoring. The right and left common (CCA) and internal carotid arteries (including bifurcations) were evaluated with the head of the subjects turned away from the sonographer and the neck extended with mild rotation. The IMT, defined as the distance between intimal-luminal interface and medial—adventitial interface, was measured as previously described [24]. In posterior approach and with the sound beam set perpendicular to the arterial surface, 1 cm from the bifurcation, three longitudinal measurements of IMT were completed on the right and left common carotid arteries far-wall, at sites free of any discrete plaques. The mean of the three right and left longitudinal measurements was then calculated. Then, we calculated and used for statistical analysis the mean CIMT between right and left CCA. The coefficient variation of the methods was 3.3%.

3. Statistical Analysis

Data is reported as mean ± SD. Thirty subjects for each group are required to detect a significant difference of RQ greater than 2% (21–26) with 80% power on a two-sided level of significance of 0.05. A chi-square test was performed to analyze the prevalence of the cardiovascular risk factors and medications. ANOVA was performed to compare the means between groups with a Fisher's LSD test as a post-hoc analysis. REE and RQ values were eventually adjusted according to the difference in FFM between groups or if RQ and REE correlated with FFM.

The Pearson's correlation was used to identify the variables correlated with RQ given that the continuous variables were normally distributed. We analyzed the correlation with the following variables: REE, FFM, age, BMI, WC, glucose, LDL, HDL, triglycerides, PAS, PAD, HOMA-IR. Stepwise multivariable linear regression analysis was used to test the association between RQ and the variables selected among those correlated with RQ in the univariate analysis, with $p < 0.1$. When we tested the association with HOMA-IR and cardiometabolic risk factors, glucose was excluded since it was considered as part of HOMA-IR. Significant differences were assumed to be present at $p < 0.05$ (two-tailed). All comparisons were performed using SPSS 20.0 for Windows (IBM Corporation, New York, NY, USA).

4. Results

Among the participants, we enrolled 80, 58, and 34 individuals who were overweight/obese, with MS and Type 2 Diabetes, respectively. Since we did not find any difference of RQ between gender and between individuals taking medications or not (data not shown) we presented the data altogether.

The demographic and anthropometric characteristics, the prevalence of cardiovascular risk factors, and medications use of the population are indicated in Table 1. Healthy overweight/obese had a lower RQ than those with MS and Type 2 diabetes ($p = 0.04$; ANOVA, Table 2). In particular, healthy overweight/obese had a lower RQ than MS ($p = 0.04$; post-hoc analysis) and a lower RQ than T2DM ($p = 0.03$; *post-hoc* analysis; Table 2), respectively. FFM did not differ between groups ($p = 0.92$). Furthermore, RQ and FFM (as absolute value) did not correlate ($r = 0.11$ and $p = 0.27$). As expected, CIMT were significantly higher in T2DM than in MS ($p = 0.03$; post-hoc analysis) and the healthy overweight/obese ($p = 0.02$; post-hoc analysis).

Table 3 shows the factors significantly associated with RQ in the univariate analysis, which were the following: HOMA-IR, glucose, triglycerides, SBP. In the multivariable analysis, RQ remained still associated with HOMA-IR, while triglycerides and SBP were not associated (Table 4).

5. Discussion

In this investigation, we find that fasting RQ, an index of nutrient utilization assessed by indirect calorimetry, is significantly lower in individuals with metabolically healthy overweight/obesity than in those with MS and T2DM. This suggests that individuals who are healthy overweight/obese are still able, to some extent, to utilize fat in the fasting state while fat utilization is significantly reduced in individuals with unhealthy obesity (Table 2). These results could help to hypothesize that new factors are involved in the pathogenesis of T2DM and potential new therapeutic goals exist. Furthermore, in this population, we demonstrated the association between RQ and HOMA-IR, which is widely utilized as an insulin resistance index (Table 4). This result could have important implications in predicting diabetes, which must be confirmed by longitudinal studies. The mechanisms underlying the switch in phenotype from healthy overweight/obese to T2DM are still unknown and our study was not designed to investigate these mechanisms. However, our study may be useful in generating intriguing hypotheses. Whether [34,35] or not [36–39] increase in fatty acid β-oxidation leads to insulin resistance is still a subject of debate. There is evidence that obesity-associated glucose intolerance might develop from an overload of fatty acid in muscle mitochondria [40]. It has been demonstrated that the excessive availability of fatty acids may exert an insulin-desensitizing action in muscle mitochondria [8]. Furthermore, it has been demonstrated that a HF diet and/or obesity can increase the expression of several β-oxidative enzymes [41] and reduce RQ [8]. It is interesting that these events precede the onset of insulin resistance [8]. Our findings are in line with these studies since we find that individuals who are metabolically healthy overweight/obese have, to some extent, a greater ability to burn fat (lower RQ) in comparison to those with MS and T2DM. However, it has also been demonstrated that an unhealthy lifestyle, including HF feeding and the absence of physical activity, favors incomplete β-oxidation caused by the mismatch between β-oxidation and tricarboxylic acid cycle activity, contributing to mitochondrial damage [41,42]. Incomplete fatty acid oxidation also facilitates the production of reactive oxygen species (ROS) which can cause damage to mitochondrial enzymes [42]. Furthermore, the production of ROS represents a common pathway in the cascade of events that finally results in β-cell failure [43]. Consequently, as confirmed by other investigations, both glucose-tolerance and fat oxidation are decreased [9–11,44–46]. Together these studies lead us to hypothesize that a reduction in fatty acid oxidation is achieved over time, probably in the context of an unhealthy lifestyle. The significant difference of RQ (of fasting fat utilization) between metabolically healthy but overweight/obese phenotype, with MS and T2DM individuals may confirm this mechanism.

Table 1. Demographic, anthropometric and clinical characteristics of the population.

Variables	Overweight/Obese (OO) (n = 80)	Metabolic Syndrome (MS) (n = 58)	T2 Diabetes (T2DM) (n = 34)	P ANOVA	p Post-Hoc Analysis
Females (%)	31.3	34.5	35.3	0.63	/
Age (years)	56 ± 10	58 ± 9	62 ± 10	0.016	OO *vs.* T2DM 0.004
Weight (Kg)	83 ± 17	87 ± 21	85 ± 20	0.505	/
BMI (Kg/m^2)	33 ± 6	34 ± 7	34 ± 6	0.514	/
WC (cm)	102 ± 14	106 ± 15	108 ± 13	0.120	/
HC (cm)	109 ± 15	110 ± 12	110 ± 11	0.905	/
SBP (mmHg)	122 ± 11	133 ± 15	130 ± 13	<0.001	OO *vs.* MS < 0.001 OO *vs.* T2DM 0.003
DBP (mmHg)	78 ± 8	80 ± 11	77 ± 9	0.161	/
Glucose-mg/dL (mmol/L)	91 ± 9 (5.06 ± 0.5)	100 ± 10 (5.56 ± 0.5)	130 ± 45 (7.22 ± 2.5)	<0.001	OO *vs.* MS 0.019 OO *vs.* T2DM < 0.001 MS *vs.* T2DM < 0.001
Insulin-mU/L (pmol/L)	16 ± 8 (114.7 ± 57)	23 ± 20 (164.9 ± 143)	35 ± 26 (250.9 ± 186)	0.039	OO *vs.* T2D 0.012
HOMA-IR	3.7 ± 2	6 ± 5	12 ± 11	0.004	OO *vs.* T2DM 0.001 MS *vs.* T2DM 0.017
TotCholesterol-mg/dL (mmol/L)	199 ± 38 (5.14 ± 0.98)	213 ± 42 (5.5 ± 1.09)	195 ± 47 (5.04 ± 1.2)	0.055	OO *vs.* MS 0.042 MS *vs.* T2DM 0.037
HDL (mmol/L)	1.52 ± 0.41	1.16 ± 0.36	1.37 ± 0.44	<0.001	OO *vs.* MS < 0.001 OO *vs.* T2DM 0.017 MS *vs.* T2DM 0.046
LDL (mmol/L)	3.18 ± 0.83	3.39 ± 0.96	2.97 ± 1.06	0.141	/
Triglycerides (mmol/L)	91 ± 28 (1.03 ± 0.32)	201 ± 81 (2.27 ± 0.91)	151 ± 85 (1.70 ± 0.96)	<0.001	OO *vs.* MS < 0.001 OO *vs.* T2D < 0.001 MS *vs.* T2D < 0.001
		Prevalence			
Hypertension (%)	12	26	52	0.001	/
Dyslipidemia (%)	19	29	30	0.129	/
Smokers (%)	38	46	24	0.390	/
Antidiabetic agents (%)	0	0	56	<0.001	/
Antihypertensive agents (%)	0	0	56	<0.001	/
Lipid lowering agents (%)	0	0	44	<0.001	/

Legend: BMI, body mass index; DBP, diastolic blood pressure; HC, hip circumferences; HDL, high density lipoprotein; HOMA IR, Homeostasis Model Assessment of Insulin Resistance; LDL, low density lipoprotein; SBP, systolic blood pressure; Tot Cholesterol, total cholesterol; WC, Waist circumferences.

Table 2. Respiratory quotient, resting energy expenditure, body composition, and carotid intima-media thickness according to groups (Overweight/Obese, with Metabolic Syndrome, with Type 2 Diabetes Mellitus).

Variables	Overweight/Obese (OO) (n = 80)	Metabolic Syndrome (MS) (n = 58)	T2 Diabetes (T2DM) (n = 34)	P ANOVA	p Post-Hoc Analysis
REE (FFM adjusted; kcal)	1371 ± 33	1392 ± 42	1383 ± 45	0.93	/
RQ	0.85 ± 0.05	0.87 ± 0.06	0.88 ± 0.05	0.042	OO *vs.* MS 0.044 OO *vs.* T2DM 0.033
TBW (%)	45 ± 10	47 ± 9	47 ± 8	0.596	/
ECW (%)	31 ± 15	32 ± 14	37 ± 14	0.272	/
FFM (%)	59 ± 12	61 ± 12	61 ± 10	0.707	/
MM (%)	38 ± 8	40 ± 8	39 ± 9	0.665	/
FM (%)	36 ± 9	36 ± 8	36 ± 8	0.943	/
FFM (%)	59 ± 12	61 ± 12	61 ± 10	0.707	/
FFM(kg)	50.4 ± 18	52.4 ± 25	51.8 ± 18	0.92	/
CIMT (mm)	0.7 ± 0.2	0.7 ± 0.2	0.8 ± 0.2	0.054	OO *vs.* T2D 0.024 MS *vs.* T2D 0.038

Legend: CIMT, carotid intima-media thickness; ECW, extracellular water; FFM, free fat mass; FM, fat mass; MM, muscle mass; REE, resting energy expenditure; RQ, respiratory quotient; TBW, total body water.

Table 3. Pearson correlation-factors correlated to respiratory quotient.

Variable	Correlation Parameters	Age	REE	BMI	WC	FFM	HOMA-IR	Glucose	LDL	Triglycerides	HDL	SBP	DBP
RQ	r	0.07	0.04	−0.03	0.02	0.92	0.42	0.16	−0.03	0.19	−0.11	0.18	0.08
	p	0.35	0.53	0.65	0.79	0.27	0.005	0.03	0.62	0.01	0.13	0.01	0.25

Legend: BMI, body mass index; DBP, diastolic blood pressure; FFM, free fat mass; HDL, high density lipoprotein; HOMA IR, Homeostasis Model Assessment of Insulin Resistance; LDL, low density lipoprotein; REE, resting energy expenditure; RQ, respiratory quotient; SBP, systolic blood pressure; WC, Waist circumference.

Table 4. Multivariate linear regression analysis—factors associated with respiratory quotient.

Dependent Variable RQ	B	SE	β	t	p	95% C.I.	
						Lower Limit	Upper Limit
HOMA-IR	0.004	0.001	0.42	2.98	0.005	0.001	0.006
Triglycerides	0.001	0.001	0.20	1.37	0.17	−0.002	0.002
SBP	0.001	0.001	0.05	0.34	0.73	−0.001	0.001

Legend: RQ, respiratory quotients; HOMA-IR, Homeostasis Model Assessment of Insulin Resistance; SBP, systolic blood pressure.

Furthermore, it is well recognized that despite the substantial research efforts in the last 10–15 years, many individuals unavoidably progress to T2DM [47] thus, longitudinal studies are needed to clarify the eventual role of RQ in predicting the risk of diabetes. Additional studies are also needed to find appropriate intervention (dietetic, pharmacological) to maintain the healthy phenotype by increasing fat oxidation [48].

In this study, some strengths and weaknesses must be pointed out. For some researchers, it is important to consider HOMA-IR to define metabolically healthy obese individuals [49]. However, at present there is a lack of consensus on this definition [50–52]. According to previous investigations, we used the NCEP ATP III criteria to define individual who were "metabolically healthy" [53,54], taking the CVD risk into account [55]. Our study was limited by cross-sectional design, thus, it is impossible to infer causality. Nevertheless, cross-sectional studies indicate associations that may exist and are therefore useful in generating hypotheses for future research. In addition, in our study the statistical analysis is robust and adequate. Our results were not purely random as established by previous investigations [9–16,20–26] and were confirmed by multiple statistical analyses. The investigation was carried out on representative samples of the population which originates from a Mediterranean context, potentially increasing knowledge on this issue from a geographical perspective. Finally, our results are in line with those of other authors who demonstrated the association between metabolic inflexibility, which is independently associated with fasting RQ, and insulin resistance [56]. However, to our knowledge, this is the first time that a difference in fasting RQ has been found between individuals who are metabolically healthy but overweight/obese who have MS and T2DM.

6. Conclusions

We find that fasting fat utilization is significantly lower in individuals who are metabolically healthy overweight/obese than in those who are metabolically unhealthy. These results can help to hypothesize the factors involved in the pathogenesis of T2DM.

Acknowledgments: Acknowledgments: This research did not receive any specific grant from any funding agency in the public, commercial or not-for-profit sector.

Author Contributions: Author Contributions: Tiziana Montalcini, Arturo Pujia and Carmine Gazzaruso were responsible for study design, data analysis, for writing manuscript and approved the final version. Yvelise Ferro and Samantha Maurotti were responsible for enrollment and integrity of data. Elisa Mazza performed instrumental assessment; Stefano Romeo, Cristina Russo and Veronica Lazzaro contributed to interpretation of the data. All authors gave their final approval of the submitted version.

References

1. Calori, G.; Lattuada, G.; Piemonti, L.; Garancini, M.P.; Ragogna, F.; Villa, M.; Mannino, S.; Crosignani, P.; Bosi, E.; Luzi, L.; *et al.* Prevalence, metabolic features, and prognosis of metabolically healthy obese Italian individuals: The cremona study. *Diabetes Care* **2011**, *34*, 210–215. [CrossRef] [PubMed]
2. Kip, K.E.; Marroquin, O.C.; Kelley, D.E.; Johnson, B.D.; Kelsey, S.F.; Shaw, L.J.; Rogers, W.J.; Reis, S.E. Clinical importance of obesity *versus* the metabolic syndrome in cardiovascular risk in women: A report from the Women's Ischemia Syndrome Evaluation (WISE) study. *Circulation* **2004**, *109*, 706–713. [CrossRef] [PubMed]

3. Stefan, N.; Haring, H.U.; Hu, F.B.; Schulze, M.B. Metabolically healthy obesity: Epidemiology, mechanisms, and clinical implications. *Lancet Diabetes Endocrinol.* **2013**, *1*, 152–162. [CrossRef]
4. Meigs, J.B.; Wilson, P.W.F.; Fox, C.S.; Vasan, R.S.; Nathan, D.M.; Sullivan, L.M.; D'Agostino, R.B. Body mass index, metabolic syndrome, and risk of type 2 diabetes or cardiovascular disease. *J. Clin. Endocrinol. Metab.* **2006**, *91*, 2906–2912. [CrossRef] [PubMed]
5. Appleton, S.L.; Seaborn, C.J.; Visvanathan, R.; Hill, C.L.; Gill, T.K.; Taylor, A.W.; Adams, R.J. North West Adelaide Health Study Team. Diabetes and cardiovascular disease outcomes in the metabolically healthy obese phenotype: A cohort study. *Diabetes Care* **2013**, *36*, 2388–2394. [CrossRef] [PubMed]
6. DeBoer, M.D. Obesity, systemic inflammation, and increased risk for cardiovascular disease and diabetes among adolescents: A need for screening tools to target interventions. *Nutrition* **2013**, *29*, 379–386. [CrossRef] [PubMed]
7. Arner, P. Regional differences in protein production by human adipose tissue. *Biochem. Soc. Trans.* **2001**, *29*, 72–75. [CrossRef] [PubMed]
8. Koves, T.R.; Ussher, J.R.; Noland, R.C.; Slentz, D.; Mosedale, M.; Ilkayeva, O.; Bain, J.; Stevens, R.; Dyck, J.R.; Newgard, C.B.; *et al.* Mitochondrial overload and incomplete fatty acid oxidation contribute to skeletal muscle insulin resistance. *Cell Metab.* **2008**, *7*, 45–56. [CrossRef] [PubMed]
9. Bandyopadhyay, G.K.; Yu, J.G.; Ofrecio, J.; Olefsky, J.M. Increased malonyl-CoA levels in muscle from obese and type 2 diabetic subjects lead to decreased fatty acid oxidation and increased lipogenesis; thiazolidinedione treatment reverses these defects. *Diabetes* **2006**, *55*, 2277–2285. [CrossRef] [PubMed]
10. Kelley, D.E.; Goodpaster, B.; Wing, R.R.; Simoneau, J.A. Skeletal muscle fatty acid metabolism in association with insulin resistance, obesity, and weight loss. *Am. J. Physiol.* **1999**, *277*, E1130–E1141. [PubMed]
11. Blaak, E.E. Basic disturbances in skeletal muscle fatty acid metabolism in obesity and type 2 diabetes mellitus. *Proc. Nutr. Soc.* **2004**, *63*, 323–330. [CrossRef] [PubMed]
12. Toft-Nielsen, M.B.; Damholt, M.B.; Madsbad, S.; Hilsted, L.M.; Hughes, T.E.; Michelsen, B.K.; Holst, J.J. Determinants of the impaired secretion of glucagon-like peptide-1 in type 2 diabetic patients. *J. Clin. Endocrinol. Metab.* **2001**, *86*, 3717–3723. [CrossRef] [PubMed]
13. Vilsbøll, T.; Krarup, T.; Deacon, C.F.; Madsbad, S.; Holst, J.J. Reduced postprandial concentrations of intact biologically active glucagon-like peptide 1 in type 2 diabetic patients. *Diabetes* **2001**, *50*, 609–613. [CrossRef] [PubMed]
14. De León, D.D.; Crutchlow, M.F.; Ham, J.Y.; Stoffers, D.A. Role of glucagon-like peptide-1 in the pathogenesis and treatment of diabetes mellitus. *Int. J. Biochem. Cell Biol.* **2006**, *38*, 845–859. [CrossRef] [PubMed]
15. Pannacciulli, N.; Bunt, J.C.; Koska, J.; Bogardus, C.; Krakoff, J. Higher fasting plasma concentrations of glucagon-like peptide 1 are associated with higher resting energy expenditure and fat oxidation rates in humans. *Am. J. Clin. Nutr.* **2006**, *84*, 556–560. [PubMed]
16. Conarello, S.L.; Li, Z.; Ronan, J.; Roy, R.S.; Zhu, L.; Jiang, G.; Liu, F.; Woods, J.; Zycband, E.; Moller, D.E.; *et al.* Mice lacking dipeptidyl peptidase IV are protected against obesity and insulin resistance. *Proc. Natl. Acad. Sci. USA* **2003**, *100*, 6825–6830. [CrossRef] [PubMed]
17. McNeill, G.; Bruce, A.C.; Ralph, A.; James, W.P. Inter-individual differences in fasting nutrient oxidation and the influence of diet composition. *Int. J. Obes.* **1988**, *12*, 455–463. [PubMed]
18. Schutz, Y. Abnormalities of fuel utilization as predisposing to the development of obesity in humans. *Obes. Res.* **1995**, *3* (Suppl. 2), S173–S178. [CrossRef]
19. Schutz, Y.; Flatt, J.P.; Jéquier, E. Failure of dietary fat intake to promote fat oxidation: A factor favoring the development of obesity. *Am. J. Clin. Nutr.* **1989**, *50*, 307–314. [PubMed]
20. Zurlo, F.; Lillioja, S.; Esposito-Del Puente, A.; Nyomba, B.L.; Raz, I.; Saad, M.F.; Swinburn, B.A.; Knowler, W.C.; Bogardus, C.; Ravussin, E. Low ratio of fat to carbohydrate oxidation as predictor of weight gain: Study of 24-h RQ. *Am. J. Physiol.* **1990**, *259*, E650–E657. [PubMed]
21. Ferro, Y.; Gazzaruso, C.; Coppola, A.; Romeo, S.; Migliaccio, V.; Giustina, A.; Pujia, A.; Montalcini, T. Fat utilization and arterial hypertension in overweight/obese subjects. *J. Transl. Med.* **2013**, *11*, 159. [CrossRef] [PubMed]
22. Lorenz, M.W.; Markus, H.S.; Bots, M.L.; Rosvall, M.; Sitzer, M. Prediction of clinical cardiovascular events with carotid intima-media thickness: A systematic review and meta-analysis. *Circulation* **2007**, *115*, 459–467. [CrossRef] [PubMed]

23. Di Bello, V.; Carerj, S.; Perticone, F.; Benedetto, F.; Palombo, C.; Talini, E.; Giannini, D.; la Carrubba, S.; Antonini-Canterin, F.; di Salvo, G.; *et al.* Carotid intima-media thickness in asymptomatic patients with arterial hypertension without clinical cardiovascular disease: Relation with left ventricular geometry and mass and coexisting risk factors. *Angiology* **2009**, *60*, 705–713. [CrossRef] [PubMed]
24. Montalcini, T.; Gazzaruso, C.; Ferro, Y.; Migliaccio, V.; Rotundo, S.; Castagna, A.; Pujia, A. Metabolic fuel utilization and subclinical atherosclerosis in overweight/obese subjects. *Endocrine* **2013**, *44*, 380–385. [CrossRef] [PubMed]
25. Montalcini, T.; Lamprinoudi, T.; Morrone, A.; Mazza, E.; Gazzaruso, C.; Romeo, S.; Pujia, A. Nutrients utilization in obese individuals with and without hypertriglyceridemia. *Nutrients* **2014**, *21*, 790–798. [CrossRef] [PubMed]
26. Montalcini, T.; Lamprinoudi, T.; Gorgone, G.; Ferro, Y.; Romeo, S.; Pujia, A. Subclinical cardiovascular damage and fat utilization in overweight/obese individuals receiving the same dietary and pharmacological interventions. *Nutrients* **2014**, *6*, 5560–5571. [CrossRef] [PubMed]
27. Centers for Disease Control and Prevention. Tobacco use among adults—United States. *MMWR* **2006**, *55*, 1145–1148.
28. Psaty, B.M.; Furberg, C.D.; Kuller, L.H.; Bild, D.E.; Rautaharju, P.M.; Polak, J.F.; Bovill, E.; Gottdiener, J.S. Traditional risk factors and subclinical disease measures as predictors of first myocardial infarction in older adults: The cardiovascular health study. *Arch. Intern. Med.* **1999**, *59*, 1339–1347. [CrossRef]
29. Expert Panel on Detection, Evaluation, and Treatment of High Blood Cholesterol in Adults. Executive summary of The Third Report of The National Cholesterol Education Program (NCEP) Expert Panel on Detection, Evaluation, and Treatment of High Blood Cholesterol in Adults (Adult Treatment Panel III). *JAMA* **2001**, *285*, 2486–2497.
30. Montalcini, T.; Gorgone, G.; Fava, A.; Romeo, S.; Gazzaruso, C.; Pujia, A. Carotid and brachial arterial enlargement in postmenopausal women with hypertension. *Menopause* **2012**, *9*, 145–149. [CrossRef] [PubMed]
31. Montalcini, T.; Gorgone, G.; Garzaniti, A.; Gazzaruso, C.; Pujia, A. Artery remodelling and abdominal adiposity in nonobese postmenopausal women. *Eur. J. Clin. Nutr.* **2010**, *64*, 1022–1024. [CrossRef] [PubMed]
32. Talluri, T.; Lietdke, R.J.; Evangelisti, A.; Talluri, J.; Maggia, G. Fat-free mass qualitative assessment with bioelectric impedance analysis (BIA). *Ann. N. Y. Acad. Sci.* **1999**, *873*, 94–98. [CrossRef] [PubMed]
33. Zemel, M.B.; Bruckbauer, A. Effects of a leucine and pyridoxine-containing nutraceutical on fat oxidation, and oxidative and inflammatory stress in overweight and obese subjects. *Nutrients* **2012**, *4*, 529–541. [CrossRef] [PubMed]
34. Mazumder, P.K.; O'Neill, B.T.; Roberts, M.W.; Buchanan, J.; Yun, U.J.; Cooksey, R.C.; Boudina, S.; Abel, E.D. Impaired cardiac efficiency and increased fatty acid oxidation in insulin-resistant *ob/ob* mouse hearts. *Diabetes* **2004**, *53*, 2366–2374. [CrossRef] [PubMed]
35. Young, M.E.; Guthrie, P.H.; Razeghi, P.; Leighton, B.; Abbasi, S.; Patil, S.; Youker, K.A.; Taegtmeyer, H. Impaired long-chain fatty acid oxidation and contractile dysfunction in the obese Zucker rat heart. *Diabetes* **2002**, *51*, 2587–2595. [CrossRef] [PubMed]
36. Choi, C.S.; Savage, D.B.; Abu-Elheiga, L.; Liu, Z.X.; Kim, S.; Kulkarni, A.; Distefano, A.; Hwang, Y.J.; Reznick, R.M.; Codella, R.; *et al.* Continuous fat oxidation in acetyl-CoA carboxylase 2 knockout mice increases total energy expenditure, reduces fat mass, and improves insulin sensitivity. *Proc. Natl. Acad. Sci. USA* **2007**, *104*, 16480–16485. [CrossRef] [PubMed]
37. Turner, N.; Bruce, C.R.; Beale, S.M.; Hoehn, K.L.; So, T.; Rolph, M.S.; Cooney, G.J. Excess lipid availability increases mitochondrial fatty acid oxidative capacity in muscle: Evidence against a role for reduced fatty acid oxidation in lipid-induced insulin resistance in rodents. *Diabetes* **2007**, *56*, 2085–2092. [CrossRef] [PubMed]
38. Aasum, E.; Belke, D.D.; Severson, D.L.; Riemersma, R.A.; Cooper, M.; Andreassen, M.; Larsen, T.S. Cardiac function and metabolism in Type 2 diabetic mice after treatment with BM 17.0744, a novel PPAR-alpha activator. *Am. J. Physiol. Heart Circ. Physiol.* **2002**, *283*, H949–H957. [CrossRef] [PubMed]
39. Belke, D.D.; Larsen, T.S.; Gibbs, E.M.; Severson, D.L. Altered metabolism causes cardiac dysfunction in perfused hearts from diabetic (*db/db*) mice. *Am. J. Physiol. Endocrinol. Metab.* **2000**, *279*, E1104–E1113. [PubMed]

40. An, J.; Muoio, D.M.; Shiota, M.; Fujimoto, Y.; Cline, G.W.; Shulman, G.I.; Koves, T.R.; Stevens, R.; Millington, D.; Newgard, C.B. Hepatic expression of malonyl-CoA decarboxylase reverses muscle, liver and whole-animal insulin resistance. *Nat. Med.* **2004**, *10*, 268–274. [CrossRef] [PubMed]
41. Yechoor, V.K.; Patti, M.E.; Saccone, R.; Kahn, C.R. Coordinated patterns of gene expression for substrate and energy metabolism in skeletal muscle of diabetic mice. *Proc. Natl. Acad. Sci. USA* **2002**, *99*, 10587–10592. [CrossRef] [PubMed]
42. Roden, M. Muscle triglycerides and mitochondrial function: Possible mechanisms for the development of type 2 diabetes. *Int. J. Obes. (Lond.)* **2005**, *2* (Suppl. 2), S111–S115. [CrossRef]
43. Ma, Z.A.; Zhao, Z.; Turk, J. Mitochondrial dysfunction and β-cell failure in type 2 diabetes mellitus. *Exp. Diabetes Res.* **2012**, *2012*. [CrossRef] [PubMed]
44. Robitaille, J.; Houde, A.; Lemieux, S.; Pérusse, L.; Gaudet, D. Variants within the muscle and liver isoforms of the carnitine palmitoyltransferase I (CPT_1) gene interact with fat intake to modulate indices of obesity in French-Canadians. *J. Mol. Med.* **2007**, *85*, 129–137. [PubMed]
45. Wolfgang, M.J.; Kurama, T.; Dai, Y.; Suwa, A.; Asaumi, M.; Matsumoto, S.I.; Cha, S.H.; Shimokawa, T.; Lane, M.D. The brain-specific carnitine palmitoyltransferase-1c regulates energy homeostasis. *Proc. Natl. Acad. Sci. USA* **2006**, *103*, 7282–7287. [PubMed]
46. Kim, T.; Moore, J.F.; Sharer, J.D.; Yang, K.; Wood, P.A.; Yang, Q. Carnitine Palmitoyltransferase 1b Deficient Mice Develop Severe Insulin Resistance after Prolonged High Fat Diet Feeding. *J. Diabetes Metab.* **2014**, *5*, 1000401. [CrossRef] [PubMed]
47. Bergman, M. Inadequacies of current approaches to prediabetes and diabetes prevention. *Endocrine* **2013**, *44*, 623–633. [PubMed]
48. Den Besten, G.; Bleeker, A.; Gerding, A.; van Eunen, K.; Havinga, R.; van Dijk, T.H.; Oosterveer, M.H.; Jonker, J.W.; Groen, A.K.; Reijngoud, D.J.; *et al.* Short-Chain Fatty Acids Protect against High-Fat Diet-Induced Obesity via a PPARγ-Dependent Switch from Lipogenesis to Fat Oxidation. *Diabetes* **2015**, *64*, 2398–2408. [CrossRef] [PubMed]
49. Hinnouho, G.M.; Czernichow, S.; Dugravot, A.; Batty, G.D.; Kivimaki, M.; Singh-Manoux, A. Metabolically healthy obesity and risk of mortality: Does the definition of metabolic health matter? *Diabetes Care* **2013**, *36*, 2294–2300. [PubMed]
50. Rey-López, J.P.; de Rezende, L.F.; Pastor-Valero, M.; Tess, B.H. The prevalence of metabolically healthy obesity: A systematic review and critical evaluation of the definitions used. *Obes. Rev.* **2014**, *15*, 781–790. [CrossRef] [PubMed]
51. Phillips, C.M. Metabolically healthy obesity: Definitions, determinants and clinical implications. *Rev. Endocr. Metab. Disord.* **2013**, *14*, 219–227. [PubMed]
52. Blüher, M. Are there still healthy obese patients? *Curr. Opin. Endocrinol. Diabetes Obes.* **2012**, *19*, 341–346. [CrossRef] [PubMed]
53. Katzmarzyk, P.T.; Church, T.S.; Janssen, I.; Ross, R.; Blair, S.N. Metabolic syndrome, obesity, and mortality: Impact of cardiorespiratory fitness. *Diabetes Care* **2005**, *28*, 391–397. [CrossRef] [PubMed]
54. Voulgari, C.; Tentolouris, N.; Dilaveris, P.; Tousoulis, D.; Katsilambros, N.; Stefanadis, C. Increased heart failure risk in normal-weight people with metabolic syndrome compared with metabolically healthy obese individuals. *J. Am. Coll. Cardiol.* **2011**, *58*, 1343–1350. [CrossRef] [PubMed]
55. Song, Y.; Manson, J.E.; Meigs, J.B.; Ridker, P.M.; Buring, J.E.; Liu, S. Comparison of usefulness of body mass index *versus* metabolic risk factors in predicting 10-year risk of cardiovascular events in women. *Am. J. Cardiol.* **2007**, *100*, 1654–1658. [CrossRef] [PubMed]
56. Di Sarra, D.; Tosi, F.; Bonin, C.; Fiers, T.; Kaufman, J.M.; Signori, C.; Zambotti, F.; Dall'Alda, M.; Caruso, B.; Zanolin, M.E.; *et al.* Metabolic inflexibility is a feature of women with polycystic ovary syndrome and is associated with both insulin resistance and hyperandrogenism. *J. Clin. Endocrinol. Metab.* **2013**, *98*, 2581–2588. [CrossRef] [PubMed]

7

Usability and Engagement Evaluation of an Unguided Online Program for Promoting a Healthy Lifestyle and Reducing the Risk for Eating Disorders and Obesity in the School Setting

Martina Nitsch [1,†], Tanja Adamcik [1,†], Stefanie Kuso [1], Michael Zeiler [2] and Karin Waldherr [1,*]

1 FernFH Distance Learning University of Applied Sciences, Ferdinand Porsche Ring 3, 2700 Wiener Neustadt, Austria; martina.nitsch@fernfh.ac.at (M.N.); tanja.adamcik@fernfh.ac.at (T.A.); stefanie.kuso@fernfh.ac.at (S.K.)

2 Department for Child and Adolescent Psychiatry, Medical University of Vienna, Waehringer Guertel 18-20, 1090 Vienna, Austria; michael.zeiler@meduniwien.ac.at

* Correspondence: karin.waldherr@fernfh.ac.at

† Both authors contributed equally to this work.

Abstract: Implementing integrated online prevention to reduce the risk of both obesity and eating disorders, in the school setting, is a promising approach. The challenge is to develop highly user-friendly and motivating programs, to foster adherence and effectiveness. The purpose of this study was to evaluate the usability of such a universal prevention program for students aged 14–19 years, and to address engagement issues. A mixed-methods approach was chosen, consisting of a think-aloud task, a semi-structured interview, and a questionnaire including items on sociodemographic characteristics and the System Usability Scale (SUS). Usability tests were conducted in two rounds, with five adolescents participating per round. Mean score in the SUS was 92.5 of 100 points (range 85–100), in the second round, after some adaptations from the participants' feedback. In the course of the think-aloud tasks and interviews, five major themes emerged—visual design, navigation, mode of transfer, content, and engagement conditions. Interesting headlines, gamification, and monitoring tools are crucial for engagement. Apart from the importance of using the program during school hours, the study showed that problems currently perceived as important by the target group, need to be considered and addressed, prior to offering them prevention programs, which highlights the importance of a user-centered design.

Keywords: usability study; online health intervention; adolescents; school setting; eating disorders; overweight; prevention; engagement; E-Mental Health

1. Introduction

Prevalence rates of overweight and obesity, worldwide, have increased drastically [1,2]; consequently, the World Health Organization has labeled obesity as a "global epidemic" [3]. Over-evaluation of weight and shape, restricted eating and dieting are also on the rise [4], and are amongst the strongest risk factors for full and sub-threshold eating disorders (EDs) [5]. Whereas, EDs like anorexia nervosa and bulimia nervosa especially affect girls and young women, health implications of problematic eating and exercise habits affect both women and men, at all ages [4,6,7]. Recurring episodes of unhealthy dieting, binge eating, and purging behavior are also common in adolescents suffering from overweight and obesity [7–9], influenced by the social pressure on overweight people to reduce their weight. However, a couple of longitudinal studies have shown an association between dieting and weight gain, among adolescents [10–13].

Given the shared risk factors for eating disorders and being overweight, researchers have called for integrated approaches to prevention [14]. Such approaches are also considered to reduce the risk of unintentionally causing eating disorders with obesity prevention programs [14], and they have the potential to reduce stigma. There already exists a number of effective prevention programs addressing the full range between anorexia nervosa and obesity [15].

Due to their scalability, their potential to reach a large number of people, and relatively low costs, online programs seem to have a high potential to tackle this public health challenge [16]. Especially in group settings, like school classes, online programs offer the possibility to provide different program parts for different participants, simultaneously, within the same school class, thus allowing to tailor program content to participants' characteristics, like gender, and risk status [17]. Furthermore, it is assumed that adolescents, especially, can benefit from Internet-based interventions [18].

More than 95% of European adolescents and young adults between 16 and 24 years, are using the Internet regularly, therefore, Internet-based or mobile phone applications/platforms could be a key resource in providing health information to adolescents [19]. As for interventions promoting mental health, there is evidence of positive effects on young people's mental health, especially when implemented in the school setting [20–22]. However, the challenges of such intervention programs are poor adherence and high dropout rates [23,24]. Since these factors limit the effectiveness of Internet-based interventions, further insights into user technology interaction are urgently needed. Traditional approaches like randomized controlled trials (RCT) are not appropriate for investigating those complex phenomena, including many contextual and confounding factors. Thus, several authors suggest the application of a mixed-methods design, focusing on process variables like dropout and usage, and outcome variables like costs, health condition, or adherence [25].

Accordingly, this study aimed to evaluate the usability of a school-based online intervention program for adolescents, as well as to address engagement issues, to reduce dropout rates in the "Healthy Teens @ School" study, a multi-country cluster RCT [26]. The intervention was adapted from an evidence-based program developed in the USA, called "Staying Fit" [17,27]. The unguided online intervention program "Healthy Teens @ School" aims to promote a healthy lifestyle and reduce problematic eating behavior, eating disorder risk, and obesity risk, among adolescents aged 14 to 19 years. Prior to the conduction of the main study on "Healthy Teens @ School" in Austria, we conducted three focus groups with representatives of the target group [28], and a subsequent usability study. For the usability study we used a mixed-methods approach suggested by Nitsch et al., [29] which proved to be an appropriate design, in order to get detailed insights into users' needs and to learn more about the challenges regarding engagement at the same time. In this context, especially the evaluation of the first program modules and the users' first interaction with the program, are crucial elements for determining future engagement and adherence patterns, since most participants drop out from online interventions at this very early stage of a program [23,30,31]. This paper will present the results of the usability study and highlight the importance of investigating engagement issues, prior to the program start.

2. Materials and Methods

2.1. Recruitment

Potential participants were recruited via social media (Facebook). Girls and boys aged between 14 and 18 years, from different schools in Vienna, were invited to take part in a study aiming to test the prototype of an online program for promoting healthy habits in pupils. The inclusion criteria for this usability study reflected the target population of the "Healthy Teens @ School" program that was designed for students between 14 and 19 years. Participants were offered gift cards of € 20 for their participation.

Following the principles of usability evaluation, we conducted usability tests in two rounds, with five participants per round. A sample size of five participants per round was regarded as sufficient to detect more than 85% of usability problems. Including more participants would have required more resources in terms of time and money, while only producing repetitive information [32,33]. In the first round, five participants tested the prototype of the program on the computer. Based on the results of the first round, the program was modified and tested by another five participants in the second round.

2.2. Program/Intervention

"Healthy Teens @ School" is a ten-week online program (one online-module per week) designed to promote a healthy lifestyle and reduce eating disorder risk and obesity risk. Based on a screening questionnaire, which includes the assessment of eating behaviors, eating disorder risk, weight status, weight/shape concerns, physical activity habits, stress coping, depression, anxiety, self-esteem, and quality of life, the participants get access to the online program and are assigned to either one of two program tracks. Adolescents with normal weight (with and without eating disorder risk) are assigned to the "Healthy habits" track, overweight adolescents (>85th sex-age-specific BMI percentile) are assigned to the "Weight management" track. In ten modules, the students learn about building a healthy lifestyle, about balanced nutrition and physical activity habits, about ways of improving their body image and body satisfaction, as well as ways of improving media literacy. Whereas the content in the "Healthy habits" track is framed towards building a healthy lifestyle, the content in the "Weight management track" is framed more towards maintaining a healthy weight. In the course of the three preceding focus groups, especially stress in school turned out to be a major issue for the students [28]. As a result, we adapted the program and added elements about how to deal with difficult and challenging situations, emotions, and stress, in order to prevent mental health problems. Details on the program content are published elsewhere [26]. The program is based on principles of Cognitive Behavioral Therapy (e.g., goal setting, behavior monitoring, practical exercises to be tried out between online modules). The users are encouraged to use a "diary"-function that can be accessed via PC or an app, to monitor their habits on a daily, or at least weekly basis. Furthermore, the users receive feedback on their strengths and weaknesses, based on the results of the screening questionnaire.

The program is provided on an online platform hosted by Minddistrict GmbH. The users log on the platform via an e-mail address and a self-chosen password. From the user's dashboard, the screening questionnaire and program modules can be accessed; students can see new tasks assigned and they have the possibility to contact the study team via a messaging function. Screenshots of the user's dashboard and the program module including the app-diary are provided in Figures 1 and 2.

The program can be accessed within and outside school lessons, via different devices, like computers, tablets, and smartphones [26]. For this usability study, we used a shortened version of the screening questionnaire and feedback, the first two online modules, as well as the diary function. We decided to test those parts that are scheduled at the beginning of the program, as they may be crucial for subsequent adherence [23,29–31]. The screening questionnaire used in the usability study included about 60 items, covering sociodemographic questions (including height and weight) and standardized questionnaires, to assess stress coping, intuitive eating, self-esteem, and health-related quality of life. The KIDCOPE [34] assesses the frequency and perceived effectiveness of ten different coping strategies for a defined problem. Coping strategies are divided into active strategies (e.g., cognitive restructuring), avoiding strategies (e.g., social withdrawal) and negative strategies (e.g., self-blame). Prior to rating the frequency and effectiveness of the used coping strategies on a 4-point scale, participants were asked to define a situation or problem that has stressed them often. Coping is conceptualized as a dynamic process and not a stable personality trait, resulting in a rather limited re-test reliability, after 10 weeks ($r = 0.15$–0.43). The Intuitive Eating Scale (IES, [35]) measures the individuals' tendency to follow their physical hunger and satiety cues, by determining when, what, and how much to eat. The 23 items are rated on a five-point scale and are summed up to a total score and four subscales ("Unconditional Permission to Eat", "Eating for Physical Rather than Emotional Reasons", "Reliance on Hunger and Satiety Cues", and "Body-Food Choice Congruence"). Good internal consistencies of the total score (Cronbach Alpha 0.91 for females and 0.82 for males) and subscales (Cronbach Alphas

>0.72) were reported [36]. The Rosenberg Self-Esteem Scale [37] is a standard measure for self-esteem, consisting of ten items rated on a five-point scale. Internal consistencies are high (Cronbach Alpha = 0.88) [38]. Finally, we also used the Inventory of Life Quality for Children and Adolescents [39], which measures subjective well-being and satisfaction in seven different domains, including school, family, peers, leisure activities, physical health, psychological health, and overall health-related quality of life. The seven items are rated on a five-point scale and calculated to an overall score. The re-test reliabilities for the total score reported by the authors range from r = 0.60 to r = 0.80.

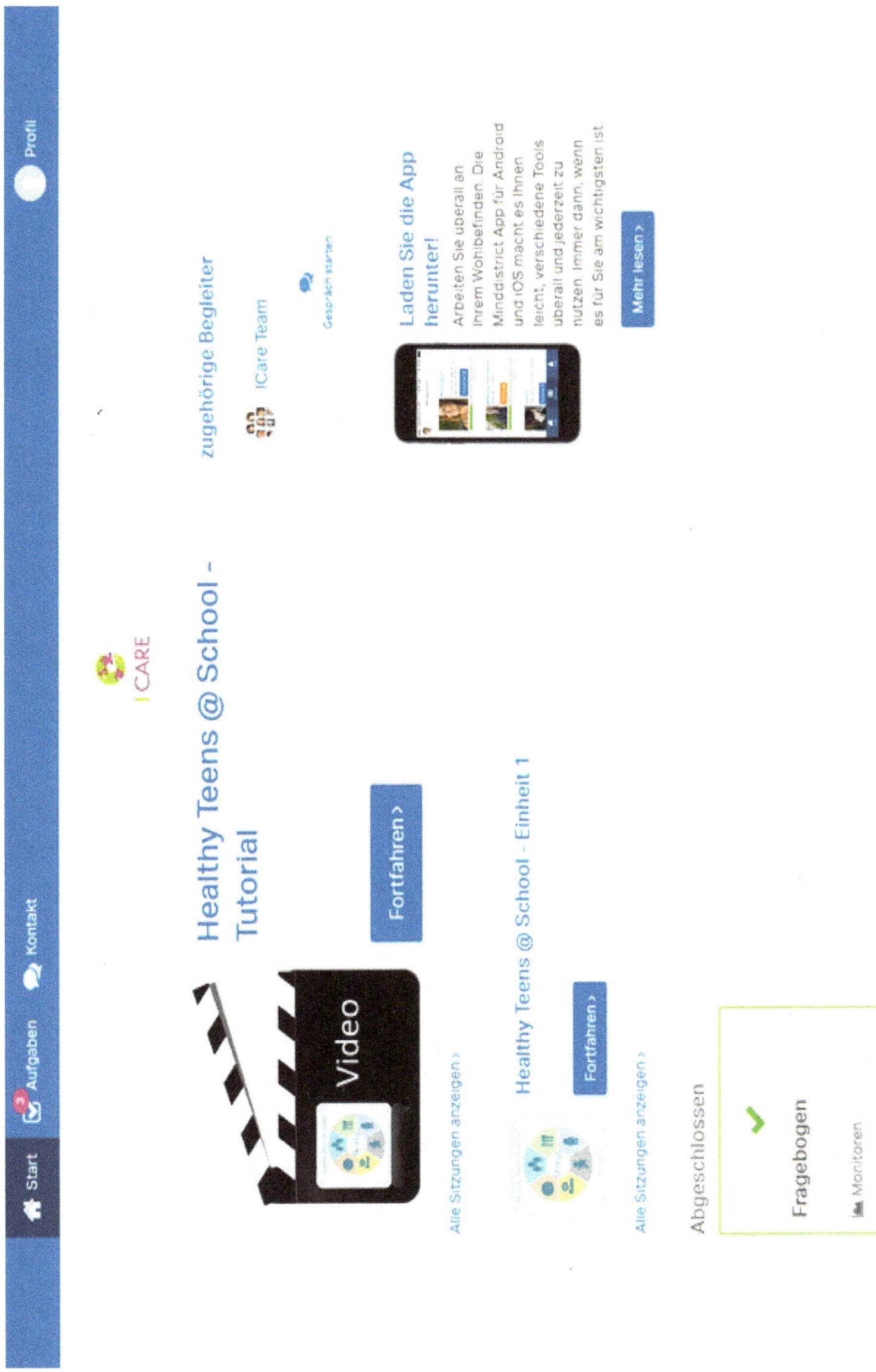

Figure 1. Screenshot of the user's dashboard on the online platform.

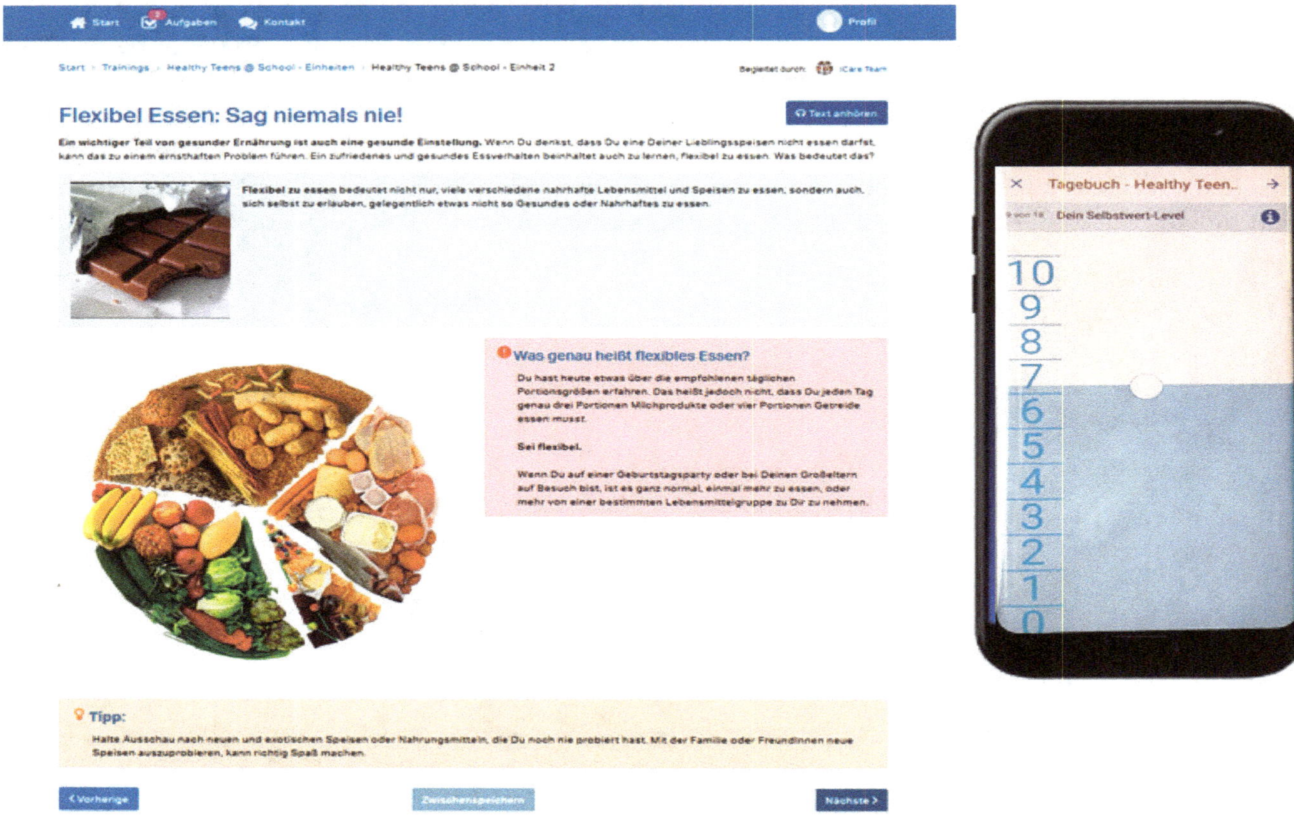

Figure 2. Screenshot of one page in module 2 of the Healthy Teens @ School program and the app-diary.

2.3. Procedure

We conducted an evaluation study focusing on aspects of usability and engagement, following the study protocol of Nitsch et al. [29].

Prior to testing, informed consents of the participants and legal representatives were obtained, and the researcher explained the procedure. The usability testing sessions consisted of three parts, (a) program use while performing the think-aloud technique, (b) a semi-structured interview, and (c) completion of a questionnaire, including sociodemographic questions and the System Usability Scale (SUS, [40]). The think-aloud process involved four tasks. First, registration on the platform and setting a password; second, completion of the online assessment and reading the feedback; third, completion of the first and the second module of the "Healthy Teens @ School" program; and fourth, to make a diary entry on the PC and via the app. Before starting the think-aloud task, the students practiced the technique by completing an Internet-based task (searching for a DVD on Amazon), which was unrelated to the "Healthy Teens @ School" program. The moderator of the test presented the different think-aloud tasks to the participant. However, participants were instructed to act as if they were alone, talking to themselves. Participants were encouraged to express anything that came into their mind, including positive and negative thoughts about the program, as the researchers on-site were not involved in the development of the original program but are only interested in improving it. There was little interaction with the researchers, only in case the participant stopped thinking aloud, the moderator motivated the student to try again. All comments and problems during the think-aloud task were recorded and protocolled by an observer. In addition, the computer screen was recorded (©Microsoft Expression Encoder 4 Screen Capture SP2), in order to capture verbal and non-verbal reactions of the participants.

Following the think-aloud task, a semi-structured interview was conducted. The interview guide included questions about expectations towards the program, impressions of the program, questions about program content, the diary, motivation for completing the program, and if the participant would recommend the program to others.

Subsequent to the semi-structured interview, the participants were asked to complete questions on sociodemographic characteristics, their current Internet use, as well as the SUS questionnaire [40]. The SUS is a method for measuring the usability of an application. It is a standardized 10-item questionnaire. The items are rated on a five-point Likert scale. A high reliability (Cronbach Alpha = 0.91) was reported for the total SUS score [41].

The usability testing sessions took 55 to 90 min, in which participants had the possibility to familiarize themselves with the program and answer the questions. The testing sessions were conducted from January till February 2017, and took place at the FernFH Distance Learning University of Applied Sciences in Vienna and at the Medical University of Vienna.

The study protocol was approved by the Ethics Commission of the Medical University of Vienna (Austria, Record Number: 2209/2015).

2.4. *Analysis*

Both, the think-aloud task and the interviews, were videotaped and audiotaped, then transcribed verbatim, including the non-verbal reactions of the participants, based on the video recordings and the observer notes. The transcripts were coded and analyzed, using NVivo 11. Thematic analysis [42] was used to identify new aspects and relations between the themes and to combine data from the think-aloud task and the semi-structured interviews. The themes and categories were discussed, reviewed, and interpreted by the research team. The SUS questionnaire was analyzed in © Microsoft Excel, as follows. After recoding the inverted items, item codings were summed up and the sum score was multiplied by 2.5. This resulted in a total SUS score that ranged from 0 (no usability) to 100 (perfect usability). Finally, we calculated an average score for each usability round. A SUS-score of higher than 70 points is regarded as an acceptable usability (representing the average SUS scores found in other usability studies) and scores higher than 85 points are regarded as excellent usability [41].

3. Results

3.1. *Participants*

All ten participants were students between 14 and 18 years old (mean age = 16.2 years, standard deviation (SD) = 1.2), attending different high schools in Vienna. In the first usability test round, four male students and one female student took part, and in the second round, four female students and one male student participated. Their BMI ranged from 18.8 to 24.2 (mean = 21.67, SD = 1.73). None of the participants had a diagnosed psychiatric disorder or received psychotherapeutic treatment. In the IES which was defined as the main outcome of the intervention, eight participants had average scores and two participants had above-average scores (mean score = 3.76, SD = 0.45).

3.2. *SUS-Questionnaire*

Regarding the SUS-questionnaire, the usability of the program was in the acceptable range (SUS-Score > 70) in the first round, and in the excellent range (SUS-Score > 85) in the second round. The average SUS score was 84 (range from 67.5 to 97.5), in the first round, and improved to an average SUS score of 92.5 (range from 85 to 100) of 100 points, in the second usability test round.

3.3. *Think-Aloud Task and Semi-Structured Interview*

By using the think-aloud tasks and the semi-structured interviews, we were able to identify five central themes, referring to visual design, navigation, mode of transfer, content, and engagement conditions.

3.3.1. Visual Design

Most of the students liked the visual design of the "Healthy Teens @ School" program, especially the pictures and graphics were highlighted as positive. The layout of the program was perceived as *"youthful"*, *"cool"*, *"pretty"*, *"appealing"*, and *"clearly arranged"* and reminded some participants of social media platforms and search engines: *"The landing page looks up-to-date, similar to social media and Facebook and instant messaging design, appealing to teenagers (...) I also liked the layout and pictures"* (male#5). The program's color design was rated ambivalent by the participants. Some liked the variation, others recommended a reduction in colors or a more targeted use of colors. *"Maybe, there should be less red, because I know, especially on a bright website, red indicates that there is something very important or wrong"* (male#7). Some students observed, that the font size was too small in some areas. All participants mentioned, that they like the layout of the diary, regardless of using it on the computer or via the app. They were also motivated to complete the diary because they liked the visualization of their improvement in healthy habits over time. Furthermore, participants liked the absence of advertising elements in the program.

3.3.2. Navigation

The majority of the students described the navigation of the program as *"easy"* and *"self-explanatory"*. However, it seemed to be a challenge to create a secure password. Only one of ten participants managed to include all demanded aspects (minimum 12 characters and one special character) at the first attempt.

In the think-aloud sessions we observed some challenges finding the next module or the diary function. Some asked for help, others found the next module or the diary after repeatedly trying. Consequently, we produced and included a tutorial video lasting five minutes for the second usability test round. This video included a short introduction to the navigation and the functions of the program and the platform. Most participants liked the tutorial video, they described it as *"helpful"*, *"reasonable for orientation"*, and *"well-illustrated"*. Others said, that they would not need such a video, stating young people prefer to try out programs and do not want to watch videos about the navigation: *"I think, it is self-explanatory (. . .). And I think, most teenagers would prefer to simply try it out instead of watching some explanation for a long time. Okay, actually, it's not so long, but I think, that most people would just try it out"* (female#6). After showing the tutorial video in the second usability round we could monitor more targeted approaches to find the diary, the different modules and an overall improvement in the platform navigation. A participant even mentioned that *"you will instantly find your way"* (male#7) in the program.

3.3.3. Mode of Transfer

This theme refers to the way the content and information is communicated to the user. After completing the screening questionnaire, some participants were irritated by certain questions of the IES, which sounded similar and felt like a repetition to them.

During the first test round, participants had to scroll to the top several times, as due to its length, the response options of the IES questionnaire did not fit on one screen, after a certain number of items. Therefore, prior to the second test round, we divided a long block of questions into two smaller parts, in order to ensure that the response options were visible at all times. Negated questions were harder to understand for some students. One person said that sometimes the wording in the IES questionnaire was unclear (e.g., "substantial food") or students indicated questions that appeared strange to them. Furthermore, some participants mentioned that the open question asking to describe a personal stress inducing problem (out of the KIDCOPE-questionnaire), was somewhat confusing, since the subsequent set of questions, directly referring to the mentioned problem, were not always fitting.

In the interviews, participants criticized the long text passages, very detailed information and suggested shorter texts and sentences: *"There was a bit too much written text, but the texts were not always the same, and addressed you directly"* (male#3). An aversion for long texts became also apparent in the think-aloud sessions, where many participants only skimmed or even skipped longer texts. On the contrary, interactive tools like quizzes and questions were always noticed and used and rated as positive: *"It is better than just reading tips, (...) that you can fill out things and instantly get feedback"* (male#1). Accordingly, the students underlined the importance of the "gamification" of the program; they liked to do quizzes to repeat the content or knowledge games, instead of reading long texts with detailed information and complex wording. For example, one girl argued that interactive tools might also be helpful with regard to concentration: *"You can't finish it [the program] in five minutes; instead you really have to take your time, sit down and read it in detail. Maybe it should be a bit shorter, so that you don't have to read that much, yeah, more quizzes, and just make it simpler, so you don't have to concentrate so hard"* (female#2). Furthermore, the participants said that they liked to explore new things in the program and that they like being addressed personally with "you" or "your". Since text passages without interesting headlines were partially only skimmed and students stated that significant headlines motivated them to read text passages, we added more headings after the first round.

The diary tool was considered as interesting and useful, especially regarding the possibility to visualize habits over time. In the second round, the diary function was available on the computer and additionally on the app. Both modes were rated as positive, but two advantages of the app were highlighted—the app appeared more game-like and chances of using the app more frequently were rated higher, since it is more convenient to use the program on the smartphone: *"It is done real quick, it takes less time than a normal diary entry. Well, on the smartphone it is quick, you can do it on the subway or on the way home, that's fine, that's convenient"* (male#7).

3.3.4. Content

In general, the students denoted the information delivered in the different parts of the "Healthy Teens @ School" program as *"helpful"*, *"informative"*, *"diversified"*, *"good to read"* and *"meaningful"*. One participant said that the program *"is cool"* because *"it is not counseling, not like at the psychologist or the doctor, you don't feel sick (...) it is a kind of help but not in an uncomfortable way (...) not bad for your self-worth"* (female#8).

The explanation and the outcome of the feedback were described as fitting to the person and very informative: *"I think, it fits me well, and it came across very personal and that I find really cool, I mean that was really cool. And for me personally, it is real fun to fill out quizzes and to get such feedback. That is fun, that is cool"* (female#6).

The provided information in the modules was described as meaningful and interesting. Some students expressed that they have already heard about some of the information, but it was also nice to hear familiar content again. Some parts of the content were new to them. For example, most participants stated that they already knew about the food pyramid or learned about it in school. The information on how many portion sizes a day is recommended for the different food groups, and how portion sizes can be measured, was perceived as new and interesting: *"I didn't know much yet, for example the daily food requirement, how many snacks you should eat, what and how much food you should eat to be balanced, in school and at home"*(male#5).

3.3.5. Engagement Conditions

The participants stated that they would use the program in their daily routine, if they feel that they need it and would recommend the program to colleagues and friends, if they had psychological or health problems or if they think the content would be interesting for them. Some students indicated that they like the program because it was informative, exciting, easy and fast to use. The motivation to complete the program was the desire for a change in daily lifestyle and the personal feedback received. For example, one participant stated that *"if you do that (the program), then you want that something changes. If you wouldn't want to change something, then you would not do it"* (male#3). The possibility to use the program, including the diary, on different devices like computer, smartphone, and tablet was very attractive for the users and might also improve the adherence of participants. Especially, the smartphone version of the program was described as *"user friendly"*, *"comfortable"* and *"always within reach"*. For example, one participant said that she would use the program *"more likely on the smartphone as it's always in reach. And I do not have to turn on the computer, enter the password and so on (...) but your smartphone is always there. You can also do it on the way"* (female#9). Another participant found that he personally would prefer doing the program *"on the computer because there is a keyboard and I prefer that, but for many others at my age the smartphone is the number one and they would prefer doing it on their smartphone"* (male#5).

Since a lack of time also seemed to be an important aspect for students, they positively highlighted the length of the program modules. The majority of the participants indicated that over the course of 10 weeks, investing 20 to 30 min once a week, seems to be feasible.

The possibility of using the program within school lessons turned out to be an important factor in terms of engagement. On the one hand, all participants stated, that if they had the chance to do the program in class, they would use it regularly. However, in most cases the program simply turned out to be a better alternative than regular school lessons: *"I would do it, I'm not sure if the other students would do it as well, but when it takes place in school instead of a regular class, then I think they would. It depends on how the first five modules are, if I would do it at home as well"* (female#10). On the other hand, although the school was generally described as an adequate setting for using the program, the school setting itself raised many issues in connection with the topic of stress. For example, in the course of the usability session, students were asked to describe a recent problem that bothered them and nine out of ten participants gave an example of school-related stress, including *"work overload"*, *"exam stress"*, stress related to bad grades and interpersonal problems with classmates. During the think-aloud task, many participants emphasized consequences of school stress, for example influencing their overall well-being: *"I'm not feeling well at the moment, because I have school stress"* (female#10). Another participant highlighted that stress has a negative effect on his leisure activities: *"I have too much schoolwork and don't have much free time to do anything else"* (male#3). This finding is especially important, since it validates and highlights the results of the pre-study, in which focus groups with students were conducted and stress turned out to be a major issue as well [28]. One participant emphasized that she *"would recommend [the program] to students experiencing stress or health problems; but rather not to others"* (female#10).

4. Discussion

The aim of this usability study was to evaluate and advance the usability and engagement aspects of an unguided online intervention program for promoting a healthy lifestyle and to reduce the risk for eating disorders and obesity among adolescents. Additionally, we aimed to validate the results of preceding focus groups with representatives of the target group. The application of a mixed methods research design not only allowed us to gain deeper insights regarding the students' perception of online health promotion and prevention programs and their media usage, but also to improve and test the program in a very effective way. In this usability study, we found five major themes—visual design, navigation, mode of transfer, content, and engagement conditions.

Especially, the findings of the current study regarding the design, navigation, and the mode of transfer of online interventions are comparable to other studies. For example, one major finding was the fact that the participants disliked reading long texts and preferred multimedia content, which was also a result in similar studies [29,43,44]. This implies that the transfer of content on prevention, via multimedia elements, might increase engagement and, therefore, is preferable to text-based information [43,45]. Furthermore, instead of presenting participants an introductory text about navigation and functions of the program, we produced a short tutorial video, in order to reduce the amount of text. Although some participants doubted the need of the tutorial video for program navigation, we observed an overall improvement regarding the navigation of the different tools, after its implementation.

Since some participants tended to skim or skip long texts, it is crucial to visually distinguish important from less important text parts [44]. We tried to highlight important information, concerning content and navigation, by putting it into boxes with prominent colors, like red and yellow. Informative headings facilitate orientation and let users choose what to read. In general, this might be a more realistic approach regarding the needs and usage habits of adolescents, than to expect them to read everything.

Similar to the study of Nitsch et al. [29], some participants expressed objections about the length of the assessments and particular questions. As a result of the standardized instruments used, a change of the questions was not possible. Based on present and previous research, there is clearly a lack of user-friendly research assessment, which have been developed to use within online programs, by considering adequate wording and format. However, a very positive mentioned tool, in conjunction with the assessment, was the subsequent personalized feedback, which all participants regarded as suitable for their needs and as very informative. Especially, the prospect of receiving a feedback turned out to be an important motivational factor to complete the assessment.

Furthermore, especially for adolescents, the integration of interactive and gamification elements seems to be an essential prerequisite [46]. Changes in the layout, navigation, and content showed improvements in the second usability round.

We observed that time was a crucial factor for using the program or recommending it to others. The length of the weekly modules was described as suitable and the daily diary was evaluated as very good and realistic, regarding regular program use. Accordingly, the participants mentioned the importance of different user devices. The possibility to use the online intervention program, including the diary, on the computer, smartphone, and the tablet increases the accessibility.

Another motivating point was that the program addressed the users personally with "you". In the diary the participants liked the possibility to visualize habits over time and mentioned this as a factor for using the diary regularly or daily.

A crucial factor in terms of engagement and regular program use was the possibility of working with the program in the school setting, and not in the free time. This result can also be confirmed by various other studies, for example Neil et al. [47] highlighted that participation in an online prevention program in the school setting, yields higher adherence than not participating in the school. Additionally, the majority of youth can be reached through the school setting and since schools are familiar settings for students, stigma, for example, associated with mental health interventions can be reduced [48]. Generally, evidence also suggests that the school is an important setting for universal prevention interventions [49,50].

However, when implementing interventions in particular settings, confounding or contextual factors concerning the setting itself need to be considered as well. The present study showed that the school setting raised various issues related to the topic of stress. For example, when students were asked about a recent problem, the majority of the participants mentioned a school-related problem. Accordingly, the problems currently perceived as important by the target group, need to be considered and addressed, prior to offering them programs for health-related issues, which they might not even think of, or are interested in. The results of this study, as well as our previous research on engagement issues, suggest that framing a program, primarily designed to reduce eating disorder and obesity risk, towards stress and stress reduction, might help to improve engagement. Stress turned out to be a major issue for adolescents who participated in our study, and this might also motivate them to use the program. Furthermore, program content covering a balanced nutrition, physical activity, and body image, can easily be linked to the topic of stress, for example, by highlighting the association between high levels of stress and fast eating or the benefits of regular physical activity for stress reduction. On the other hand, providing adolescents with helpful coping strategies, might prevent them from resorting to negative behavioral patterns, like self-blame or emotional eating. Furthermore, participating in a program labeled as a stress-reduction program might also be less stigmatizing than participating in a program for preventing eating disorders and obesity, since almost every adolescent experiences stress in some way or another. This was also an issue in another study where adolescents said that the terms describing mental disorders sounded daunting. They recommended that the program title and content should be framed positively (e.g., "improving healthy habits" instead of "reducing risk for eating disorders and obesity") [28]. Generally, we suggest evaluating the potential users' needs, prior to the program start, since addressing their needs might contribute to adherence and engagement. However, for students in a different context, other topics might be more relevant.

In this context, the value of user-centered design needs to be highlighted, since it does not only allow us to tailor interventions to the users' needs, but also offers a high potential to improve the translation of evidence-based health research into particular settings [51]. Moreover, the design of online (mental) health programs affects their uptake and use [25,52–54]. Accordingly, future research needs to address this gap, by highlighting the value of integrating aspects from different interdisciplinary fields. In this context, especially a combination of different methods from the broader field of implementation science and human computer-interaction, is suggested [52,53].

Besides the usability and engagement issues, which were addressed in the present study, further steps are necessary to ensure a successful and sustainable implementation of online prevention programs in school settings. Strong evidence for the effectiveness and cost-effectiveness of such programs are an important prerequisite for long-term implementation, not only according to various stakeholders in the school setting, but also from an ethical point of view [28]. Therefore, the "Healthy Teens @ School" program is currently being tested for its effectiveness and cost-effectiveness, as part of a cluster RCT, involving more than 800 adolescents in two European countries [26,55]. Since adherence to an online prevention program and consequently its effectiveness are not only affected by usability issues but also by other contextual factors, such as participant, setting, and intervention characteristics, we also aim to investigate a variety of moderators and mediators potentially influencing outcome [56]. Furthermore, we aim to evaluate the potential public health impact of this program by applying the Reach-Effectiveness-Adoption-Implementation-Maintenance (RE-AIM) framework [57]. RE-AIM encourages the researcher not only to focus on effectiveness but also to obtain a number of indicators—reach of adolescents, adoption (willingness of schools to offer the intervention to their students), implementation (e.g., adherence, adaptations to be made), and maintenance (both on the individual and organizational level). Overall, these research steps will help us to develop an online prevention program for EDs and obesity, which is well-accepted by schools and adolescents and which can be further disseminated to a wide range of schools.

Limitations

The participants completed only the first part of the assessments and the program modules. Therefore, results can only partly be generalized to the other assessment questionnaires or modules. However, the evaluation of engagement and usability issues of the users' first interaction with the program proved to be a suitable method, in order to determine future participant behavior [29]. Moreover, most participants drop-out during the very early stage of an online program, which indicates that the first impression is crucial for future adherence [23,30,31]. Furthermore, since the usability testing took place in a lab, it is possible, that the students were influenced by the situation itself. However, we addressed this issue and gave the participants the opportunity to test the think-aloud method, before we started with the actual study.

Not all of the feedback of the participants could be implemented in the second round and subsequently for the actual clinical trial, due to multiple reasons. Although much of the criticism about some questions seemed legitimate, the used questionnaires were standardized questionnaires that could not be changed, simplified, or shortened. Some problems or barriers were related to the navigation which was not intuitive in some aspects and led to the need to try out a few times. Since our possibilities to change these aspects, which were linked to the functions of the Minddistrict platform, were limited, we tried to tackle these issues by providing the tutorial video and additional information on the navigation in the text.

Another major limitation might be the gender imbalance of the test rounds. In the first round, four boys and one girl participated and in the second round four girls and one boy took part. We tried to reach a balance of gender per round, but due to time collisions and short-term illness of two participants, this was not feasible.

5. Conclusions

This usability and engagement study was conducted in preparation for a randomized controlled trial of the unguided online program "Healthy Teens @ School", taking place in the school setting. This study helped us to improve the usability of our online program, prior to the program start, in five major areas—visual design, navigation, mode of transfer, content, and engagement conditions. Furthermore, the results of this study contribute towards a wider research base, showing that usability and engagement issues in this first phase of the users' interaction with the program is not only inextricably linked, but is essential for identifying future engagement and adherence issues. Especially, the users' current needs have to be evaluated and addressed. As the results of this study showed, the engagement issues of this particular target group were closely linked to specific setting-related issues, such as stress in school or the possibility to use the program during school hours. This implies that the involvement and participation of the target group in the development of online interventions, should be an essential part in future research designs. Especially for prevention interventions, intrinsic motivation plays a major role, since members of the potential target group usually do not feel a certain urge or level of suffering that motivates them to use an online program. Additionally, from a public health perspective, it is important to point out the benefits of such programs for the target group. In this context, user centered-designs do not only help to improve the usability and adherence of online programs but also their overall effectiveness.

Author Contributions: Conceptualization, M.N., K.W.; methodology, M.N., T.A., and M.Z.; software, M.Z. and S.K.; formal analysis, T.A. and S.K.; investigation, T.A., M.Z., and S.K.; resources, Medical University of Vienna, FernFH Distance Learning University of Applied Sciences.; writing—original draft preparation, T.A. and M.N.; writing—review and editing, M.N., T.A., K.W., M.Z., and S.K.; visualization, M.Z and T.A.; supervision, K.W.; project administration, M.Z. and S.K.; funding acquisition, ICare Consortium.

Acknowledgments: We would like to thank the participants, without whom this study would not be possible and Ursula Fitsch for transcribing the interviews.

References

1. Hales, C.M.; Carroll, M.D.; Fryar, C.D.; Ogden, C.L. Prevalence of obesity among adults and youth: United States, 2015-2016. *NCHS Data Brief* **2017**, *288*.
2. Ahluwalia, N.; Dalmasso, P.; Rasmussen, M.; Lipsky, L.; Currie, C.; Haug, E.; Kelly, C.; Damsgaard, M.T.; Due, P.; Tabak, I.; et al. Trends in overweight prevalence among 11-, 13- and 15-year-olds in 25 countries in Europe, Canada and USA from 2002 to 2010. *Eur. J. Public Health* **2015**, *25* (Suppl. 2), 28–32. [CrossRef] [PubMed]
3. World Health Organization. *Obesity: Preventing and Managing the Global Epidemic*; 2000. Available online: https://www.who.int/nutrition/publications/obesity/WHO_TRS_894/en/ (accessed on 14 February 2019).
4. Hay, P.J.; Mond, J.; Buttner, P.; Darby, A. Eating disorder behaviors are increasing: Findings from two sequential community surveys in South Australia. *PLoS ONE* **2008**, *3*, e1541. [CrossRef] [PubMed]
5. Jacobi, C.; Hütter, K.; Fittig, E. Psychosocial risk factors for eating disorders. In *The Oxford Handbook of Eating Disorders*, 2nd ed.; Agras, W.S., Robinson, A., Eds.; Oxford University Press: New York, NY, USA, 2017.
6. Shisslak, C.M.; Crago, M.; Estes, L.S. The spectrum of eating disturbances. *Int. J. Eat. Disord.* **1995**, *18*, 209–219. [CrossRef]

7. Zeiler, M.; Waldherr, K.; Philipp, J.; Nitsch, M.; Dür, W.; Karwautz, A.; Wagner, G. Prevalence of eating disorder risk and associations with health-related quality of life: results from a large school-based population screening. *Eur. Eat. Disord. Rev.* **2016**, *24*, 9–18. [CrossRef]
8. French, S.A.; Jeffery, R.W.; Sherwood, N.E.; Neumark-Sztainer, D. Prevalence and correlates of binge eating in a nonclinical sample of women enrolled in a weight gain prevention program. *Int. J. Obes. Relat. Metab. Disord. J. Int. Assoc. Study Obes.* **1999**, *23*, 576–585. [CrossRef]
9. Boutelle, K.; Neumark-Sztainer, D.; Story, M.; Resnick, M. Weight control behaviors among obese, overweight, and nonoverweight adolescents. *J. Pediatr. Psychol.* **2002**, *27*, 531–540. [CrossRef]
10. Field, A.E.; Austin, S.B.; Taylor, C.B.; Malspeis, S.; Rosner, B.; Rockett, H.R.; Gillman, M.W.; Colditz, G.A. Relation between dieting and weight change among preadolescents and adolescents. *Pediatrics* **2003**, *112*, 900–906. [CrossRef] [PubMed]
11. Stice, E.; Cameron, R.P.; Killen, J.D.; Hayward, C.; Taylor, C.B. Naturalistic weight-reduction efforts prospectively predict growth in relative weight and onset of obesity among female adolescents. *J. Consult. Clin. Psychol.* **1999**, *67*, 967–974. [CrossRef]
12. Neumark-Sztainer, D.; Wall, M.; Guo, J.; Story, M.; Haines, J.; Eisenberg, M. Obesity, disordered eating, and eating disorders in a longitudinal study of adolescents: How do dieters fare 5 years later? *J. Am. Diet. Assoc.* **2006**, *106*, 559–568. [CrossRef] [PubMed]
13. Neumark-Sztainer, D.; Wall, M.; Story, M.; Standish, A.R. Dieting and unhealthy weight control behaviors during adolescence: associations with 10-year changes in body mass index. *J. Adolesc. Health* **2012**, *50*, 80–86. [CrossRef]
14. Haines, J.; Neumark-Sztainer, D. Prevention of obesity and eating disorders: A consideration of shared risk factors. *Health Educ. Res.* **2006**, *21*, 770–782. [CrossRef] [PubMed]
15. Sánchez-Carracedo, D.; Neumark-Sztainer, D.; López-Guimerà, G. Integrated prevention of obesity and eating disorders: Barriers, developments and opportunities. *Public Health Nutr.* **2012**, *15*, 2295–2309. [CrossRef]
16. Kazdin, A.E.; Fitzsimmons-Craft, E.E.; Wilfley, D.E. Addressing critical gaps in the treatment of eating disorders. *Int. J. Eat. Disord.* **2017**, *50*, 170–189. [CrossRef] [PubMed]
17. Jones, M.; Taylor Lynch, K.; Kass, A.E.; Burrows, A.; Williams, J.; Wilfley, D.E.; Taylor, C.B. Healthy weight regulation and eating disorder prevention in high school students: A universal and targeted Web-based intervention. *J. Med. Internet Res.* **2014**, *16*, e57. [CrossRef] [PubMed]
18. Hollis, C.; Falconer, C.J.; Martin, J.L.; Whittington, C.; Stockton, S.; Glazebrook, C.; Davies, E.B. Annual Research Review: Digital health interventions for children and young people with mental health problems—A systematic and meta-review. *J. Child Psychol. Psychiatry* **2017**, *58*, 474–503. [CrossRef]
19. European Commission Internet Access and Use Statistics—Households and Individuals 2017. Available online: https://ec.europa.eu/eurostat/statistics-explained/index.php?title=Internet_access_and_use_statistics_-_households_and_individuals&oldid=324579#Internet_use_by_individuals (accessed on 14 February 2019).
20. Lee, Y.Y.; Barendregt, J.J.; Stockings, E.A.; Ferrari, A.J.; Whiteford, H.A.; Patton, G.A.; Mihalopoulos, C. The population cost-effectiveness of delivering universal and indicated school-based interventions to prevent the onset of major depression among youth in Australia. *Epidemiol. Psychiatr. Sci.* **2017**, *26*, 545–564. [CrossRef]
21. Werner-Seidler, A.; Perry, Y.; Calear, A.L.; Newby, J.M.; Christensen, H. School-based depression and anxiety prevention programs for young people: A systematic review and meta-analysis. *Clin. Psychol. Rev.* **2017**, *51*, 30–47. [CrossRef]
22. Dray, J.; Bowman, J.; Campbell, E.; Freund, M.; Wolfenden, L.; Hodder, R.K.; McElwaine, K.; Tremain, D.; Bartlem, K.; Bailey, J.; et al. Systematic review of universal resilience-focused interventions targeting child and adolescent mental health in the school setting. *J. Am. Acad. Child Adolesc. Psychiatry* **2017**, *56*, 813–824. [CrossRef]
23. Eysenbach, G. The law of attrition. *J. Med. Internet Res.* **2005**, *7*, e11. [CrossRef]
24. Kelders, S.M.; Kok, R.N.; Ossebaard, H.C.; Gemert-Pijnen, J.E.V. Persuasive system design does matter: A systematic review of adherence to web-based interventions. *J. Med. Internet Res.* **2012**, *14*, e152. [CrossRef] [PubMed]

25. Van Gemert-Pijnen, J.E.; Nijland, N.; van Limburg, M.; Ossebaard, H.C.; Kelders, S.M.; Eysenbach, G.; Seydel, E.R. A holistic framework to improve the uptake and impact of ehealth technologies. *J. Med. Internet Res.* **2011**, *13*, e111. [CrossRef]
26. Jones Bell, M.; Zeiler, M.; Herrero, R.; Kuso, S.; Nitsch, M.; Etchemendy, E.; Fonseca-Baeza, S.; Oliver, E.; Adamcik, T.; Karwautz, A.; et al. Healthy Teens @ School: Evaluating and disseminating transdiagnostic preventive interventions for eating disorders and obesity for adolescents in school settings. *Internet Interv.* **2019**, *16*, 65–75. [CrossRef]
27. Taylor, C.B.; Taylor, K.; Jones, M.; Shorter, A.; Yee, M.; Genkin, B.; Burrows, A.; Kass, A.E.; Rizk, M.; Redman, M.; et al. Obesity prevention in defined (high school) populations. *Int. J. Obes. Suppl.* **2012**, *2*, S30–S32. [CrossRef]
28. Zeiler, M.; Kuso, S.; Nitsch, M.; Simek, M.; Adamcik, T.; Herrero, R.; Etchemendy, E.; Mira, A.; Oliver, E.; Jones Bell, M.; et al. Online Interventions to prevent mental health problems implemented in school settings: The perspectives from key stakeholders in Austria and Spain. *Eur. J. Public Health* **2019**, in press.
29. Nitsch, M.; Dimopoulos, C.N.; Flaschberger, E.; Saffran, K.; Kruger, J.F.; Garlock, L.; Wilfley, D.E.; Taylor, C.B.; Jones, M. A Guided online and mobile self-help program for individuals with eating disorders: An iterative engagement and usability study. *J. Med. Internet Res.* **2016**, *18*, e7. [CrossRef]
30. Wangberg, S.C.; Bergmo, T.S.; Johnsen, J.-A.K. Adherence in Internet-based interventions. *Patient Prefer. Adherence* **2008**, *2*, 57–65.
31. Wanner, M.; Martin-Diener, E.; Bauer, G.; Braun-Fahrländer, C.; Martin, B.W. Comparison of trial participants and open access users of a web-based physical activity intervention regarding adherence, attrition, and repeated participation. *J. Med. Internet Res.* **2010**, *12*, e3. [CrossRef] [PubMed]
32. Nielsen, J. Iterative user-interface design. *Computer* **1993**, *26*, 32–41. [CrossRef]
33. Nielsen, J.; Landauer, T.K. A Mathematical Model of the Finding of Usability Problems. In Proceedings of the INTERACT '93 and CHI '93 Conference on Human Factors in Computing Systems, Amsterdam, The Netherlands, 24–29 April 1993; ACM: New York, NY, USA, 1993; pp. 206–213.
34. Spirito, A.; Stark, L.J.; Williams, C. Development of a brief coping checklist for use with pediatric populations. *J. Pediatr. Psychol.* **1988**, *13*, 555–574. [CrossRef]
35. Tylka, T.L.; Kroon Van Diest, A.M. The Intuitive Eating Scale-2: Item refinement and psychometric evaluation with college women and men. *J. Couns. Psychol.* **2013**, *60*, 137–153. [CrossRef] [PubMed]
36. Van Dyck, Z.; Herbert, B.M.; Happ, C.; Kleveman, G.V.; Vögele, C. German version of the intuitive eating scale: Psychometric evaluation and application to an eating disordered population. *Appetite* **2016**, *105*, 798–807. [CrossRef] [PubMed]
37. Rosenberg, M. *Society and the Adolescent Self-Image*; Princeton University Press: Princeton, NJ, USA, 1965.
38. Roth, M.; Decker, O.; Herzberg, P.Y.; Brähler, E. Dimensionality and Norms of the Rosenberg Self-esteem Scale in a German General Population Sample. *Eur. J. Psychol. Assess.* **2008**, *24*, 190–197. [CrossRef]
39. Mattejat, F.; Remschmidt, H. *ILK-Inventar zur Erfassung der Lebensqualität bei Kindern und Jugendlichen: Ratingbogen für Kinder, Jugendliche und Eltern: Manual*; Huber: Bern, Switzerland, 2006.
40. Brooke, J. System usability scale (SUS): A quick-and-dirty method of system evaluation user information. *Read. UK Digit. Equip. Co Ltd.* **1986**, 43.
41. Bangor, A.; Kortum, P.T.; Miller, J.T. An empirical evaluation of the system usability scale. *Int. J. Hum. Comput. Interact.* **2008**, *24*, 574–594. [CrossRef]
42. Froschauer, U.; Lueger, M. *Das Qualitative Interview*, 1st ed.; Facultas: Vienna, Austria, 1993.
43. Grieben, C.; Stassen, G.; Froböse, I. How should web-based physical activity and healthy eating interventions be designed for young office workers? A Qualitative Approach. *J. Healthc. Commun.* **2018**, *3*, 1–15.
44. Schaarup, C.; Hartvigsen, G.; Larsen, L.B.; Tan, Z.-H.; Årsand, E.; Hejlesen, O.K. Assessing the potential use of eye-tracking triangulation for evaluating the usability of an online diabetes exercise system. *Stud. Health Technol. Inform.* **2015**, *216*, 84–88. [PubMed]
45. Ludden, G.D.S.; van Rompay, T.J.L.; Kelders, S.M.; van Gemert-Pijnen, J.E.W.C. How to increase reach and adherence of web-based interventions: A design research viewpoint. *J. Med. Internet Res.* **2015**, *17*, e172. [CrossRef] [PubMed]
46. Kuosmanen, T.; Fleming, T.M.; Barry, M.M. Using computerized mental health programs in alternative education: Understanding the requirements of students and staff. *Health Commun.* **2018**, *33*, 753–761. [CrossRef]

47. Neil, A.L.; Batterham, P.; Christensen, H.; Bennett, K.; Griffiths, K.M. Predictors of adherence by adolescents to a cognitive behavior therapy website in school and community-based settings. *J. Med. Internet Res.* **2009**, *11*, e6. [CrossRef]
48. Masia-Warner, C.; Nangle, D.W.; Hansen, D.J. Bringing evidence-based child mental health services to the schools: General issues and specific populations. *Educ. Treat. Child.* **2006**, *29*, 165–172.
49. Kern, L.; Mathur, S.R.; Albrecht, S.F.; Poland, S.; Rozalski, M.; Skiba, R.J. The need for school-based mental health services and recommendations for implementation. *School Ment. Health* **2017**, *9*, 205–217. [CrossRef]
50. Arango, C.; Díaz-Caneja, C.M.; McGorry, P.D.; Rapoport, J.; Sommer, I.E.; Vorstman, J.A.; McDaid, D.; Marín, O.; Serrano-Drozdowskyj, E.; Freedman, R.; et al. Preventive strategies for mental health. *Lancet Psychiatry* **2018**, *5*, 591–604. [CrossRef]
51. Dopp, A.R.; Parisi, K.E.; Munson, S.A.; Lyon, A.R. A glossary of user-centered design strategies for implementation experts. *Transl. Behav. Med.* **2018**, in press. [CrossRef] [PubMed]
52. Mohr, D.C.; Lyon, A.R.; Lattie, E.G.; Reddy, M.; Schueller, S.M. Accelerating digital mental health research from early design and creation to successful implementation and sustainment. *J. Med. Internet Res.* **2017**, *19*, e153. [CrossRef] [PubMed]
53. Dopp, A.R.; Parisi, K.E.; Munson, S.A.; Lyon, A.R. Integrating implementation and user-centred design strategies to enhance the impact of health services: Protocol from a concept mapping study. *Health Res. Policy Syst.* **2019**, *17*, 1. [CrossRef] [PubMed]
54. Lyon, A.R.; Koerner, K. User-Centered Design for Psychosocial Intervention Development and Implementation. *Clin. Psychol. Publ. Div. Clin. Psychol. Am. Psychol. Assoc.* **2016**, *23*, 180–200. [CrossRef] [PubMed]
55. Beecham, J.; Bonin, E.-M.; Görlich, D.; Baños, R.; Beintner, I.; Buntrock, C.; Bolinski, F.; Botella, C.; Ebert, D.D.; Herrero, R.; et al. Assessing the costs and cost-effectiveness of ICare internet-based interventions (protocol). *Internet Interv.* **2019**, *16*, 12–19. [CrossRef]
56. Beintner, I.; Görlich, D.; Berger, T.; Ebert, D.D.; Zeiler, M.; Herrero Camarano, R.; Waldherr, K.; Jacobi, C. Interrelations between participant and intervention characteristics, process variables and outcomes in online interventions: A protocol for overarching analyses within and across seven clinical trials in ICare. *Internet Interv.* **2019**, *16*, 86–97. [CrossRef] [PubMed]
57. Glasgow, R.E.; Vogt, T.M.; Boles, S.M. Evaluating the public health impact of health promotion interventions: The RE-AIM framework. *Am. J. Public Health* **1999**, *89*, 1322–1327. [CrossRef]

8

Gut Microbiota and Metabolic Health: The Potential Beneficial Effects of a Medium Chain Triglyceride Diet in Obese Individuals

Sabri Ahmed Rial [1], Antony D. Karelis [2], Karl-F. Bergeron [1] and Catherine Mounier [1,*]

1 BioMed Research Center, Biological Sciences Department, University of Quebec at Montreal, Montreal, QC H2X 1Y4, Canada; rial.ahmed_sabri@courrier.uqam.ca (S.A.R.); bergeron.karl-frederik@uqam.ca (K.-F.B.)

2 Department of Exercise Science, University of Quebec at Montreal, Montreal, QC H2X 1Y4, Canada; karelis.antony@uqam.ca

* Correspondence: mounier.catherine@uqam.ca

Abstract: Obesity and associated metabolic complications, such as non-alcoholic fatty liver disease (NAFLD) and type 2 diabetes (T2D), are in constant increase around the world. While most obese patients show several metabolic and biometric abnormalities and comorbidities, a subgroup of patients representing 3% to 57% of obese adults, depending on the diagnosis criteria, remains metabolically healthy. Among many other factors, the gut microbiota is now identified as a determining factor in the pathogenesis of metabolically unhealthy obese (MUHO) individuals and in obesity-related diseases such as endotoxemia, intestinal and systemic inflammation, as well as insulin resistance. Interestingly, recent studies suggest that an optimal healthy-like gut microbiota structure may contribute to the metabolically healthy obese (MHO) phenotype. Here, we describe how dietary medium chain triglycerides (MCT), previously found to promote lipid catabolism, energy expenditure and weight loss, can ameliorate metabolic health via their capacity to improve both intestinal ecosystem and permeability. MCT-enriched diets could therefore be used to manage metabolic diseases through modification of gut microbiota.

Keywords: obesity; metabolically unhealthy obese; metabolically healthy obese; metabolic syndrome; non-alcoholic fatty liver disease; gut microbiota; *Bacteroidetes*; *Firmicutes*; endotoxemia; lipopolysaccharide; medium chain triglycerides; medium chain fatty acids

---

1. Introduction

Obesity has become an international public health problem with 2.1 billion people worldwide being overweight (body mass index (BMI) $\geqslant$ 25.0) and more than half a billion among them being obese (BMI $\geqslant$ 30.0) [1,2]. Obesity is now described as a pandemic with increased prevalence in both adult and child populations. Since the 1980s, the combined prevalence of obesity and overweight increased by 28% in adults and 47% in children [1,2]. Obesity is a multifactorial affection with broad etiology, and multiple comorbidities. Most of these comorbidities are thought to be the result of aberrant body fat distribution leading to the metabolic syndrome [3–5]. This pathology is associated with an elevated waist circumference, a progressive state of non-alcoholic fatty liver disease (NAFLD) [3,4], insulin resistance, type 2 diabetes (T2D), some types of cancers (especially in women), hypertension, cardiovascular diseases, reproductive abnormalities, dyslipidemias, psychological affections [6], and a severely reduced life expectancy [3,7,8]. Obesity is also considered a risk factor for several other diseases such as chronic respiratory diseases [9] and arthritis [3].

Some contributing factors for obesity progression are: unfavorable genetic determinants [10], lack of physical activity [11], socio-economic status [1], circadian cycle disturbance [12], sleep deprivation [13], hormonal dysregulation [14], persistent organic pollutants [15] and alteration of the gut microbiota [16,17]. However, the most powerful inducer of obesity and its associated adverse metabolic effects remains, by far, inappropriate food intake [18]. The modern prevalence of obesity and metabolic syndrome is likely due to the rise in consumption of energy-dense food, containing high amounts of fat and carbohydrates [18], especially in Western countries. In these countries, fats typically account for 33% to 42% of dietary energy intake, with a rich proportion of long chain saturated fat [18]. When the energy intake exceeds both the caloric needs of the body and its glycogen storage capacity, dietary carbohydrates and fats are first converted and stored as triglycerides (TG) in white adipose tissue (WAT) and, later on, in other tissues such as the liver [19,20]. Sustained and abusive accumulation of lipids in the liver induces NAFLD (highly concurrent with obesity) which may result in lipotoxicity, steatohepatitis, hepatocyte cell death, fibrosis and eventually liver cirrhosis as well as hepatocarcinoma [21].

We aim here to overview the underlying causes of obesity and its associated metabolic abnormalities while paying special attention to a unique subset of the obese population: the metabolically healthy but obese (MHO) individuals. We will highlight the potential involvement of the gut microbiome as one of several contributors to the MHO status. We will finally introduce the idea of a medium chain triglycerides (MCT)-based dietary intervention with the aim of improving the metabolic state of metabolically unhealthy obese (MUHO) patients, either through modification of their intestinal health or by directly influencing lipid metabolism.

2. Etiology of Obesity and Associated Metabolic Complications

The current paradigm posits that fat accumulation leading to obesity results from an imbalance between energy intake and energy expenditure. Post-World War II food processing and marketing practices (quickly available energy-dense foods) and reductions in physical activity are the two main factors often blamed for the contemporary prevalence of obesity. As such, most treatment options involve creation of a negative energy balance, achieved by consuming fewer calories than energy expended. Alternatively, pharmacological and surgical therapies also exist [22]. Nevertheless, complex interactions among heredity [23], epigenetic imprinting [24], lifestyle, feeding behavior [25], as well as environmental [26] and physiologic inflammatory factors [27,28] also contribute to the etiology of obesity.

2.1. Comorbidities Related to Obesity

Most obese individuals fall into the MUHO category and are at increased risk for several diseases. They suffer from a severely reduced life expectancy: a 5.8 years average decrease for men and 7 years for women [29]. The visceral adipose tissue (typically abundant in obese individuals) secretes pro-inflammatory cytokines [27,28] that are, in part, responsible for obesity-associated pathogenesis [27,28]. The resulting metabolic syndrome defines a group of metabolic risk factors linked to health problems associated with overweight and obesity such as elevated visceral adiposity, larger waist circumference (>102 cm in men and >88 cm in women), hyper-triglyceridemia (>150 mg/dL) [5], reduced HDL (high density lipoprotein) cholesterol levels (<40 mg/dL in men and <50 mg/dL in women), elevated blood pressure (systolic > 130 mmHg and/or diastolic > 85 mmHg) and high fasting glucose levels [30]. A patient with at least three of these risk factors is currently diagnosed with the metabolic syndrome.

High levels of glycemia, associated with insulin resistance, are a hallmark of prediabetes and T2D, common diseases occurring in obese individuals suffering from the metabolic syndrome [5]. According to the most recent criteria, prediabetes is defined by a fasting glucose ranging between 100 and 125 mg/dL or between 140 and 199 mg/dL 2 h *post-prandium*, while these two values often exceed 126 mg/dL and 200 mg/dL in T2D, respectively [5]. In addition, the latest medical updates indicate that 50%–90% of patients with TD2 have a BMI > 25.0 (the overweight threshold) while those with a BMI > 35 have a 20-fold higher risk of developing T2D than healthy lean patients [31].

Risk of cardiovascular diseases, including atherosclerosis, coronary artery disease, stroke and pulmonary embolism, is higher in obese patients [32]. Obesity is also associated with a large spectrum of liver abnormalities including NAFLD [33]. Several additional comorbid disease risks are associated with obesity such as cholelithias, pancreatic failure sleep apnea, gynecological abnormalities, osteoarthritis, psychiatric illness as well as some types of cancer (breast, endometrial, prostate and colon) [22].

2.2. *Metabolically Healthy but Obese Individuals (MHO)*

There is a large body of evidence suggesting that not all obese individuals develop such important metabolic complications [34]. A unique subtype of obese individuals has been identified as MHO [35]. Despite excessive levels of body fat mass, MHO patients present higher levels of insulin sensitivity, a normal circulating lipid profile, no pronounced hepatic steatosis nor associated inflammatory state, no hypertension, and a lower visceral, muscle and hepatic fat content compared to MUHO subjects [36]. Since there is no standard definition for the identification of the MHO phenotype, the true prevalence of MHO individuals in the obese population is currently unclear. Depending on the method and the cut-off point used for certain metabolic risk factors, the prevalence of MHO subjects may range from approximately 3% to 57% of obese adults [37,38].

The favorable metabolic profile of MHO individuals has been associated with a lower risk of developing T2D or cardiovascular disease (CVD), and having a lower mortality risk compared to MUHO individuals [39]. There is also evidence refuting the notion that MHO subjects are totally protected from metabolic diseases [40]. The fundamental mechanisms underlying the different metabolic profiles of MHO and MUHO individuals remain poorly understood [41]. However, Berezina *et al.* showed that among patients with abdominal obesity, MHO phenotype was associated with a G45G Adiponectin genotype, while the T45T genotype for Adiponectin increased metabolic disorders risks [42]. This observation is all the more interesting since Adiponectin is a potent modulator of insulin sensitivity [43]. Also, in the latter decade, a consensus has emerged, which make the gut microbial population (also called the gut microbiota) a key determinant in the host metabolic profile [17,44]. The gut microbiota should therefore be taken into consideration in dietary and clinical approaches, for both MUHO and MHO treatments.

3. The Gut Microbiota: A Determining Factor for Metabolic State

3.1. *Gut Microbiota Dysbiosis in Obesity*

Current estimations indicate that the human intestine is colonized by a large population of above 100 trillion microbial cells organized in several taxa and constituting the gut microbiota [45]. The total biomass of the gut microbiota exceeds 1kg and is mainly concentrated in the large intestine, where about 10^{12} bacteria per gram of colonic tissue are found [46]. Such an important quantity of "foreign" cells implies a tightly regulated acceptance by the immune system of the host [46]. The gut microbiota plays a symbiotic role, ensuring several metabolic functions essential to the host. It is involved in the degradation of polysaccharides and oligosaccharides into simple metabolites such as short chain fatty acids (SCFA). These SCFA were recently found to promote intestinal impermeability [47] as well as hepatic sugar and lipid anabolism [48–50]. The gut microbiota is also an indispensable source of essential vitamins B and K [51]. Gut microbiota composition and diversity are subjected to important variations between individuals but also within the same individual under the influence of several physiologic and environmental factors such as antibiotic consumption, lifestyle and diet [52].

The alteration of gut microbiota is closely linked to tissue inflammation and to a broad range of metabolic abnormalities, including obesity and insulin resistance [52,53]. First observations suggested a link between the gut microbiota and the metabolic state of the host [54,55]. Several studies have since confirmed a direct implication of gut microbiota in obesity progression [17].

Backhed and colleagues first demonstrated that germ-free mice were protected against high fat and high sugar diet-induced obesity, via enhanced expression of hepatic and muscular Pgc-1α (a PPAR coactivator) and activation of lipid catabolism via AMPK activity [56]. Subsequently, Cani and collaborators established a close link between gut microbiota-induced "metabolic endotoxemia" and obesity-related insulin resistance in mice. They established the paradigm of gut microbiota-mediated metabolic endotoxemia inducing chronic low-grade of inflammation in the host. In obese mice, a dramatic change in caecum-resident bacteria characterized by a decrease in low lipopolysaccharide (LPS)-expressing bacterial taxa (such as *Bifidobacteria*) and concomitant elevation in high LPS-expressing taxa (gram-negative bacteria) was observed. This lead to increased concentration of circulating pro-inflammatory LPS [55]. A prolonged high fat diet was also reported to induce physiologic high-grade inflammation, weight gain and T2D progression by an LPS-dependent gut microbiota-associated endotoxemia mechanism in mice [56]. In addition, it was shown that genetically obese *ob/ob* mice display a lower endotoxemia and caecal LPS content following the inactivation of CD14, a cell receptor involved in inflammation [55,57]. Concomitantly, in a randomly recruited human male cohort, a link has been observed between circulating LPS and food intake [58].

In mice fed a high-fat diet, and in genetically obese *ob/ob* mice, suppression of gut microbiota via administration of a broad range of antibiotics resulted in a significant decrease of LPS caecal content. Consequently, fat accumulation and body weight were diminished, endotoxemia and inflammation at both systemic- and tissue-specific levels were blunted, and insulin sensitivity was improved [57]. Intriguingly, administration of antibiotics to livestock trough water and food is typically used to promote cattle and swine growth and weight-gain [59,60]. The mechanisms underlying this opposite effect are not known yet support a link between enteric bacteria and host metabolism, suggesting variable responses between animal species [59,61,62].

A dysbiosis induced by obesogenic factors adversely enhances intestinal permeability by modulating the expression of epithelial junction genes *zo-1* and *occludin* [63,64]. An optimal gut microbiota helps maintain intestinal barrier impermeability via the production of SCFA, which serve as metabolic precursors for colonocytes in normal physiologic hypoxia conditions [47–49]. Colonocytes require the catabolism of SCFA to potentiate the Hypoxia-inducible factor 1-dependent expression of key genes involved in biosynthesis [47–49]. This may explain why, in metabolic diseases such as obesity, an inappropriate microbiota adversely impacts intestinal permeability, leading to infiltration of bacterial LPS from gut lumen into intestinal epithelia, bloodstream and tissue (such as the liver) contributing to metabolic endotoxemia [47–49,65]. In fact, administration of antibacterial agents targeting caecal aerobic and anaerobic bacteria with high efficiency (namely norfloxacin and ampicillin) to mice fed a high-fat diet and *ob/ob* mice significantly enhanced their global glucose tolerance, decreased their fasting glycaemia and circulating LPS levels, and improved the secretion of Adiponectin [66], known for its positive effects on insulin sensitivity [43]. The current model of obesity-associated endotoxemia posits that gut-derived LPS and free fatty acids activate M1 macrophages which, together with other immune cells, create a hepatic and physiologic inflammatory process sustaining the above-mentioned obesity-related comorbidities [67].

Gut microbiota is now considered as a key factor of metabolic health [44,64]. The relative abundance of some bacterial phyla within the gut microbiota are associated with specific metabolic states, and subjected to the influence of diets [54]. In fact, quantitative identification of bacteria using the 16S ribosomal RNA gene showed that obesity is associated to a notable decrease in the relative abundance of *Bacteroidetes vs. Firmicutes* (from a proportion of 40:60 in lean patients or non-obese mice down to a proportion of 20:80) [54,68,69]. Interestingly, this ratio is similarly decreased in *ob/ob* mice, in mice subjected to obesogenic and diabetogenic diets, as well as in obese human subjects [68,70,71]. Moreover, within these two superkingdoms, bacterial subpopulations are themselves submitted to specific changes reflecting metabolic health, diet and antiobesity medical interventions such as bariatric surgery-induced weight loss [72–74]. These changes are diverse and still not well established (see Delzenne and Cani for a detailed review [69]).

While these observations established a definitive link between gut microbiota disturbance and metabolic diseases progression, it is still unclear which one of the two events induces the other. This question was addressed by several microbiota transplantation experiments [44,75]. The transplantation of fecal microbiota from obese mice and obese patients into germ-free lean mice transformed the lean mice into obese mice, while the germ-free mice receiving microbiota from lean mice did not show any metabolic symptoms related to obesity or insulin resistance [54,75–77]. These findings revealed a microbiota-mediated transmissible effect of diets and metabolic status, demonstrating that gut microbiota is not simply a collateral unit modulated by metabolic diseases but an active and potent modulator of metabolism. The gut microbiota may therefore play a role in the determination of metabolic status.

3.2. Correlation of MHO Metabolic Status with Gut Microbiota Profile

To date, very few animal studies described a clear role for gut microbiota in the establishment of the MHO phenotype. Serino *et al.* showed that different cohorts of mice issued from the same C57BL6 genetic background became either diabetic or resistant to diabetes and metabolic disorders despite being fed the same obesogenic high-fat diet. Compared to diabetic mice, resistant mice showed higher insulin sensitivity, lower inflammation, improved intestinal impermeability (in the ileum, caecum and colon) and lower adipogenesis [78]. Moreover, the metabolic profile of resistant mice was similar to the metabolic profile observed in mice fed a high fat diet supplemented with gluco-oligosaccharidic fibers. Oligosaccharidic fibers are commonly used to prevent high fat diet-induced endotoxemia, dysbiosis and obesity [79]. Interestingly, the resistant mice harbored a distinctive gut microbiota. The gut microbiota of the diabetic mice, in comparison with resistant mice, was characterized by a 20% decrease in the abundance of *Firmicutes* to the benefit of *Bacteriodetes*, mainly resulting from a dramatic decrease of the *lachnospiraceae* bacterial family. Within the *Bacteroidetes* phylum, the family of S24-7 bacteria was specifically increased (3-fold). In addition, compared to the diabetic mice, the microbiota of resistant mice presented an important decrease of the *helicobacter* genus, while *actinobacteria* remained stable [78]. The authors suggested that the gut microbiota could represent a "signature of the metabolic phenotype independent of differences in host genetic background and diets". This suggestion is consistent with the results of a recent study performed in the brown bear (*Ursus arctos*) [80]. The bear is a mammal well known to accumulate very large amounts of adipose fat during the summer; developing hyperlipidemia while remaining metabolically healthy and resistant to atherosclerosis [81]. Sommer and colleagues showed that, during summer, bears harbored a different gut microbiota composition than during winter. Summer microbiota was enriched in *Firmicutes, Actinobacteria* and, in a lower proportion, enriched in proteobacteria while being depleted in *Bacteroidetes* [80]. Moreover, the abundance of several other bacterial families was also seasonally modulated. Interestingly, the transplantation of summer or winter microbiota from bear intestines to germ-free mice revealed a microbiota-dependent transmissible seasonal metabolic status as mice receiving summer microbiota showed a significant elevation of adiposity and body weight gain but a better glucose tolerance and a lower circulating TG level, suggesting an improved cardiometabolic state [80].

Completely ignored previously, the fungal subdivision of the gut microbiota (or "mycobiota") has recently been revealed as a determinant of human metabolic state. As for bacteria, its specific composition seems to distinguish MHO from MUHO [82]. For example, Rodriguez and collaborators showed that obese patients with relative abundance of *Eurotiomycetes* > 1% in their gut, showed improved fasting insulinemia, insulin resistance index and circulating LDL-cholesterol levels [82].

There is a definite correlation between MHO status and intestinal flora. Gut microbiota remodelling could therefore be considered as a strategy to ameliorate metabolic health. Hence, we believe that a switch from MUHO into MHO metabolic state may be possible following gut microbiota remodelling, and that dietary interventions (such as those using prebiotic or bioactive nutrients) may help in this process.

4. MHO and MUHO: From Classical Dietary Interventions to a MCT-Based One?

Obese individuals have a lower success rate of maintaining weight loss after one year compared to non-obese individuals [83]. This high risk of weight regain may lead to a pattern of weight cycling [83], and this may be associated with metabolic complications as well as CVD and mortality [84,85]. In addition, significant weight loss can increase the levels of persistent organic pollutants (POPs) in the bloodstream [86,87] and may offset the beneficial effects of weight loss. In support of this idea, a recent study showed that obese subjects with the highest POP blood levels after weight loss suffered from a delay in the improvement of lipid and liver toxicity markers [88]. Therefore, health professionals may want to favor a metabolically healthy state instead of focusing on weight loss.

4.1. Weight Management in MHO Subjects

Several studies have examined the effect of lifestyle interventions, including diet and/or exercise training in MHO individuals. These have led to contradictory findings. Some have shown that, compared to MUHO, the metabolic profile of MHO individuals after weight loss did not improve following weight loss [89–91] while other studies have reported an improvement of several metabolic risk factors [92–95]. For example, a 9-month intensive lifestyle intervention program that consisted of Mediterranean diet nutritional counselling and high intensity interval training was associated with a reduction of metabolic risk factors (e.g., blood pressure, fasting glucose level) [94]. Furthermore, weight loss following laparoscopic adjustable gastric banding in MHO patients was associated with an improvement of insulin sensitivity levels after 6 months [96]. However, a significant decrease in insulin sensitivity was observed after weight loss in a different cohort of MHO individuals [97,98]. Finally, MHO women may lose less weight than MUHO subjects after 3 months on a low fat diet [99]. Based on the current evidence, it appears difficult to prescribe an optimal lifestyle intervention program to both MUHO and MHO individuals.

4.2. The Metabolic Protective Potential of Medium Chain Triglycerides (MCTs)

4.2.1. MCTs as Bioactive Lipids

One angle of attack against metabolic diseases is the modification of the quality of dietary lipids. Such a nutritional strategy may be based on the consumption of "bioactive lipids", such as mono-unsaturated or poly-unsaturated lipids, phytosterols, and free or esterified medium chain lipids [100,101]. We will emphasize our review on the metabolic benefits of medium chain free fatty acids (MCFA) and medium chain triglycerides (MCT).

Dietary medium chain fatty acids (MCFA) range between 6 and 10 carbon-chain lengths, including hexanoate (C6:0), octanoate (C8:0) and decanoate (C10:0). Large amounts of MCFA are found, in the form of MCT, in coconut and palm kernel oils where they account for more than 50% of total lipids [102,103]. They are also found in smaller amounts in bovine milk, where they can reach 14%–15% of the total lipid mass depending on cow breeds, types of pasture and seasonal conditions [104]. MCT differ from long chain triglycerides (LCT) by several physicochemical characteristics such as their smaller molecular size. MCT are hydrolyzed both faster and more extensively during digestion. Most of the remaining non-hydrolyzed MCT are readily absorbed by intestinal cells [103]. In addition, MCFA show greater solubility in aqueous media while remaining capable of passive, non-rate-limiting diffusion across cell membranes as a result of their relative short chains [100–103,105,106]. MCFA show a low affinity for anabolic enzymes (such as diglyceride acyltransferase) therefore undergoing minimal re-esterification, a process necessary for *de novo* synthesis of TG. Once absorbed during digestion, most of MCFA and MCT are transported through the portal system directly to the liver with minimal mobilization of chylomicrons while long chain fatty acids (LCFA) are packed in chylomicrons prior to their shipment to the periphery mainly via the lymphatic system [100–103,105]. Finally, in the liver, MCFA are preferentially metabolized to generate energy [107]. In fact, MCFA are known to enter cells passively before crossing mitochondria membranes, independently of the availability of the rate-limiting carnitine palmitoyltransferase 1 (CPT-1) transport system, to fuel the β-oxidation and ATP-generating pathways [105,106], induce thermogenesis and reduce *de novo* lipogenesis [108].

Because of these properties, MCT have been used for decades to overcome many metabolic and digestive abnormalities such as pancreatic insufficiency, fat malabsorption, impaired lymphatic chylomicron transport, severe hyperchylomicronemia, and total parenteral nutrition. MCTs are also used in preterm infant formulas [106].

4.2.2. MCT-Supplemented Diets Prevent Obesity

(i) MCT and MCFA Exert Antilipogenic Effects

Using chick embryo hepatocytes, we have previously demonstrated, that free non-esterified hexanoate and octanoate significantly decrease insulin and T3 (triiodothyronine)-induced fatty acid synthase (FAS) expression and activity [108]. Activity of FAS, a key enzyme of *de novo* lipogenesis, is positively regulated in the post-prandial state by several hormones (such as insulin, ghrelin and T3) and nutrients (dietary lipid and carbohydrate derivatives) [109,110], and is an important contributor to obesity and NAFLD [20,111]. We and others have demonstrated that MCFA inhibit binding of transactivating receptors on the T3 response elements of FAS and Acetyl-CoA carboxylase (ACC) promoters [108,112–114]. Using LO2 hepatocytes, Wang and collaborators showed that the induction of cellular steatosis by LCT (esterified oleate and palmitate) is reversed by addition of either octanoate or decanoate. MCFA treatment shifts cells from global lipid anabolism to lipid catabolism and downregulates main *de novo* lipogenesis-activating transcription factors (Liver-X-receptor alpha and Sterol regulatory element binding protein-1), the lipogenic enzymes (ACC and FAS) and enzymes involved in fatty acid-uptake (Cluster of differentiation-36 and Lipoprotein lipase) [115].

(ii) The Cardiometabolic Protective Effects of Dietary MCT

The propensity of MCFA to be catabolized rather than esterified, highlights their metabolically beneficial potential. Several years ago, it was shown in rats that replacement of dietary LCT by octanoate-based MCT led to a significant attenuation of alcoholic steatosis associated with a decrease in *de novo* TG synthesis an adiposity, as well as elevated lipid oxidation [116]. Therefore, MCT-supplemented diets constitute a promising tool against adipogenic and steatogenic diseases. Feeding healthy rats with MCT-containing diets *vs.* diets containing LCT greatly decreases fat deposition without affecting whole-body protein content and assimilation [117]. Consumption of MCT is safe in regards to toxicological considerations and has been sanctioned by the FDA (Food and Drug Administration) for over 20 years [106,118]. Interestingly, dietary MCT promote post-prandial energy production. A single dose of MCT ranging between 5 and 50 g or a weeklong diet containing 40% MCT-fat systematically leads to elevated post-prandial oxygen consumption and thermogenesis, increased total lipid oxidation, higher energy expenditure and diminished energy storage in comparison with LCT administered under identical conditions [101,119–123]. Importantly, the propensity of MCT/MCFA to be degraded by oxidation is also observed in obese individuals [120,124].

Long-term replacement of LCT with TG composed of esterified MCFA and LCFA induces a measurable body fat loss without any impact on energy intake and global metabolism [101,125,126]. These specific TG, produced from the transesterification of MCT and LCT (S-MLCT) are interesting compounds because of their higher smoking temperature making them more appropriate for cooking purposes than simple mixtures of MCT and LCT. S-MLCT display a "L-M-L"-type structure (TG with LCFA in sn-1 position, MCFA in sn-2 and LCFA in sn-3), are preferable substrates for pancreatic enzymes and are therefore highly digestible [101,125,126]. Feeding healthy young volunteers for 3 months with either S-MLCT or LCT-enriched liquid formulas (1040 kJ/day) led to a bodyweight increase from the baseline in both groups [127]. Interestingly, diets supplemented with S-MLCT induced a lower increase in body fat mass compared to the LCT supplemented diets (+10% for

S-MLCT *vs.* +30% for LCT) [127]. The general metabolic profiles between the two groups were not different, with the exception of glycemia (S-MLCT = 924 *vs.* LCT = 853 mg/100 mL) [127]. A clear link was concurrently established between the propensity of MCT to increase thermogenesis and their previously reported capacity to reduce diet-induced adiposity and body weight-gain [107,128]. Wistar rats submitted to a single oral gavage of 1 g MCT or LCT showed significant elevation in oxygen consumption concomitantly with elevated thermogenesis (1.5 kcal/6 h for MCT *vs.* 0.8 kcal/6 h for LCT) [107]. Another study showed that feeding rats with a diet containing 10% MCT during 6 weeks diminished body fat mass by decreasing subcutaneous and intra-abdominal adiposity compared to a diet containing 10% LCT, suggesting that dietary-MCT lowered body fat mass by inducing thermogenesis [107]. Interestingly, MCT also lower caloric intake, compared to LCT, by improving satiety [129,130]. Octanoate, which constitutes most of the MCT used in dietary interventions, was suggested to be the main co-substrate of the Ghrelin *O*-acetyltransferase enzyme, involved in the activation of the powerful orexigenic peptide hormone Ghrelin [131–133]. However, an acute diminution of food intake induced by the consumption of MCT oil is associated with an elevation of Leptin, a hormone with a well-known anti-orexigenic effect [129]. These unsolved discrepancies between different studies highlights the necessity to better understand the molecular effects of MCT and their physiologic implications [132].

Consistent observations related to anti-obesity effects of MCT were generated through animal and human clinical studies. Daily consumption (for 12 weeks at breakfast) of bread supplemented with 14 g S-MLCT (produced by a transesterification of MCT and LCT) led, in comparison with control LCT, to a mild but significant decrease in body weight, and a decrease in subcutaneous and visceral adiposity as well as in total cholesterol level. However, the other metabolic and anthropometric parameters did not significantly vary [134]. The impact of MCT consumption on body-weight is noticeably variable depending on studies and diet protocol designs. Women on a one-month diet where 30% of total energy was supplied by MCT displayed improved fat oxidation and energy expenditure compared to women on LCT-containing meals, and showed a tendency towards decreasing body weight [135]. Interestingly, studies suggested that the catabolic effects induced by the dietary MCT may depend on BMI. In humans, MCT consumption for 4 weeks induced energy expenditure, fat oxidation and body weight loss inversely proportional to BMI [136]. A recent observation has been also made on the impact of MCFA diets on cardiac functions [137]. Compared to LCFA, a 2-week administration of a 38% fat diet containing mostly MCFA positively altered plasma lipids and potentially improved cardiac function as well as insulinemia in adult type 2 diabetics. However, this diet did not significantly impact cardiac TG load or cardiac steatosis [137].

Nevertheless, the consumption of MCT is systematically associated with higher energy expenditure compared to LCT. Solid evidences support the feasibility of using MCT preparations for nutritional trials against obesity, considering their sources, their flexible use and their safety. Compared to soybean oil (providing high amounts of LCT), coconut oil, which is the most easily obtained source of MCT, improves (in synergy with exercise) the cardiometabolic and anthropometric profiles (including waist circumference) of women presenting unhealthy abdominal obesity [138]. However, coconut oil contains other compounds such as antioxidant polyphenols also known to improve metabolic profile by lowering LDL and VLDL while increasing HDL [138,139]. St-Onge and collaborators demonstrated that consumption of a combination of MCT, phytosterols and omega-3-enriched flaxseed oil for 1 month compared to olive oil or beef tallow-based diets, led to improvement in plasma lipid profile in both healthy and overweight women as well as in MHO men [140,141]. In addition, MCT oils can be incorporated into a weight loss program without any adverse effects on metabolic health [142]. Table 1 summarizes the main studies that have revealed the antiobesity potential of MCT.

Consistent with these observations, a recent meta-analysis of randomized controlled trials, combining a broad spectrum of publication resources, showed that MCT administered for 3 weeks or more reduced body weight (−0.51 kg average), waist circumference (−1.46 cm average), hip circumference (−0.79 cm average), total body fat, total subcutaneous fat and visceral fat in comparison with LCT and despite high heterogeneity [143]. Such observations strongly support the relevance of using MCT to modulate body weight and metabolic profile in MUHO patients.

Table 1. Antiobesity effects of MCT and MCFA.

Model	Main Reported Effects for MCT or MCFA	References
Hepatocyte	Downregulated expression of genes involved in DNL and fatty acid uptake; promoted lipid catabolism; reduced steatosis; prevented deleterious lipid accumulation	[108,113,115]
Rat	Lowered TG accumulation in the liver; reduced alcoholic steatosis	[116]
Rat	Decreased body weight gain and body fat mass; lowered fat accumulation and visceral adiposity; did not affect protein assimilation nor metabolism	[107,117]
Rat	Resulted in a higher induction of oxygen consumption and thermogenesis	[107]
Human	Significantly increased postprandial oxygen consumption, energy expenditure, and fat oxidation, in a MCT dose-dependent manner and at a greater extend for lower BMIs	[119–122,135,136,142,144]
Human	Decreased global adiposity, body fat, and whole-body subcutaneous adipose tissue loss, waist circumference; significantly lowered rate of variation of body fat percentage	[127,130,134]
Human	Did not improve global adiposity	[135]
Human	Did not elevate postprandial circulating TG; did not modulate glucose response, insulinemia and circulating TG levels; lowered LDL/HDL ratio, total and HDL-cholesterol; improved cardiometabolic profile	[129,134,136,138,141]
Human	Promoted rise in leptin and peptide YY	[129]

MCT: medium chain triglyceride; MCFA: medium chain fatty acid; DNL: *de novo* lipogenesis; TG: triglyceride; BMI: body mass index; LDL: low density lipoprotein; HDL: high density lipoprotein; Peptide YY: peptide tyrosine tyrosine.

4.2.3. MCT-Supplemented Diets Improve Gut Microbiota and Intestinal Health

MCT are known for their antimicrobial properties. MCT, as well as their constituent MCFA, when provided by maternal milk (along with endogenous long chain unsaturated monoglycerides), exerted antimicrobial effects on the gastro-intestinal tract of suckling neonates and contributed to reduce pathogen transmission [145–147]. Moreover, MCT and MCFA were also shown to reduce proliferation of certain species of *Malassezia*, an infectious fungus widespread in hospitals [148].

Kono and collaborators demonstrated that MCT could prevent LPS-mediated endotoxemia. Rats were fed MCT or corn oil (a source of LCT) by daily gavage for 1 week, prior to an intravenously acute dose of endotoxic LPS. Interestingly, while LPS injection led to mortality in corn oil-fed animals, this mortality was prevented in MCT-fed rats [149]. Furthermore, in contrast with the corn oil/LPS group, the MCT/LPS group showed a lower liver injury and inflammation as revealed by a significant decrease in CD14 and tumor necrosis factor alpha (TNF-α) expression in Kupffer cells. In parallel with this, while the corn oil/LPS combination induced a significant increase of intestinal permeability compared to corn oil without LPS, the MCT/LPS combination was associated with a significant improvement of intestinal permeability [149]. In addition, MCT gavage prevented intestinal atrophy (a current problem occurring during parenteral nutrition) and massively reduced (10-fold) the bacterial fecal content [149]. This study showed that MCT administration prevented CD14-activation dependent endotoxemia mediated by LPS, a model consensually associated to obesity and metabolic syndrome.

Most studies on juvenile models use piglets because of their similarities with humans during intestinal development [150–153]. MCT supplements can be used as alternatives to antibiotics against certain types of porcine colitis [152,154,155]. MCT-fed piglets had a better gastro-intestinal health, with improved intestinal apoptotic index and mucosal turnover, and lowered intraepithelial lymphocyte infiltration (reflecting reduced local inflammation and diminished immune response) compared to controls [152,153]. Furthermore, piglets fed with MCT supplements display a marked modulation of microbial gastric and intestinal populations [152,153,156]. This contributed to a decrease in intestinal inflammation and to an improvement of gut health and integrity [157] with a direct impact on the gut bacteria from Gram-positive (low LPS) and Gram-negative (high LPS) subdivisions [156]. Another study showed that dietary organic acids (OA) and MCFA changed the gut microbiota of weaning piglets [151]. MCFA were shown to reduce the pH of the digesta because of diminished bacterial acid production. OA and MCFA altered the population distribution of *Bacteroidetes/Porphyromonas/Prevotella* phyla and *Clostridia/Streptococcus* genus in a tissue specific manner (stomach, jejunum, ileum and colon). MCFA specifically modulated the bacterial populations in specific regions such as jejunum and colon by promoting the growth of *Escherichia/Hafnia/Shigella* bacteria and *Clostridia* genus [151]. Combining SCFA and MCFA may constitute a potent tool for the management of optimal gut microbiota. This combination as well as other sources of MCT including coconuts oils, functional mixed oils, or purified MCT oils may be therefore useful for remodelling MUHO gut microbiota and improving metabolically unhealthy obesity. Table 2 summarizes these advances.

Table 2. Antimicrobial and gut-managing effects of MCT.

Model	Main Reported Effects	References
Malassezia	Supressed growth of *M. sympodialis* and *M. furfur*	[148]
Rats	Prevented acute LPS administration-induced mortality, liver injury, liver inflammation, gut impermeability and injury; blunted LPS-induced endotoxemia	[149]
Rats	Significantly blunted TNBS-induced colitis; improved both colonic MPO activity and colonocytes-expressed inflammatory markers	[155]
Rats	Improved gut integrity; modulated immune response to LPS; improved intestinal secretion of IgA	[158]
Piglets	Lowered intestinal pH, in synergy with OA; modulated several gut microbial taxa, potentially preventing postweaning diarrhea	[151]

M. sympodialis: *Malassezia sympodialis*; *M. furfur*: *Malassezia furfur*; LPS: lipopolysaccharide; TNBS: 2,4,6-trinitrobenzene sulphonic acid; MPO: myeloperoxidase.

5. Synthesis and Conclusions

This review aimed to highlight several aspects underlying the condition of obese subjects, which can be either metabolically unhealthy obese (MUHO) or metabolically healthy obese (MHO). While a panel of criteria serves to define the MUHO state, those defining metabolically healthy obesity remain the subject of current discussions. We underline the necessity of better defining the potential role of gut microbiota in the establishment of MUHO or MHO states. Moreover, we believe that gut microbiota structure may not only serve as a biomarker of those metabolic states, but can also be subjected to a diet-induced remodelling, modifying in turn the metabolic status of patients (MUHO *vs.* MHO or lean state). Dietary MCT, taken alone or with other supplements (such as prebiotics, probiotics, organic acids, *etc.*) could be used as anti-obesity interventions, in regards to their capacity to prevent intestinal permeability/endotoxemia by remodeling gut microbiota, and to prevent unhealthy storage by improving the lipid catabolism/anabolism balance. Figure 1 illustrates this concept.

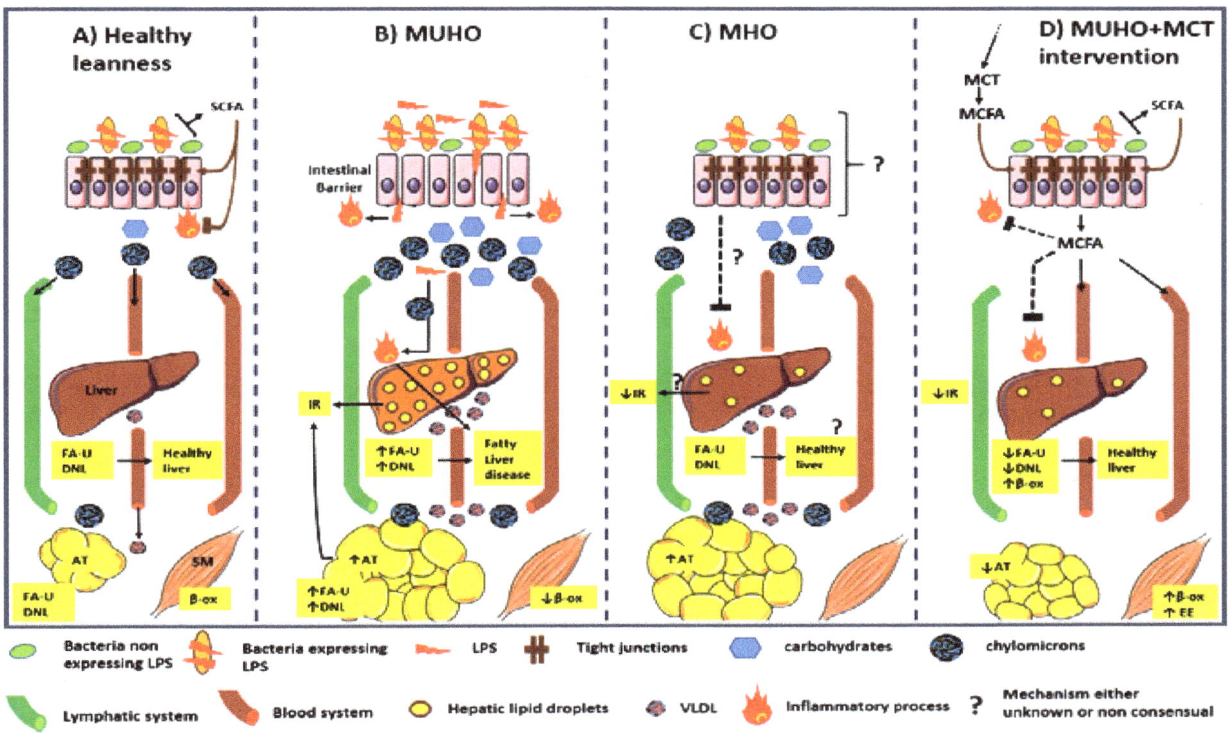

Figure 1. Crosstalk between gut, liver and peripheral metabolic tissues under 4 metabolic states. Under condition of healthy leanness (**A**) an optimal relative abundance of LPS-expressing *vs.* non-expressing bacteria contribute to gut impermeability, low intestinal and hepatic inflammation, and non-obesogenic/steatogenic nutrient supply. Under MUHO conditions (**B**), an elevation in the relative abundance of LPS-expressing bacteria (Gram-negative) induces LPS infiltration and leads to altered intestinal barrier integrity, local inflammation, liver injury and endotoxemia. At the same time, a high fat and carbohydrate supply contributes to adiposity, hepatic steatosis and peripheral insulin resistance. In MHO subjects (**C**), despite an adiposity sustained by a rich diet, a balanced gut microbiota would contribute to maintain intestinal and systemic metabolic health, prevent endotoxemia, and lower hepatic injury and peripheral insulin resistance. Our hypothetical model (**D**) suggests that diet MCT supplementation for MUHO subjects may facilitate a shift towards an MHO-like profile by improving lipid catabolism and lowering adiposity in part, but also by remodelling the gut microbiota into a metabolically beneficial structure. SCFA: short chain fatty acids; FA-U: Fatty acid uptake; AT: adipose tissue; DNL: *de novo* lipogenesis; SM: skeletal muscle; MUHO: metabolically unhealthy obese (or obesity); IR: Insulin resistance; β-ox: beta-oxidation; MHO: metabolically healthy obese (or obesity); MCT: medium chain triglycerides; MCFA: medium chain fatty acids; LPS: lipopolysaccharides; VLDL: very low density lipoproteins.

Acknowledgments: The authors are grateful to Rodolphe Soret and Quentin Escoula (UQAM, Canada) for suggestions, corrections and advice. Finally, authors are grateful to SERVIER Medical Art [159] creators for allowing free access to their images bank, which was used to construct Figure 1.

Author Contributions: S.A.R., A.D.K., K.F.B., and C.M. conceived, designed, revised and illustrated the ideas and the manuscript, and all approved its final version.

References

1. Smith, K.B.; Smith, M.S. Obesity statistics. *Prim. Care* **2016**, *43*, 121–135. [CrossRef] [PubMed]
2. Ng, M.; Fleming, T.; Robinson, M.; Thomson, B.; Graetz, N.; Margono, C.; Mullany, E.C.; Biryukov, S.; Abbafati, C.; Abera, S.F.; *et al.* Global, regional, and national prevalence of overweight and obesity in children and adults during 1980–2013: A systematic analysis for the global burden of disease study 2013. *Lancet* **2014**, *384*, 766–781. [CrossRef]
3. Haslam, D.W.; James, W.P. Obesity. *Lancet* **2005**, *366*, 1197–1209. [CrossRef]
4. Graffy, P.M.; Pickhardt, P.J. Quantification of hepatic and visceral fat by ct and mr imaging: Relevance to the obesity epidemic, metabolic syndrome and nafld. *Br. J. Radiol.* **2016**, *89*, 20151024. [CrossRef] [PubMed]
5. Grundy, S.M. Metabolic syndrome update. *Trends Cardiovasc. Med.* **2016**, *26*, 364–373. [CrossRef] [PubMed]
6. Hryhorczuk, C.; Sharma, S.; Fulton, S.E. Metabolic disturbances connecting obesity and depression. *Front. Neurosci.* **2013**, *7*, 177. [CrossRef] [PubMed]
7. Reuter, C.P.; Silva, P.T.; Renner, J.D.; Mello, E.D.; Valim, A.R.; Pasa, L.; Silva, R.D.; Burgos, M.S. Dyslipidemia is associated with unfit and overweight-obese children and adolescents. *Arq. Brasil. Cardiol.* **2016**. [CrossRef] [PubMed]
8. Elmaogullari, S.; Tepe, D.; Ucakturk, S.A.; Karaca Kara, F.; Demirel, F. Prevalence of dyslipidemia and associated factors in obese children and adolescents. *J. Clin. Res. Pediatr. Endocrinol.* **2015**, *7*, 228–234. [CrossRef] [PubMed]
9. Cho, Y.; Shore, S.A. Obesity, asthma, and the microbiome. *Physiology* **2016**, *31*, 108–116. [CrossRef] [PubMed]
10. Payab, M.; Amoli, M.M.; Qorbani, M.; Hasani-Ranjbar, S. Adiponectin gene variants and abdominal obesity in an iranian population. *Eat. Weight Disord.* **2016**. [CrossRef] [PubMed]
11. Waleh, M.Q. Impacts of physical activity on the obese. *Prim. Care* **2016**, *43*, 97–107. [CrossRef] [PubMed]
12. Scott, E.M. Circadian clocks, obesity and cardiometabolic function. *Diabetes Obes. Metab.* **2015**, *17*, 84–89. [CrossRef] [PubMed]
13. Klingenberg, L.; Sjodin, A.; Holmback, U.; Astrup, A.; Chaput, J.P. Short sleep duration and its association with energy metabolism. *Obes. Rev. Off. J. Int. Assoc. Stud. Obes.* **2012**, *13*, 565–577. [CrossRef] [PubMed]
14. Choudhury, S.M.; Tan, T.M.; Bloom, S.R. Gastrointestinal hormones and their role in obesity. *Curr. Opin. Endocrinol. Diabetes Obes.* **2016**, *23*, 18–22. [CrossRef] [PubMed]
15. Lee, D.H.; Porta, M.; Jacobs, D.R., Jr.; Vandenberg, L.N. Chlorinated persistent organic pollutants, obesity, and type 2 diabetes. *Endocr. Rev.* **2014**, *35*, 557–601. [CrossRef] [PubMed]
16. Nova, E.; Perez de Heredia, F.; Gomez-Martinez, S.; Marcos, A. The role of probiotics on the microbiota: Effect on obesity. *Nutr. Clin. Pract.* **2016**. [CrossRef] [PubMed]
17. Patterson, E.; Ryan, P.M.; Cryan, J.F.; Dinan, T.G.; Ross, R.P.; Fitzgerald, G.F.; Stanton, C. Gut microbiota, obesity and diabetes. *Postgrad. Med. J.* **2016**. [CrossRef] [PubMed]
18. Drewnowski, A.; Almiron-Roig, E. Frontiers in neuroscience human perceptions and preferences for fat-rich foods. In *Fat Detection: Taste, Texture, and Post Ingestive Effects*; Montmayeur, J.P., Le Coutre, J., Eds.; CRC Press/Taylor & Francis Group, LLC.: Boca Raton, FL, USA, 2010.
19. Strable, M.S.; Ntambi, J.M. Genetic control of *de novo* lipogenesis: Role in diet-induced obesity. *Crit. Rev. Biochem. Mol. Biol.* **2010**, *45*, 199–214. [CrossRef] [PubMed]
20. Ameer, F.; Scandiuzzi, L.; Hasnain, S.; Kalbacher, H.; Zaidi, N. *De novo* lipogenesis in health and disease. *Metabol. Clin. Exp.* **2014**, *63*, 895–902. [CrossRef] [PubMed]
21. Povero, D.; Feldstein, A.E. Novel molecular mechanisms in the development of non-alcoholic steatohepatitis. *Diabetes Metabol. J.* **2016**, *40*, 1–11. [CrossRef] [PubMed]
22. Kaila, B.; Raman, M. Obesity: A review of pathogenesis and management strategies. *Can. J. Gastroenterol.* **2008**, *22*, 61–68. [CrossRef] [PubMed]
23. Rankinen, T.; Zuberi, A.; Chagnon, Y.C.; Weisnagel, S.J.; Argyropoulos, G.; Walts, B.; Perusse, L.; Bouchard, C. The human obesity gene map: The 2005 update. *Obesity* **2006**, *14*, 529–644. [CrossRef] [PubMed]
24. Waterland, R.A.; Travisano, M.; Tahiliani, K.G.; Rached, M.T.; Mirza, S. Methyl donor supplementation prevents transgenerational amplification of obesity. *Int. J. Obes.* **2008**, *32*, 1373–1379. [CrossRef] [PubMed]
25. McAllister, E.J.; Dhurandhar, N.V.; Keith, S.W.; Aronne, L.J.; Barger, J.; Baskin, M.; Benca, R.M.; Biggio, J.; Boggiano, M.M.; Eisenmann, J.C.; *et al.* Ten putative contributors to the obesity epidemic. *Crit. Rev. Food Sci. Nutr.* **2009**, *49*, 868–913. [CrossRef] [PubMed]

26. Kanayama, T.; Kobayashi, N.; Mamiya, S.; Nakanishi, T.; Nishikawa, J. Organotin compounds promote adipocyte differentiation as agonists of the peroxisome proliferator-activated receptor gamma/retinoid X receptor pathway. *Mol. Pharmacol.* **2005**, *67*, 766–774. [CrossRef] [PubMed]
27. Trayhurn, P.; Beattie, J.H. Physiological role of adipose tissue: White adipose tissue as an endocrine and secretory organ. *Proc. Nutr. Soc.* **2001**, *60*, 329–339. [CrossRef] [PubMed]
28. Maachi, M.; Pieroni, L.; Bruckert, E.; Jardel, C.; Fellahi, S.; Hainque, B.; Capeau, J.; Bastard, J.P. Systemic low-grade inflammation is related to both circulating and adipose tissue tnfalpha, leptin and il-6 levels in obese women. *Int. J. Obes. Relat. Metab. Disord.* **2004**, *28*, 993–997. [CrossRef] [PubMed]
29. Grover, S.A.; Kaouache, M.; Rempel, P.; Joseph, L.; Dawes, M.; Lau, D.C.; Lowensteyn, I. Years of life lost and healthy life-years lost from diabetes and cardiovascular disease in overweight and obese people: A modelling study. *Lancet Diabetes Endocrinol.* **2015**, *3*, 114–122. [CrossRef]
30. Roberts, C.K.; Hevener, A.L.; Barnard, R.J. Metabolic syndrome and insulin resistance: Underlying causes and modification by exercise training. *Compr. Physiol.* **2013**, *3*, 1–58. [PubMed]
31. Kyrou, I.; Randeva, H.S.; Weickert, M.O. Clinical problems caused by obesity. In *Endotext*; De Groot, L.J., Beck-Peccoz, P., Chrousos, G., Dungan, K., Grossman, A., Hershman, J.M., Koch, C., McLachlan, R., New, M., Rebar, R., *et al.*, Eds.; MDText.com, Inc.: South Dartmouth, MA, USA, 2000.
32. Poirier, P.; Giles, T.D.; Bray, G.A.; Hong, Y.; Stern, J.S.; Pi-Sunyer, F.X.; Eckel, R.H. Obesity and cardiovascular disease: Pathophysiology, evaluation, and effect of weight loss: An update of the 1997 american heart association scientific statement on obesity and heart disease from the obesity committee of the council on nutrition, physical activity, and metabolism. *Circulation* **2006**, *113*, 898–918. [PubMed]
33. Fabbrini, E.; Sullivan, S.; Klein, S. Obesity and nonalcoholic fatty liver disease: Biochemical, metabolic, and clinical implications. *Hepatology* **2010**, *51*, 679–689. [CrossRef] [PubMed]
34. Samocha-Bonet, D.; Dixit, V.D.; Kahn, C.R.; Leibel, R.L.; Lin, X.; Nieuwdorp, M.; Pietilainen, K.H.; Rabasa-Lhoret, R.; Roden, M.; Scherer, P.E.; *et al.* Metabolically healthy and unhealthy obese—The 2013 stock conference report. *Obes. Rev.* **2014**, *15*, 697–708. [CrossRef] [PubMed]
35. Karelis, A.D. Metabolically healthy but obese individuals. *Lancet* **2008**, *372*, 1281–1283. [CrossRef]
36. Primeau, V.; Coderre, L.; Karelis, A.D.; Brochu, M.; Lavoie, M.E.; Messier, V.; Sladek, R.; Rabasa-Lhoret, R. Characterizing the profile of obese patients who are metabolically healthy. *Int. J. Obes.* **2011**, *35*, 971–981. [CrossRef] [PubMed]
37. Velho, S.; Paccaud, F.; Waeber, G.; Vollenweider, P.; Marques-Vidal, P. Metabolically healthy obesity: Different prevalences using different criteria. *Eur. J. Clin. Nutr.* **2010**, *64*, 1043–1051. [CrossRef] [PubMed]
38. Wildman, R.P.; Muntner, P.; Reynolds, K.; McGinn, A.P.; Rajpathak, S.; Wylie-Rosett, J.; Sowers, M.R. The obese without cardiometabolic risk factor clustering and the normal weight with cardiometabolic risk factor clustering: Prevalence and correlates of 2 phenotypes among the US population (NHANES 1999–2004). *Arch. Intern. Med.* **2008**, *168*, 1617–1624. [CrossRef] [PubMed]
39. Plourde, G.; Karelis, A.D. Current issues in the identification and treatment of metabolically healthy but obese individuals. *Nutr. Metab. Cardiovasc. Dis.* **2014**, *24*, 455–459. [CrossRef] [PubMed]
40. Eckel, N.; Meidtner, K.; Kalle-Uhlmann, T.; Stefan, N.; Schulze, M.B. Metabolically healthy obesity and cardiovascular events: A systematic review and meta-analysis. *Eur. J. Prev. Cardiol.* **2015**. [CrossRef] [PubMed]
41. Loos, R.J. Integrating publicly available genome-wide association data to study the genetic basis of metabolically healthy obese and metabolically obese but normal-weight individuals. *Diabetes* **2014**, *63*, 4004–4007. [CrossRef] [PubMed]
42. Berezina, A.; Belyaeva, O.; Berkovich, O.; Baranova, E.; Karonova, T.; Bazhenova, E.; Brovin, D.; Grineva, E.; Shlyakhto, E. Prevalence, risk factors, and genetic traits in metabolically healthy and unhealthy obese individuals. *Biomed. Res. Int.* **2015**, *2015*, 548734. [CrossRef] [PubMed]
43. Kandasamy, A.D.; Sung, M.M.; Boisvenue, J.J.; Barr, A.J.; Dyck, J.R. Adiponectin gene therapy ameliorates high-fat, high-sucrose diet-induced metabolic perturbations in mice. *Nutr. Diabetes* **2012**, *2*, e45. [CrossRef] [PubMed]
44. Hur, K.Y.; Lee, M.S. Gut microbiota and metabolic disorders. *Diabetes Metab. J.* **2015**, *39*, 198–203. [CrossRef] [PubMed]
45. Guinane, C.M.; Cotter, P.D. Role of the gut microbiota in health and chronic gastrointestinal disease: Understanding a hidden metabolic organ. *Ther. Adv. Gastroenterol.* **2013**, *6*, 295–308. [CrossRef] [PubMed]

46. Chow, J.; Lee, S.M.; Shen, Y.; Khosravi, A.; Mazmanian, S.K. Host-bacterial symbiosis in health and disease. *Adv. Immunol.* **2010**, *107*, 243–274. [PubMed]
47. Kelly, C.J.; Zheng, L.; Campbell, E.L.; Saeedi, B.; Scholz, C.C.; Bayless, A.J.; Wilson, K.E.; Glover, L.E.; Kominsky, D.J.; Magnuson, A.; *et al.* Crosstalk between microbiota-derived short-chain fatty acids and intestinal epithelial hif augments tissue barrier function. *Cell Host Microb.* **2015**, *17*, 662–671. [CrossRef] [PubMed]
48. Den Besten, G.; Lange, K.; Havinga, R.; van Dijk, T.H.; Gerding, A.; van Eunen, K.; Muller, M.; Groen, A.K.; Hooiveld, G.J.; Bakker, B.M.; *et al.* Gut-derived short-chain fatty acids are vividly assimilated into host carbohydrates and lipids. *Am. J. Physiol. Gastrointest. Liver Physiol.* **2013**, *305*, G900–G910. [CrossRef] [PubMed]
49. Den Besten, G.; van Eunen, K.; Groen, A.K.; Venema, K.; Reijngoud, D.J.; Bakker, B.M. The role of short-chain fatty acids in the interplay between diet, gut microbiota, and host energy metabolism. *J. Lipid Res.* **2013**, *54*, 2325–2340. [CrossRef] [PubMed]
50. Singh, V.; Chassaing, B.; Zhang, L.; San Yeoh, B.; Xiao, X.; Kumar, M.; Baker, M.T.; Cai, J.; Walker, R.; Borkowski, K.; *et al.* Microbiota-dependent hepatic lipogenesis mediated by stearoyl coa desaturase 1 (scd1) promotes metabolic syndrome in tlr5-deficient mice. *Cell Metab.* **2015**, *22*, 983–996. [CrossRef] [PubMed]
51. LeBlanc, J.G.; Milani, C.; de Giori, G.S.; Sesma, F.; van Sinderen, D.; Ventura, M. Bacteria as vitamin suppliers to their host: A gut microbiota perspective. *Curr. Opin. Biotechnol.* **2013**, *24*, 160–168. [CrossRef] [PubMed]
52. Janssen, A.W.; Kersten, S. The role of the gut microbiota in metabolic health. *Fed. Am. Soc. Exp. Biol. J.* **2015**, *29*, 3111–3123. [CrossRef] [PubMed]
53. Everard, A.; Cani, P.D. Diabetes, obesity and gut microbiota. *Best Pract. Res. Clin. Gastroenterol.* **2013**, *27*, 73–83. [CrossRef] [PubMed]
54. Turnbaugh, P.J.; Ley, R.E.; Mahowald, M.A.; Magrini, V.; Mardis, E.R.; Gordon, J.I. An obesity-associated gut microbiome with increased capacity for energy harvest. *Nature* **2006**, *444*, 1027–1031. [CrossRef] [PubMed]
55. Cani, P.D.; Amar, J.; Iglesias, M.A.; Poggi, M.; Knauf, C.; Bastelica, D.; Neyrinck, A.M.; Fava, F.; Tuohy, K.M.; Chabo, C.; *et al.* Metabolic endotoxemia initiates obesity and insulin resistance. *Diabetes* **2007**, *56*, 1761–1772. [CrossRef] [PubMed]
56. Backhed, F.; Manchester, J.K.; Semenkovich, C.F.; Gordon, J.I. Mechanisms underlying the resistance to diet-induced obesity in germ-free mice. *Proc. Natl. Acad. Sci. USA* **2007**, *104*, 979–984. [CrossRef] [PubMed]
57. Cani, P.D.; Bibiloni, R.; Knauf, C.; Waget, A.; Neyrinck, A.M.; Delzenne, N.M.; Burcelin, R. Changes in gut microbiota control metabolic endotoxemia-induced inflammation in high-fat diet-induced obesity and diabetes in mice. *Diabetes* **2008**, *57*, 1470–1481. [CrossRef] [PubMed]
58. Amar, J.; Burcelin, R.; Ruidavets, J.B.; Cani, P.D.; Fauvel, J.; Alessi, M.C.; Chamontin, B.; Ferrieres, J. Energy intake is associated with endotoxemia in apparently healthy men. *Am. J. Clin. Nutr.* **2008**, *87*, 1219–1223. [PubMed]
59. Maron, D.F.; Smith, T.J.S.; Nachman, K.E. Restrictions on antimicrobial use in food animal production: An international regulatory and economic survey. *Glob. Health* **2013**, *9*, 48. [CrossRef] [PubMed]
60. Cazer, C.L.; Volkova, V.V.; Grohn, Y.T. Use of pharmacokinetic modeling to assess antimicrobial pressure on enteric bacteria of beef cattle fed chlortetracycline for growth promotion, disease control, or treatment. *Foodborne Pathog. Dis.* **2014**, *11*, 403–411. [CrossRef] [PubMed]
61. Van Boeckel, T.P.; Brower, C.; Gilbert, M.; Grenfell, B.T.; Levin, S.A.; Robinson, T.P.; Teillant, A.; Laxminarayan, R. Global trends in antimicrobial use in food animals. *Proc. Natl. Acad. Sci. USA* **2015**, *112*, 5649–5654. [CrossRef] [PubMed]
62. Johnson, T.A.; Stedtfeld, R.D.; Wang, Q.; Cole, J.R.; Hashsham, S.A.; Looft, T.; Zhu, Y.G.; Tiedje, J.M. Clusters of antibiotic resistance genes enriched together stay together in swine agriculture. *mBio* **2016**. [CrossRef] [PubMed]
63. Cani, P.D.; Possemiers, S.; Van de Wiele, T.; Guiot, Y.; Everard, A.; Rottier, O.; Geurts, L.; Naslain, D.; Neyrinck, A.; Lambert, D.M.; *et al.* Changes in gut microbiota control inflammation in obese mice through a mechanism involving glp-2-driven improvement of gut permeability. *Gut* **2009**, *58*, 1091–1103. [CrossRef] [PubMed]
64. Arslan, N. Obesity, fatty liver disease and intestinal microbiota. *World J. Gastroenterol.* **2014**, *20*, 16452–16463. [CrossRef] [PubMed]

65. Cani, P.D. Crosstalk between the gut microbiota and the endocannabinoid system: Impact on the gut barrier function and the adipose tissue. *Clin. Microbiol. Infect.* **2012**, *18*, 50–53. [CrossRef] [PubMed]
66. Membrez, M.; Blancher, F.; Jaquet, M.; Bibiloni, R.; Cani, P.D.; Burcelin, R.G.; Corthesy, I.; Mace, K.; Chou, C.J. Gut microbiota modulation with norfloxacin and ampicillin enhances glucose tolerance in mice. *Fed. Am. Soc. Exp. Biol. J.* **2008**, *22*, 2416–2426. [CrossRef] [PubMed]
67. Pereira, S.S.; Alvarez-Leite, J.I. Low-grade inflammation, obesity, and diabetes. *Curr. Obes. Rep.* **2014**, *3*, 422–431. [CrossRef] [PubMed]
68. Ley, R.E.; Backhed, F.; Turnbaugh, P.; Lozupone, C.A.; Knight, R.D.; Gordon, J.I. Obesity alters gut microbial ecology. *Proc. Natl. Acad. Sci. USA* **2005**, *102*, 11070–11075. [CrossRef] [PubMed]
69. Delzenne, N.M.; Cani, P.D. Interaction between obesity and the gut microbiota: Relevance in nutrition. *Annu. Rev. Nutr.* **2011**, *31*, 15–31. [CrossRef] [PubMed]
70. Abdallah Ismail, N.; Ragab, S.H.; Abd Elbaky, A.; Shoeib, A.R.; Alhosary, Y.; Fekry, D. Frequency of firmicutes and bacteroidetes in gut microbiota in obese and normal weight egyptian children and adults. *Arch. Med. Sci.* **2011**, *7*, 501–507. [CrossRef] [PubMed]
71. Clarke, S.F.; Murphy, E.F.; Nilaweera, K.; Ross, P.R.; Shanahan, F.; O'Toole, P.W.; Cotter, P.D. The gut microbiota and its relationship to diet and obesity: New insights. *Gut Microb.* **2012**, *3*, 186–202. [CrossRef] [PubMed]
72. Delzenne, N.M.; Neyrinck, A.M.; Backhed, F.; Cani, P.D. Targeting gut microbiota in obesity: Effects of prebiotics and probiotics. *Nat. Rev. Endocrinol.* **2011**, *7*, 639–646. [CrossRef] [PubMed]
73. Delzenne, N.M.; Neyrinck, A.M.; Cani, P.D. Modulation of the gut microbiota by nutrients with prebiotic properties: Consequences for host health in the context of obesity and metabolic syndrome. *Microb. Cell Fact.* **2011**, *10*, S10. [CrossRef] [PubMed]
74. Furet, J.P.; Kong, L.C.; Tap, J.; Poitou, C.; Basdevant, A.; Bouillot, J.L.; Mariat, D.; Corthier, G.; Dore, J.; Henegar, C.; *et al.* Differential adaptation of human gut microbiota to bariatric surgery-induced weight loss: Links with metabolic and low-grade inflammation markers. *Diabetes* **2010**, *59*, 3049–3057. [CrossRef] [PubMed]
75. Blaut, M. Gut microbiota and energy balance: Role in obesity. *Proc. Nutr. Soc.* **2015**, *74*, 227–234. [CrossRef] [PubMed]
76. Turnbaugh, P.J.; Ridaura, V.K.; Faith, J.J.; Rey, F.E.; Knight, R.; Gordon, J.I. The effect of diet on the human gut microbiome: A metagenomic analysis in humanized gnotobiotic mice. *Sci. Transl. Med.* **2009**, *1*, 6ra14. [CrossRef] [PubMed]
77. Ridaura, V.K.; Faith, J.J.; Rey, F.E.; Cheng, J.; Duncan, A.E.; Kau, A.L.; Griffin, N.W.; Lombard, V.; Henrissat, B.; Bain, J.R.; *et al.* Gut microbiota from twins discordant for obesity modulate metabolism in mice. *Science* **2013**, *341*, 1241214. [CrossRef] [PubMed]
78. Serino, M.; Luche, E.; Gres, S.; Baylac, A.; Berge, M.; Cenac, C.; Waget, A.; Klopp, P.; Iacovoni, J.; Klopp, C.; *et al.* Metabolic adaptation to a high-fat diet is associated with a change in the gut microbiota. *Gut* **2012**, *61*, 543–553. [CrossRef] [PubMed]
79. Neyrinck, A.M.; Van Hee, V.F.; Piront, N.; De Backer, F.; Toussaint, O.; Cani, P.D.; Delzenne, N.M. Wheat-derived arabinoxylan oligosaccharides with prebiotic effect increase satietogenic gut peptides and reduce metabolic endotoxemia in diet-induced obese mice. *Nutr. Diabetes* **2012**, *2*, e28. [CrossRef] [PubMed]
80. Sommer, F.; Stahlman, M.; Ilkayeva, O.; Arnemo, J.M.; Kindberg, J.; Josefsson, J.; Newgard, C.B.; Frobert, O.; Backhed, F. The gut microbiota modulates energy metabolism in the hibernating brown bear *Ursus arctos*. *Cell Rep.* **2016**, *14*, 1655–1661. [CrossRef] [PubMed]
81. Arinell, K.; Sahdo, B.; Evans, A.L.; Arnemo, J.M.; Baandrup, U.; Frobert, O. Brown bears (*Ursus arctos*) seem resistant to atherosclerosis despite highly elevated plasma lipids during hibernation and active state. *Clin. Transl. Sci.* **2012**, *5*, 269–272. [CrossRef] [PubMed]
82. Mar Rodriguez, M.; Perez, D.; Javier Chaves, F.; Esteve, E.; Marin-Garcia, P.; Xifra, G.; Vendrell, J.; Jove, M.; Pamplona, R.; Ricart, W.; *et al.* Obesity changes the human gut mycobiome. *Sci. Rep.* **2015**, *5*, 14600. [CrossRef] [PubMed]
83. McGuire, M.T.; Wing, R.R.; Hill, J.O. The prevalence of weight loss maintenance among american adults. *Int. J. Obes. Relat. Metab. Disord.* **1999**, *23*, 1314–1319. [CrossRef] [PubMed]
84. Field, A.E.; Malspeis, S.; Willett, W.C. Weight cycling and mortality among middle-aged or older women. *Arch. Intern. Med.* **2009**, *169*, 881–886. [CrossRef] [PubMed]

85. Hamm, P.; Shekelle, R.B.; Stamler, J. Large fluctuations in body weight during young adulthood and twenty-five-year risk of coronary death in men. *Am. J. Epidemiol.* **1989**, *129*, 312–318. [PubMed]
86. Chevrier, J.; Dewailly, E.; Ayotte, P.; Mauriege, P.; Despres, J.P.; Tremblay, A. Body weight loss increases plasma and adipose tissue concentrations of potentially toxic pollutants in obese individuals. *Int. J. Obes. Relat. Metab. Disord.* **2000**, *24*, 1272–1278. [CrossRef] [PubMed]
87. Hue, O.; Marcotte, J.; Berrigan, F.; Simoneau, M.; Dore, J.; Marceau, P.; Marceau, S.; Tremblay, A.; Teasdale, N. Increased plasma levels of toxic pollutants accompanying weight loss induced by hypocaloric diet or by bariatric surgery. *Obes. Surg.* **2006**, *16*, 1145–1154. [CrossRef] [PubMed]
88. Kim, M.J.; Marchand, P.; Henegar, C.; Antignac, J.P.; Alili, R.; Poitou, C.; Bouillot, J.L.; Basdevant, A.; Le Bizec, B.; Barouki, R.; *et al.* Fate and complex pathogenic effects of dioxins and polychlorinated biphenyls in obese subjects before and after drastic weight loss. *Environ. Health Perspect.* **2011**, *119*, 377–383. [CrossRef] [PubMed]
89. Kantartzis, K.; Machann, J.; Schick, F.; Rittig, K.; Machicao, F.; Fritsche, A.; Haring, H.U.; Stefan, N. Effects of a lifestyle intervention in metabolically benign and malign obesity. *Diabetologia* **2011**, *54*, 864–868. [CrossRef] [PubMed]
90. Shin, M.J.; Hyun, Y.J.; Kim, O.Y.; Kim, J.Y.; Jang, Y.; Lee, J.H. Weight loss effect on inflammation and ldl oxidation in metabolically healthy but obese (mho) individuals: Low inflammation and ldl oxidation in mho women. *Int. J. Obes.* **2006**, *30*, 1529–1534. [CrossRef] [PubMed]
91. McLaughlin, T.; Abbasi, F.; Lamendola, C.; Liang, L.; Reaven, G.; Schaaf, P.; Reaven, P. Differentiation between obesity and insulin resistance in the association with c-reactive protein. *Circulation* **2002**, *106*, 2908–2912. [CrossRef] [PubMed]
92. Janiszewski, P.M.; Ross, R. Effects of weight loss among metabolically healthy obese men and women. *Diabetes Care* **2010**, *33*, 1957–1959. [CrossRef] [PubMed]
93. Cui, Z.; Truesdale, K.P.; Bradshaw, P.T.; Cai, J.; Stevens, J. Three-year weight change and cardiometabolic risk factors in obese and normal weight adults who are metabolically healthy: The atherosclerosis risk in communities study. *Int. J. Obes.* **2015**, *39*, 1203–1208. [CrossRef] [PubMed]
94. Dalzill, C.; Nigam, A.; Juneau, M.; Guilbeault, V.; Latour, E.; Mauriege, P.; Gayda, M. Intensive lifestyle intervention improves cardiometabolic and exercise parameters in metabolically healthy obese and metabolically unhealthy obese individuals. *Can. J. Cardiol.* **2014**, *30*, 434–440. [CrossRef] [PubMed]
95. Liu, R.H.; Wharton, S.; Sharma, A.M.; Ardern, C.I.; Kuk, J.L. Influence of a clinical lifestyle-based weight loss program on the metabolic risk profile of metabolically normal and abnormal obese adults. *Obesity* **2013**, *21*, 1533–1539. [CrossRef] [PubMed]
96. Sesti, G.; Folli, F.; Perego, L.; Hribal, M.L.; Pontiroli, A.E. Effects of weight loss in metabolically healthy obese subjects after laparoscopic adjustable gastric banding and hypocaloric diet. *PLoS ONE* **2011**, *6*, e17737. [CrossRef] [PubMed]
97. Gilardini, L.; Vallone, L.; Cottafava, R.; Redaelli, G.; Croci, M.; Conti, A.; Pasqualinotto, L.; Invitti, C. Insulin sensitivity deteriorates after short-term lifestyle intervention in the insulin sensitive phenotype of obesity. *Obes. Facts* **2012**, *5*, 68–76. [CrossRef] [PubMed]
98. Karelis, A.D.; Messier, V.; Brochu, M.; Rabasa-Lhoret, R. Metabolically healthy but obese women: Effect of an energy-restricted diet. *Diabetologia* **2008**, *51*, 1752–1754. [CrossRef] [PubMed]
99. Evangelou, P.; Tzotzas, T.; Christou, G.; Elisaf, M.S.; Kiortsis, D.N. Does the presence of metabolic syndome influence weight loss in obese and overweight women? *Metab. Syndr. Relat. Disord.* **2010**, *8*, 173–178. [CrossRef] [PubMed]
100. Nagao, K.; Yanagita, T. Bioactive lipids in metabolic syndrome. *Prog. Lipid Res.* **2008**, *47*, 127–146. [CrossRef] [PubMed]
101. Nagao, K.; Yanagita, T. Medium-chain fatty acids: Functional lipids for the prevention and treatment of the metabolic syndrome. *Pharmacol. Res.* **2010**, *61*, 208–212. [CrossRef] [PubMed]
102. Babayan, V.K. Medium chain triglycerides and structured lipids. *Lipids* **1987**, *22*, 417–420. [CrossRef] [PubMed]
103. Bach, A.C.; Babayan, V.K. Medium-chain triglycerides: An update. *Am. J. Clin. Nutr.* **1982**, *36*, 950–962. [PubMed]
104. Jensen, R.G. The composition of bovine milk lipids: January 1995 to december 2000. *J. Dairy Sci.* **2002**, *85*, 295–350. [CrossRef]

105. Papamandjaris, A.A.; MacDougall, D.E.; Jones, P.J. Medium chain fatty acid metabolism and energy expenditure: Obesity treatment implications. *Life Sci.* **1998**, *62*, 1203–1215. [CrossRef]
106. Marten, B.; Pfeuffer, M.; Schrezenmeir, J. Medium-chain triglycerides. *Int. Dairy J.* **2006**, *16*, 1374–1382. [CrossRef]
107. Noguchi, O.; Takeuchi, H.; Kubota, F.; Tsuji, H.; Aoyama, T. Larger diet-induced thermogenesis and less body fat accumulation in rats fed medium-chain triacylglycerols than in those fed long-chain triacylglycerols. *J. Nutr. Sci. Vitaminol.* **2002**, *48*, 524–529. [CrossRef] [PubMed]
108. Akpa, M.M.; Point, F.; Sawadogo, S.; Radenne, A.; Mounier, C. Inhibition of insulin and t3-induced fatty acid synthase by hexanoate. *Lipids* **2010**, *45*, 997–1009. [CrossRef] [PubMed]
109. Kersten, S. Mechanisms of nutritional and hormonal regulation of lipogenesis. *EMBO Rep.* **2001**, *2*, 282–286. [CrossRef] [PubMed]
110. Ambati, S.; Li, Q.; Rayalam, S.; Hartzell, D.L.; Della-Fera, M.A.; Hamrick, M.W.; Baile, C.A. Central leptin *versus* ghrelin: Effects on bone marrow adiposity and gene expression. *Endocrine* **2010**, *37*, 115–123. [CrossRef] [PubMed]
111. Berlanga, A.; Guiu-Jurado, E.; Porras, J.A.; Auguet, T. Molecular pathways in non-alcoholic fatty liver disease. *Clin. Exp. Gastroenterol.* **2014**, *7*, 221–239. [PubMed]
112. Goodridge, A.G.; Thurmond, D.C.; Baillie, R.A.; Hodnett, D.W.; Xu, G. Nutritional and hormonal regulation of the gene for malic enzyme. *Z. Ernahrungswissenschaft* **1998**, *37*, 8–13.
113. Roncero, C.; Goodridge, A.G. Hexanoate and octanoate inhibit transcription of the malic enzyme and fatty acid synthase genes in chick embryo hepatocytes in culture. *J. Biol. Chem.* **1992**, *267*, 14918–14927. [PubMed]
114. Thurmond, D.C.; Baillie, R.A.; Goodridge, A.G. Regulation of the action of steroid/thyroid hormone receptors by medium-chain fatty acids. *J. Biol. Chem.* **1998**, *273*, 15373–15381. [CrossRef] [PubMed]
115. Wang, B.; Fu, J.; Li, L.; Gong, D.; Wen, X.; Yu, P.; Zeng, Z. Medium-chain fatty acid reduces lipid accumulation by regulating expression of lipid-sensing genes in human liver cells with steatosis. *Int. J. Food Sci. Nutr.* **2016**, *67*, 288–297. [CrossRef] [PubMed]
116. Lieber, C.S.; Lefevre, A.; Spritz, N.; Feinman, L.; DeCarli, L.M. Difference in hepatic metabolism of long- and medium-chain fatty acids: The role of fatty acid chain length in the production of the alcoholic fatty liver. *J. Clin. Investig.* **1967**, *46*, 1451–1460. [CrossRef] [PubMed]
117. Ling, P.R.; Hamawy, K.J.; Moldawer, L.L.; Istfan, N.; Bistrian, B.R.; Blackburn, G.L. Evaluation of the protein quality of diets containing medium- and long-chain triglyceride in healthy rats. *J. Nutr.* **1986**, *116*, 343–349. [PubMed]
118. Traul, K.A.; Driedger, A.; Ingle, D.L.; Nakhasi, D. Review of the toxicologic properties of medium-chain triglycerides. *Food Chem. Toxicol.* **2000**, *38*, 79–98. [CrossRef]
119. Hill, J.O.; Peters, J.C.; Yang, D.; Sharp, T.; Kaler, M.; Abumrad, N.N.; Greene, H.L. Thermogenesis in humans during overfeeding with medium-chain triglycerides. *Metab. Clin. Exp.* **1989**, *38*, 641–648. [CrossRef]
120. Seaton, T.B.; Welle, S.L.; Warenko, M.K.; Campbell, R.G. Thermic effect of medium-chain and long-chain triglycerides in man. *Am. J. Clin. Nutr.* **1986**, *44*, 630–634. [PubMed]
121. Scalfi, L.; Coltorti, A.; Contaldo, F. Postprandial thermogenesis in lean and obese subjects after meals supplemented with medium-chain and long-chain triglycerides. *Am. J. Clin. Nutr.* **1991**, *53*, 1130–1133. [PubMed]
122. Dulloo, A.G.; Fathi, M.; Mensi, N.; Girardier, L. Twenty-four-hour energy expenditure and urinary catecholamines of humans consuming low-to-moderate amounts of medium-chain triglycerides: A dose-response study in a human respiratory chamber. *Eur. J. Clin. Nutr.* **1996**, *50*, 152–158. [PubMed]
123. Ishizawa, R.; Masuda, K.; Sakata, S.; Nakatani, A. Effects of different fatty acid chain lengths on fatty acid oxidation-related protein expression levels in rat skeletal muscles. *J. Oleo Sci.* **2015**, *64*, 415–421. [CrossRef] [PubMed]
124. Binnert, C.; Pachiaudi, C.; Beylot, M.; Hans, D.; Vandermander, J.; Chantre, P.; Riou, J.P.; Laville, M. Influence of human obesity on the metabolic fate of dietary long- and medium-chain triacylglycerols. *Am. J. Clin. Nutr.* **1998**, *67*, 595–601. [PubMed]
125. Nagata, J.; Kasai, M.; Watanabe, S.; Ikeda, I.; Saito, M. Effects of highly purified structured lipids containing medium-chain fatty acids and linoleic acid on lipid profiles in rats. *Biosci. Biotechnol. Biochem.* **2003**, *67*, 1937–1943. [CrossRef] [PubMed]

126. Nagata, J.; Kasai, M.; Negishi, S.; Saito, M. Effects of structured lipids containing eicosapentaenoic or docosahexaenoic acid and caprylic acid on serum and liver lipid profiles in rats. *BioFactors* **2004**, *22*, 157–160. [CrossRef] [PubMed]
127. Matsuo, T.; Matsuo, M.; Kasai, M.; Takeuchi, H. Effects of a liquid diet supplement containing structured medium- and long-chain triacylglycerols on bodyfat accumulation in healthy young subjects. *Asia Pac. J. Clin. Nutr.* **2001**, *10*, 46–50. [CrossRef] [PubMed]
128. Tsuji, H.; Kasai, M.; Takeuchi, H.; Nakamura, M.; Okazaki, M.; Kondo, K. Dietary medium-chain triacylglycerols suppress accumulation of body fat in a double-blind, controlled trial in healthy men and women. *J. Nutr.* **2001**, *131*, 2853–2859. [PubMed]
129. St-Onge, M.P.; Mayrsohn, B.; O'Keeffe, M.; Kissileff, H.R.; Choudhury, A.R.; Laferrere, B. Impact of medium and long chain triglycerides consumption on appetite and food intake in overweight men. *Eur. J. Clin. Nutr.* **2014**, *68*, 1134–1140. [CrossRef] [PubMed]
130. St-Onge, M.P.; Ross, R.; Parsons, W.D.; Jones, P.J. Medium-chain triglycerides increase energy expenditure and decrease adiposity in overweight men. *Obes. Res.* **2003**, *11*, 395–402. [CrossRef] [PubMed]
131. Lemarie, F.; Beauchamp, E.; Dayot, S.; Duby, C.; Legrand, P.; Rioux, V. Dietary caprylic acid (c8:0) does not increase plasma acylated ghrelin but decreases plasma unacylated ghrelin in the rat. *PLoS ONE* **2015**, *10*, e0133600. [CrossRef] [PubMed]
132. Lemarie, F.; Beauchamp, E.; Legrand, P.; Rioux, V. Revisiting the metabolism and physiological functions of caprylic acid (c8:0) with special focus on ghrelin octanoylation. *Biochimie* **2016**, *120*, 40–48. [CrossRef] [PubMed]
133. Li, Z.; Mulholland, M.; Zhang, W. Ghrelin o-acyltransferase (goat) and energy metabolism. *Sci. China Life Sci.* **2016**, *59*, 281–291. [CrossRef] [PubMed]
134. Kasai, M.; Nosaka, N.; Maki, H.; Negishi, S.; Aoyama, T.; Nakamura, M.; Suzuki, Y.; Tsuji, H.; Uto, H.; Okazaki, M.; *et al.* Effect of dietary medium- and long-chain triacylglycerols (mlct) on accumulation of body fat in healthy humans. *Asia Pac. J. Clin. Nutr.* **2003**, *12*, 151–160. [PubMed]
135. St-Onge, M.P.; Bourque, C.; Jones, P.J.; Ross, R.; Parsons, W.E. Medium- *versus* long-chain triglycerides for 27 days increases fat oxidation and energy expenditure without resulting in changes in body composition in overweight women. *Int. J. Obes. Relat. Metab. Disord.* **2003**, *27*, 95–102. [CrossRef] [PubMed]
136. St-Onge, M.P.; Jones, P.J. Greater rise in fat oxidation with medium-chain triglyceride consumption relative to long-chain triglyceride is associated with lower initial body weight and greater loss of subcutaneous adipose tissue. *Int. J. Obes. Relat. Metab. Disord.* **2003**, *27*, 1565–1571. [CrossRef] [PubMed]
137. Airhart, S.; Cade, W.T.; Jiang, H.; Coggan, A.R.; Racette, S.B.; Korenblat, K.; Spearie, C.A.; Waller, S.; O'Connor, R.; Bashir, A.; *et al.* A diet rich in medium-chain fatty acids improves systolic function and alters the lipidomic profile in patients with type 2 diabetes: A pilot study. *J. Clin. Endocrinol. Metab.* **2016**, *101*, 504–512. [CrossRef] [PubMed]
138. Assuncao, M.L.; Ferreira, H.S.; dos Santos, A.F.; Cabral, C.R., Jr.; Florencio, T.M. Effects of dietary coconut oil on the biochemical and anthropometric profiles of women presenting abdominal obesity. *Lipids* **2009**, *44*, 593–601. [CrossRef] [PubMed]
139. Rimbach, G.; Melchin, M.; Moehring, J.; Wagner, A.E. Polyphenols from cocoa and vascular health—A critical review. *Int. J. Mol. Sci.* **2009**, *10*, 4290–4309. [CrossRef] [PubMed]
140. Bourque, C.; St-Onge, M.P.; Papamandjaris, A.A.; Cohn, J.S.; Jones, P.J. Consumption of an oil composed of medium chain triacyglycerols, phytosterols, and *n*-3 fatty acids improves cardiovascular risk profile in overweight women. *Metabol. Clin. Exp.* **2003**, *52*, 771–777. [CrossRef]
141. St-Onge, M.P.; Lamarche, B.; Mauger, J.F.; Jones, P.J. Consumption of a functional oil rich in phytosterols and medium-chain triglyceride oil improves plasma lipid profiles in men. *J. Nutr.* **2003**, *133*, 1815–1820. [PubMed]
142. St-Onge, M.P.; Bosarge, A.; Goree, L.L.; Darnell, B. Medium chain triglyceride oil consumption as part of a weight loss diet does not lead to an adverse metabolic profile when compared to olive oil. *J. Am. Coll. Nutr.* **2008**, *27*, 547–552. [CrossRef] [PubMed]
143. Mumme, K.; Stonehouse, W. Effects of medium-chain triglycerides on weight loss and body composition: A meta-analysis of randomized controlled trials. *J. Acad. Nutr. Diet.* **2015**, *115*, 249–263. [CrossRef] [PubMed]

144. Mori, N.; Nakanishi, S.; Shiomi, S.; Kiyokawa, S.; Kakimoto, S.; Nakagawa, K.; Hosoe, K.; Minami, K.; Nadamoto, T. Enhancement of fat oxidation by licorice flavonoid oil in healthy humans during light exercise. *J. Nutr. Sci. Vitaminol.* **2015**, *61*, 406–416. [CrossRef] [PubMed]
145. Isaacs, C.E. The antimicrobial function of milk lipids. *Adv. Nutr. Res.* **2001**, *10*, 271–285. [PubMed]
146. Rios-Covian, D.; Ruas-Madiedo, P.; Margolles, A.; Gueimonde, M.; de Los Reyes-Gavilan, C.G.; Salazar, N. Intestinal short chain fatty acids and their link with diet and human health. *Front. Microbiol.* **2016**, *7*, 185. [CrossRef] [PubMed]
147. Schanler, R.J.; Goldblum, R.M.; Garza, C.; Goldman, A.S. Enhanced fecal excretion of selected immune factors in very low birth weight infants fed fortified human milk. *Pediatr. Res.* **1986**, *20*, 711–715. [CrossRef] [PubMed]
148. Papavassilis, C.; Mach, K.K.; Mayser, P.A. Medium-chain triglycerides inhibit growth of malassezia: Implications for prevention of systemic infection. *Crit. Care Med.* **1999**, *27*, 1781–1786. [CrossRef] [PubMed]
149. Kono, H.; Fujii, H.; Asakawa, M.; Yamamoto, M.; Matsuda, M.; Maki, A.; Matsumoto, Y. Protective effects of medium-chain triglycerides on the liver and gut in rats administered endotoxin. *Ann. Surg.* **2003**, *237*, 246–255. [CrossRef] [PubMed]
150. Zentek, J.; Buchheit-Renko, S.; Ferrara, F.; Vahjen, W.; Van Kessel, A.G.; Pieper, R. Nutritional and physiological role of medium-chain triglycerides and medium-chain fatty acids in piglets. *Anim. Health Res. Rev.* **2011**, *12*, 83–93. [CrossRef] [PubMed]
151. Zentek, J.; Ferrara, F.; Pieper, R.; Tedin, L.; Meyer, W.; Vahjen, W. Effects of dietary combinations of organic acids and medium chain fatty acids on the gastrointestinal microbial ecology and bacterial metabolites in the digestive tract of weaning piglets. *J. Anim. Sci.* **2013**, *91*, 3200–3210. [CrossRef] [PubMed]
152. Dierick, N.; Michiels, J.; Van Nevel, C. Effect of medium chain fatty acids and benzoic acid, as alternatives for antibiotics, on growth and some gut parameters in piglets. *Commun. Agric. Appl. Biol. Sci.* **2004**, *69*, 187–190. [PubMed]
153. Jacobi, S.K.; Odle, J. Nutritional factors influencing intestinal health of the neonate. *Adv. Nutr.* **2012**, *3*, 687–696. [CrossRef] [PubMed]
154. Kono, H.; Fujii, H.; Ogiku, M.; Tsuchiya, M.; Ishii, K.; Hara, M. Enteral diets enriched with medium-chain triglycerides and *n*-3 fatty acids prevent chemically induced experimental colitis in rats. *Transl. Res. J. Lab. Clin. Med.* **2010**, *156*, 282–291. [CrossRef] [PubMed]
155. Kono, H.; Fujii, H.; Ishii, K.; Hosomura, N.; Ogiku, M. Dietary medium-chain triglycerides prevent chemically induced experimental colitis in rats. *Transl. Res. J. Lab. Clin. Med.* **2010**, *155*, 131–141. [CrossRef] [PubMed]
156. Decuypere, J.A.; Dierick, N.A. The combined use of triacylglycerols containing medium-chain fatty acids and exogenous lipolytic enzymes as an alternative to in-feed antibiotics in piglets: Concept, possibilities and limitations. An overview. *Nutr. Res. Rev.* **2003**, *16*, 193–210. [CrossRef] [PubMed]
157. Liu, Y. Fatty acids, inflammation and intestinal health in pigs. *J. Anim. Sci. Biotechnol.* **2015**, *6*, 41. [CrossRef] [PubMed]
158. Kono, H.; Fujii, H.; Asakawa, M.; Maki, A.; Amemiya, H.; Hirai, Y.; Matsuda, M.; Yamamoto, M. Medium-chain triglycerides enhance secretory iga expression in rat intestine after administration of endotoxin. *Am. J. Physiol. Gastrointest. Liver Physiol.* **2004**, *286*, G1081–G1089. [CrossRef] [PubMed]
159. Servier Medical Art (Servier). Available online: http://www.servier.fr/smart/banque-dimages-powerpoint/ (acessed on 21 March 2016).

9

Cultural Features Influencing Eating, Overweight and Obesity in the Roma People of South Bohemia

Věra Olišarová [1,*], Valérie Tóthová [1], Sylva Bártlová [1], František Dolák [1], Alena Kajanová [2], Dita Nováková [1], Radka Prokešová [3] and Lenka Šedová [1]

1 Institute of Nursing, Midwifery and Emergency Care, Faculty of Health and Social Sciences, University of South Bohemia in Ceske Budejovice, J. Boreckeho 1167/27, 370 05 Ceske Budejovice, Czech Republic; tothova@zsf.jcu.cz (V.T.); sbartlova@zsf.jcu.cz (S.B.); fdolak@zsf.jcu.cz (F.D.); novakovad@zsf.jcu.cz (D.N.); lsedova@zsf.jcu.cz (L.Š.)

2 Institute of Social and Special-paedagogical Sciences, Faculty of Health and Social Sciences, University of South Bohemia in Ceske Budejovice, J. Boreckeho 1167/27, 370 05 Ceske Budejovice, Czech Republic; kajanova@zsf.jcu.cz

3 Institute of Legal Branches, Management and Economics, Faculty of Health and Social Sciences, University of South Bohemia in Ceske Budejovice, J. Boreckeho 1167/27, 370 05 Ceske Budejovice, Czech Republic; rprokes@zsf.jcu.cz

* Correspondence: volisarova@zsf.jcu.cz

Abstract: This article describes the important cultural specifics that impact on treatment of overweight and obesity for the Roma people of South Bohemia. Methods: Data on health and nutrition were collected using a semi-structured interview of 302 Roma adults (quantitative phase). A further 25 participants received in-depth interviews regarding their eating and lifestyle habits and perceptions about obesity and overweight (qualitative phase). Height and weight were measured with calibrated scales and stadiometer. Qualitative data were analyzed with the "grounded theory" method. Results: The participants reported a relatively high consumption of high-sugar drinks and foods compared to fruits and vegetables. Lifestyle factors increasing risk of overweight identified from the qualitative interview included unemployment, socially isolating housing, poor transport, poverty, inactivity, tobacco smoking, and for women weight gain after childbirth. Also identified was the need for better health literacy. Conclusions: Effective health education may help to address risk factors for overweight and obesity in Roma peoples. Other measures include improved socioeconomic status and housing security, and improved health literacy of the Roma people.

Keywords: the Roma; nurse; overweight; obesity; health education; lifestyle factors; nutrition; cultural features

---

1. Introduction

Determinants of obesity include genetic predisposition, environmental factors, and the social-cultural environment [1–3].

Overweight and obesity date perhaps as far back as prehistoric times, i.e., as long as people have dealt with both an excess and a scarcity of food. However, over the course of societal development and with advances in scientific and medical knowledge, the social and cultural interpretations of diagnoses of overweight and obesity have changed as well. Although they are symbols of affluence in some societies, they also indisputably impact on health. According to available data, more than half of the population (52%) of the European Union are overweight or obese, and in the Czech Republic, 61.7% of the population have a body mass index (BMI) ≥ 25 kg/m^2 [4]. Although the number of adult individuals with a BMI ≥ 25 kg/m^2 seems to have levelled off, the proportion of people suffering from obesity is still rising [5].

The high rates of overweight are also evident in minority groups such as the Roma, who are one of the largest minorities of the Czech Republic [6,7]. Their number is estimated at 250–280,000 persons [8]. Studies designed to monitor the health status of the Roma show that, in spite of government efforts across Europe, they suffer from poorer access to health care and are often discriminated against [9]. Vazarova de Courten et al. [10] confirmed a potential link between the high prevalence of obesity with unhealthy lifestyles and improper eating habits. One study that looked at the incidence of overweight and obesity in Roma women in Slovakia found similar results. It was found that Roma suffer from extreme degrees of obesity much more often than the rest of the population. In these cases, the genetic predispositions of susceptible individuals are also supported by unhealthy lifestyles [11].

Together with external determinants, persistent cultural characteristics of the Roma can notably influence the efficiency of the public and other health interventions [12,13]. The Roma are a distinctive group with distinctive cultural features, language, and a singular cultural identity, setting them apart from the majority of the population [14]. Over the course of the centuries, they spread all over the world thanks to their nomadic lifestyle. Due to encounters with the dominant culture, there have been changes in their traditional way of life, but some particularities persist [15,16]. These particularities are evident primarily in the way of life, eating habits, experiences and perceptions of time, socio-economic status, and poorer access to services or health [14]. Preventive programs, in order to be effective, need to consider diverse cultural determinants of health and, above all, the individual needs of the target group [17]. At the same time, the level of nutritional acculturation or the level of adoption of the nutritional habits of the majority population by immigrants or other minority groups should be taken into account [18]. The preventive programs implemented at present with focus on overweight and obesity is developed for the dominant population in the Czech Republic. Their effectiveness for the Roma appears to be very low.

This article aims at to explore cultural features of the Roma that could be associated with their high prevalence of overweight and obesity and the inefficiency of currently implemented interventions. First, the anthropometrics status, nutritional intake, and eating patterns of a group of Roma participants were investigated. This was followed by exploratory interviews investigating lifestyle, intake, and sociodemographic features of a subsample of respondents.

2. Materials and Methods

2.1. Quantitative Phase

Participants were sourced from the Roma population in the South Bohemian Region between 1 June 2014 and 31 March 2015. General nurses from the Centre for Prevention of Life Style Diseases in České Budějovice recruited participants at community events and in the respondents' natural environment with the assistance of contact persons. Because census data is not available for the Roma minority in the Czech Republic, respondents were selected using the snowball method aiming to ensure an equal representation of men and women (as in the general population in the Czech Republic). Further, the respondents from the Roma minority were selected based on their subjectively perceived Roma identity.

Face-to-face semi-structured interviews were conducted using a prepared non-standardized questionnaire. The communication with the respondents was performed in Czech. The respondents were given primarily close-ended questions with employment of scaled answers. Further, the following anthropometric values were obtained: weight (determined with electronic flat scale SECA 813); height (determined with a SECA 213 folding height meter); waist and hip circumference (measured with tape measure); and body fat content (measured with OMRON BF306 Body Composition Monitor). Body mass index (BMI; kg/m^2) was subsequently calculated.

BMI reference values for obesity were applied according to those of the World Health Organization (WHO), i.e., BMI 18.5–24.9 kg/m^2 normal, BMI 25–29.9 kg/m^2 overweight, and $\geq$30 kg/m^2 obese [19]. Reference values suggesting risk metabolic complications were applied for waist circumference:

men, ≥94 cm, suggesting increased risk, and ≥102 cm, suggesting very high risk; women, ≥80 cm, suggesting increased risk, and ≥88 cm, suggesting very high risk [19].

Three hundred and two Roma individuals over 18 years of age participated; males and females were equally represented. Most were aged 18–29 years (132, i.e., 43.8%); 56 (18.6%) were aged 40–49 years, 49 (16.3%) were aged 30–39 years, 39 (13%) were aged 50–59 years, 20 (6.6%) were aged 60–69 years (20, i.e., 6.6%), and only 5 (1.7%) were aged ≥70 years. There were more respondents who had three or more children (n = 134, 44.3%) than those who had no children (n = 77, 25.6%). One hundred and forty-nine (50.1%) persons were unemployed and only 51 (17.2%) were practicing a profession. The others received a disability or old age pension or were on maternity leave.

2.2. Analyses

Data analysis was carried out with using the SASD (Statistical Analysis of 129 Social Data) program and SPSS program (in version 13.1). Statistical associations were tested with the Pearson Chi-square test—X^2) and significance levels of $\alpha < 0.05$, $\alpha < 0.01$ and $\alpha < 0.001$. In case of insufficient observations, Yates correction was applied.

2.3. Qualitative Phase

The qualitative research was aimed at acquiring more in-depth information regarding attitudes the Roma minority to overweight and obesity. It was also aimed at mapping the nutritional habits and describing the risk factors with respect to culturally conditioned behavior patterns occurring in the natural environment (Roma households and communities). The qualitative research set consisted of 25 Roma respondents over 18 years of age (8 males and 17 females). The male sample included six overweight individuals (BMI ≥ 25 kg/m^2) and two obese ones (BMI ≥ 30 kg/m^2); ages ranged from 19 to 64 years. The female sample included eight overweight individuals and nine obese individuals; ages ranged from 29 to 64 years.

Participants received a semi-structured interview; this comprised a circle of 35 basic questions with 90 sub questions in advance, and their order could be changed to achieve the highest possible interview efficiency. The interview scheme prepared in this manner included 35 basic questions divided into four circles: eating habits, physical and leisure-time activities (lifestyle), and self-perception and perceptions of overweight and obesity. The interviews took place from April 2014 to April 2015 in the community, primarily in individual's homes. They were conducted in Czech and complemented by anthropometric measurement (height, weight, calculation of BMI, waistline and body fat measurements as above). The interviews made particular use of open-ended questions. The interviews were subsequently digitalized and transcribed verbatim. The MAXQDA 11 (Software for Qualitative and Mixed Methods Research) program was chosen for the text analysis. One thousand and eight-two segments in total were marked in the transcribed interviews, subsequently exported, and further processed. To analyze the data, we used "grounded theory" including open, axial, and selective coding. Finally, we identified the central category—lifestyle. From among other categories, we identified eating habits, motivation, attitude and body image. To ensure anonymity, the respondents were given randomly selected names when processing the data.

3. Results

3.1. Quantitative Phase

The analysis of the data related to the assessment of the basic health indicators suggests that in the research set including 302 Roma from the South Bohemian Region, 61.8% persons had BMI ≥ 25 kg/m^2. Overweight (BMI 25.0–29.9 kg/m^2) was found in 29.7% of participants and obesity (BMI ≥ 30 kg/m^2) in 32.1% of respondents. It was proved that there were statistically significant differences between males and females in terms of BMI index ($p < 0.01$; $X^2 = 11.17$; df = 2). The males had lower

BMI index significantly more often, while the females were overweight (BMI 25.0–29.9 kg/m^2) and obese (BMI $\geq$ 30 kg/m^2) more often.

From among further indicators of overweight and obesity, the waistline values were observed. Increased values were recorded. One-third of the examined Roma (n = 152) had a waistline exceeding 102 cm. It should be stated here that males' waistline values over 102 cm are related with noticeable metabolic complications. Waistline values related to noticeable metabolic complications (over 88 cm for females) were also found in Roma women (63.3%, n = 150). Also, the measured values of body fat correspond to the above stated indicators. The difference between genders was minimal, but the higher values of body fat of the Roma (found in 67.55% of respondents) in the South Bohemian Region were measured.

From the perspective of prevention of overweight and obesity, the information related to consumption, selection, preparation and intake frequency of foodstuffs is important. We show the preference of selected foodstuff types in the Roma minority (Table 1) below.

Table 1. Preference of selected foodstuffs in the Roma minority per week (n = 302).

	Intake Frequency, n (%)						
Selected Foodstuff	**Not at All**	**1–2 Times a Week**	**3–4 Times a Week**	**5–6 Times a Week**	**Every Day**	**Several Times a Day**	**Did Not Answer**
Pork	28 (10.3%)	112 (41.3%)	96 (35.5%)	21 (7.7%)	10 (3.7%)	4 (1.5%)	31 (10.3%)
Beef	82 (32.0%)	148 (57.8%)	19 (7.4%)	5 (2.0%)	1 (0.4%)	1 (0.4%)	46 (15.23%)
Fish	158 (56.2%)	106 (37.7%)	10 (3.6%)	2 (0.7%)	3 (1.1%)	2 (0.7%)	21 (6.95%)
Chicken	16 (5.8%)	125 (45.3%)	98 (35.5%)	25 (9.1%)	7 (2.5%)	5 (1.8%)	26 (8.61%)
Potatoes	14 (5.0%)	157 (56.4%)	79 (28.3%)	14 (5.0%)	11 (3.9%)	4 (1.4%)	23 (7.62%)
Pasta	17 (6.3%)	191 (70.4%)	40 (14.8%)	15 (5.5%)	7 (2.6%)	1 (0.4%)	31 (10.26)
Rice	24 (8.9%)	186 (68.9%)	42 (15.6%)	12 (4.4%)	4 (1.5%)	2 (0.7%)	32 (10.6%)
Dumplings	22 (8.1%)	181 (67.1%)	49 (18.1%)	11 (4.1%)	6 (2.2%)	1 (0.4%)	32 (10.6%)
Sweet baked goods	53 (18.5%)	126 (44.2%)	57 (19.9%)	8 (2.8%)	39 (13.6%)	3 (1.0%)	16 (5.3%)
Sweets	46 (15.9%)	125 (43.3%)	46 (15.9%)	15 (5.2%)	50 (17.3%)	7 (2.4%)	13 (4.3%)
Sweet drinks	52 (18.1%)	80 (27.8%)	53 (18.4%)	19 (6.6%)	75 (26.0%)	9 (3.1%)	14 (4.64%)
Fruits	38 (13.5%)	122 (43.4%)	61 (21.7%)	9 (3.2%)	37 (13.2%)	14 (5.0%)	21 (7.95%)
Vegetables	30 (10.8%)	96 (34.7%)	64 (23.1%)	23 (8.3%)	53 (19.1%)	11 (4.0%)	25 (8.27%)

As shown on Table 1, chicken was the most frequently consumed meat, followed by pork and then beef. More than half of the respondents (56.2% persons) did not eat fish. "Side dishes" of potatoes, pasta, rice and dumplings were most commonly eaten 1–2 times a week, followed by 3–4 times a week. Fruits and vegetables were consumed at a lower frequency: most often either not at all or only 1–2 times a week. With respect to sweet baked goods, those most frequently consumed were cakes and doughnuts, but also pies, and cakes. Sweets included different types of wafers, ice cream, biscuits, chocolate and candies.

In relation to the energy balance, we also consider significant the findings related to consumption of sweet drinks (like cola, juices, water with squash, energy drinks, etc.). In this case, analysis showed that the members of the Roma minority drink soft drinks in higher frequency.

3.2. *Qualitative Phase*

The qualitative phase was implemented to explore motivational factors and culturally conditioned behavior patterns with respect to prevention and treatment of overweight and obesity. The qualitative data were analyzed by the MAXQDA 11 program. We worked with transcribed interviews. In this study, 1082 interview segments were marked in total, exported and analyzed. The analysis was made using "grounded theory" use of open, axial and selective coding [20]. The terms found were grouped by their potential belonging to categories (open coding). However, at that point, the categories could not be considered final, as their belonging to any given phenomenon was only apparent. The conceptual range of the categories gave base to their contents. We show an example in the table (Table 2).

Table 2. Open coding.

Category	Subcategory	Characteristic
Food intake	Motivation for foodstuff selection Preferred foodstuff preparation Place of alimentation Number of meals a day Frequency of alimentation	
	Regularity	Breakfast Morning snack Lunch Afternoon snack Dinner

The open coding allowed us to divide the acquired data and to determine some categories and their characteristics. Axial coding allowed us to put the data together in a new way by creating links between the categories and their subcategories. As an example, we show the embedding of the "body image" category into the paradigmatic model (Table 3).

Table 3. Application of paradigmatic model.

Causal Conditions	Phenomenon	Context	Intervening Conditions	Action Strategy	Consequences
Weight Health condition Self-perception Subjective assessment of own figure Life satisfaction	Body image	Feeling Body proportions Health complications Weight deviations Nature Family Housing	Unemployment Housing conditions Culturally conditioned behavior patterns Insufficient health literacy Number of children	Exercise Dietary measures	Temporary weight reduction Improvement of health complications Better self-feeling

Visual inspection of the paradigmatic model showed that the circular dimension best explains phenomena, as consequences sometimes may mingle with causal conditions.

Based on the acquired overview of the relations among individual categories and subcategories, the codes found were subjected to a deeper analysis. The analysis helped to identify the central category of "lifestyle", to which all other categories are related. Lifestyle constitutes the phenomenon that is closely related to eating habits, motivation, and attitude to overweight and obesity, as well as to body image. It is connected not only with the way of spending leisure time, risk behaviors, and the way of spending weekdays, but it also reflects the cultural perspective. Its characteristics influence individual areas of eating habits (e.g., choice of foodstuffs, regularity of eating, etc.). The factors resulting from it are reflected in the motivation to reduce weight, and in the individual's attitude to overweight and obesity. In this point, they are closely related to self-perception and to body image, as well as to life satisfaction.

To achieve integration of the findings, the story skeleton was interpreted, and, upon this basis, a scheme of the relations found was created (Supplementary Figure S1).

3.2.1. Story Skeleton

Remedial risk factors for overweight and obesity are related to lifestyle in the Roma population. The vast majority of the respondents were unemployed, women who were at home with children, and some men receiving the disability or old-age pension. This factor undoubtedly plays a role in the distribution of activities during the day. Their weekdays are related primarily to cleaning, eating, caring for children, and community life. Most of those Roma live in socially excluded localities, in residence halls far from the town center. They have poor transport access. Their life is noted for risk behaviors like heavy smoking and inactivity. Consumption of alcohol is rather occasional, although there are exceptions too. Poor access to transport influences their eating habits, primarily due to the accessibility of groceries.

The above-stated distribution of daily activities, normal times of getting up, and factors of social life in broader family living in the given community influence eating habits such as frequency and regularity of eating. The Roma report eating at home and in the homes of relatives whom they visit. Some of them have even multiple main dishes. Nevertheless, they have problems with describing their meals. It is difficult for them to tell how many times a day they eat. Great differences can be seen when they describe their meals of the previous day. It is effective to make use of the opportunity to describe the course of the day and to encourage them to recount what they did from the time they woke up in the morning. Then they are able to approximately describe the foodstuffs and liquids they took in. As for foodstuffs and liquids, they use illustrative comparison and examples, which they can grasp better. Their composition of foodstuffs does not essentially differ. They show a tendency to give more healthy foodstuffs (fruits and vegetables) to their children. The socioeconomic perspective is often mentioned here. We can see the financial issue. They prefer to buy something for the children, and if some money is left, they buy something for themselves too. They agree in the traditional Roma meals. However, they report their intake in a frequency of several times a month.

They are aware of the causal relation between eating and increasing weight. The women often restrict food intake to decrease their weight. However, they do not show long-lasting eating changes or dietary measures related to other diseases they suffer from. They observe regime recommendations only until the acute symptoms subside; as for medicines, they take them only until they finish the package. They do not go to the physician to ask for more. Women do not include significant amounts of exercise in their lifestyle; they exercise primarily if the physician has suggested so because of backache. On the contrary, men make use of short-term exercise in fitness centers, trying to improve their physical condition. Some of them are aware of the positive effect of exercise and sports. The increased weight of women is primarily related to childbirths after which they did not succeed in reducing their weight, although many desire to lose weight. When assessing their own figure, particularly the women tend to be undervalue their weight; they perceive themselves slimmer than they actually are. On the contrary, men are usually more objective.

The self-perception is related to life satisfaction that is reflected also in the lifestyle and affects motivation. The Roma are rather satisfied with their family lives; they perceive themselves as cheerful and quick-tempered persons. However, their life satisfaction is affected by housing, primarily by the life in communities and socially excluded localities. Many of them are not satisfied with such a lifestyle. They do not perceive the difference between overweight and obesity, they relate them rather to a disease or overeating. Most of them do not take any attitude do such people; they do not criticize them, but some feel sorry for them. Some motivation to reduce the weight consists primarily in weight reduction recommended by physicians, and women also consider the aesthetic side, if they cannot dress what they like or if they feel they compare poorly next to their partner.

3.2.2. Diagram 1 Visualization of Relations

The visualized relations helped us to create the following categories: lifestyle, eating habits, motivation, attitude, and body image. Lifestyle was identified as the central category (Table 4). Based on the connections found, we came to the conclusion that the prevention and treatment of Roma overweight and obesity are influenced by culturally conditioned influenceable risk factors resulting from their lifestyle. To eliminate them, adequate motivation and efficient education should be used. Indispensable measures include motivation to long-lasting changes, to increasing health literacy of the Roma and regular monitoring of basic health indicators. However, the impact of the other risk factors cannot be omitted in the given context. The risk factors include primarily lack of exercise, risk behaviors (smoking), socioeconomic factors related to financial security, and housing and life in socially excluded localities.

Table 4. Resulting categories.

Category	Subcategory
Life style	Weekday Leisure time activities Prevention Risky behavior
Eating habits	Food components Traditional cuisine Food intake
Motivation	Reduction efforts Consequences
Attitude	Perception of overweight and obesity Preference of figures
Body image	Weight Life satisfaction

4. Discussion

The prevalence of obesity in Europe is regularly confirmed in a range of 10–40% of the population. In addition to a genetic predisposition, the main causes include lifestyle and underestimation of the seriousness of the complications related to this disease [21]. Further determinants are: influence of the environment, improved economic situation of individuals or ethnic differentiation. The economic situation is closely related to education and income level of the population. Thus, it can be stated that the obesity in highly developed countries, including the Czech Republic, is more frequent in inhabitants with lower education and lower income, as well as in rural populations. On the contrary, the obesity in developing countries is rather related with higher social status and social prestige [5,22]. With regards to ethnicity, it is assumed that ethnicity is often a more significant predictor for overweight and obesity in children than social class or other socio-economic variables [23–26]. The results of the present study clearly suggest that, according to the above stated indicators, the Roma are at increased risk of obesity.

Normal waistline values were found in 21.4% of Roma females in the examination. In the present study the majority of the Roma participants had increased waist measurements and high BMI. Reported lifestyle factors such as unemployment and late rising (often at 10–11 a.m.) likely also contribute to obesity risk. Similarly, the qualitative findings found Roma to be underemployed with a lifestyle of sedentary activities (sitting at the computer, watching TV, contact with friends and relatives, or sleeping). However, some were aware of the positive effect of exercise and reported that when they exercised, they had less backache or pains of legs and arms.

Risk behaviors—primarily smoking—are determined by lifestyle to some degree. The respondents of the qualitative phase included more than one half of smokers; the smokers could be divided into two groups. The first group included persons who smoked less than 10 cigarettes a day; the second (comparably large) group would include person who smoke more than a pack of cigarettes a day. A distinct representation of smokers among the Roma is reported also by Urban and Kajanová [27]. They examined a sample of 164 Czech Roma and found 63.5% of males were smokers, and 58% of females. They add that the respondents started smoking at 14 years of age on average. The results related to consumption of alcohol were a little more positive. Occasional or no consumption prevailed among the respondents.

The area of nutrition of the Roma minority is described well in the following quotation [28]: "The Roma may be as poor as a church mouse, but must have enough food, even if there may be nothing left for tomorrow." These words suggest the usual eating habits. Eating is not a regular ritual, but it is closely related to the status of the family [12,29]. At present, the Roma families cook a lot, particularly after the payment of wages of social or other benefits. The parents often try to give their children everything they were deprived of. Children's food is usually not distinguished from the adults' food; meat, smoked meat products, and sweets are mostly consumed. Fruits and vegetables are not frequently consumed [30]. A very low intake of fruits and vegetables is confirmed also by Stávková and Derflerová Brázdová [31]. They also reflect on the issue of nutrition literacy, as their study showed that only 15.7% of the Roma respondents (n = 102) knew the recommendations with respect to minimum fruit and vegetable intake. Consumption of fruits and vegetables was also low, and most were cooked: "Well, yes, I eat them. We always have them. Raw, no. Not even salad, nothing. Only in meals. No, not every day, about twice a week" (Jolana). The most frequently consumed vegetables included tomatoes, peppers, cucumbers and carrots. In contrast, the traditional Roma meals constitute an integral part of the Roma diet. Oláhová [28] includes goja and flour pancakes among them. Very thick soups are reported by Davidová [30]. Our respondents reported, additionally to goja, also halusky, filled cabbage, pork with dumplings and fasulja, a traditional thick soup. They also reported eating such meals only several times a month, i.e., they did not perceive their consumption as too frequent. One of the female respondents characterized the Roma cuisine as follows: "The Gypsies have the marikl'a, halušky, fasulja (that is bean soup). We love meat. You can see meat, schnitzel, pork on Gypsy tables. Just meat, fatback, dumplings, pork, yeah. Meals of that kind. Pishot is a Gypsy meal too. Sweet triangles with cream cheese and marmalade. And the Gypsies have four to five meals, just a lot of food. And the Gypsies are used to put food on the table, if they have it. You know, we like eating. But attention, the Gypsies love oil, fat." (Irena). The above stated characteristics of traditional Roma cuisine may explain, to some degree, the preference for some side dishes (e.g., potatoes, dumplings, etc.). The analysis of the qualitative data also suggested the importance of attitude to overweight and obesity. This is primarily a result of the respondents' own experiences and health conditions, and is influenced by sociocultural background. A possible relationship between the social pressure directed at the preferred physical appearance across different cultures, and between the determinants like education, degree of acculturation, or BMI is confirmed also by Cachelin et al. [32]. Although our respondents did not perceive the difference between overweight and obesity, many of them had their own experience of the consequences of such conditions. They most frequently reported leg pain, breathlessness (primarily when climbing stairs and running to catch the bus), and backache. Some women mentioned also the impact on the individual's appearance, which is, however, not necessarily sufficient motivation for change: "Well, great. Primarily appearance. Health impact not much, well, the legs, nothing. But only when I looked at the mirror, nothing suited me. I took it off." (Irma), "Well, you cannot dress everything; although now I have lost some weight." (Irena).

The Roma may be at increased risk of eating disorders as well as higher weight through factors such as less regular eating and a culture of moderate overconsumption. Culturally-based behavior patterns appear to be very important determinants of eating habits. Also evident is the impact of perception of overweight and obesity, body image, lifestyle, and in living in socially excluded localities. On the other hand, the decreased regard for health benefits of weight loss may be protective. Further studies are needed to examine disordered eating behaviors such as binge eating in Roma and whether increased exposure to the 'mainstream' attitudes to weight and shape may result in an increase in eating disorders.

5. Conclusions

Remedial risk factors for overweight and obesity in the Roma respondents we approached included primarily inactivity, lifestyle, and inappropriate structure of food together with eating habits and, to some degree, socioeconomic factors such as living in socially excluded localities. It has also been found that the Roma do not differentiate between overweight and obesity. They call both conditions "fat" and they often related increased weight primarily to a disease or to overeating. It is unknown to what degree these attitudes may however protect them from eating disorders common in the other European populations.

Author Contributions: V.O. performed the experiments, analyzed the data and wrote the paper; V.T. conceived and designed the experiments, analyzed data, and wrote the paper; S.B. conceived and designed the experiments, analyzed data and wrote the paper; F.D. performed the experiments, analyzed the data; A.K. performed the experiments, analyzed the data; D.N. performed the experiments, analyzed the data; R.P. analyzed the data, contributed analysis tools; L.Š. performed the experiments, analyzed the data and wrote the paper.

Acknowledgments: The article is related to research grant project No. LD14114, implemented with financial support from the Ministry of Education, Youth and Physical Education within COST (Cooperation on Scientific and Technical Research) and designated for the study of Obesity and Overweight in the Roma Minority in South Bohemian Region.

References

1. Kasalický, M. Tabulizace Žaludku. In *Chirurgická Léčba Obezity*; Triton: Praha, Czech Republic, 2007.
2. World Health Organization (WHO). Obesity and Overweight. Key Fact. 2017. Available online: http://www.who.int/en/news-room/fact-sheets/detail/obesity-and-overweight (accessed on 30 April 2018).
3. OECD/European Union. Health at a Glance: Europe. 2012. Available online: http://www.oecd-ilibrary.org/sites/9789264183896-en/02/07/index.html?itemId=/content/chapter/9789264183896-26-en (accessed on 11 January 2017).
4. World Health Organization (WHO). Global Health Observatory Data Repository. Overweight (Body Mass Index >= 25). Data by Country. 2008. Available online: http://apps.who.int/gho/data/node.main.A897 (accessed on 11 January 2017).
5. Kasalický, M. *Chirurgická Léčba Obezity*; Ottova Tiskárna: Praha, Czech Republic, 2011.
6. Vláda České Republiky. Koncepce Romské Integrace na Období 2010–2013. Available online: http://www.romadecade.org/cms/upload/file/9323_file8_roma_czech_republic_strategy_cs.pdf (accessed on 11 January 2017).
7. Mačeková, S.; Bernasovský, I.; Gabriková, D.; Bôžiková, A.; Bernasovská, J.; Boroňová, I.; Behulová, R.; Svíčková, P.; Petrejčíková, E.; Soták, M.; et al. Association of the FTO rs9939609 polymorphism with obesity in Roma/Gypsy population. *Am. J. Phys. Anthropol.* **2012**, *1*, 30–34. [CrossRef] [PubMed]
8. Kalibová, K. Kolik Romů žije v Česku? *Geogr. Rozhl.* **2008**, *17*, 8–9.
9. Šedová, L.; Olišarová, V.; Tóthová, V. Romové a specifika zdravotní edukace. *Stud. Kinanthropol.* **2014**, *15*, 259–267.
10. Vazarova de Courten, B.; de Courten, M.; Hanson, R.L.; Zahorakova, A.; Egyenes, H.P.; Tataranni, P.A.; Bennett, P.H.; Vozar, J. Higher prevalence of type 2 diabetes, metabolit syndrome and cardiovascular diseases in gypsies that in non-gypsies in Slovakia. *Diabetes Res. Clin. Pract.* **2003**, *62*, 95–103. [CrossRef]
11. Dolinska, S.; Kudlackova, M.; Ginter, E. The prevalence of female obesity in the world and in the Slovak Gypsy women. *Bratisl. Lek. Listy* **2007**, *108*, 207–211. [PubMed]
12. Prokešová, M. Romové. In *Otázky a Hledání Odpovědí*; Repronis: Ostrava, Czech Republic, 2010.
13. Šlechtová, D.; Bürgerová, O. Specifika romského etnika ve vztahu k poskytování zdravotní a ošetřovatelské péče. *Kontakt* **2009**, *11*, 189–192.
14. Ippolito, F.; Sánchez, S.I. *Protecting Vulnerable Groups: The European Human Rights Framework*; Modern Studies in European Law; Bloomsbury Publishing: London, UK, 2015.
15. O'Nions, H. *Minority Rights Protection in International Law: The Roma of Europe*; Research in Migration and Ethnic Relations Series; Ashgate Publishing: Farnham, UK, 2012.
16. Strielkowski, W. *Roma Migrations*; Faculty of Social Science, Charles University in Prague: Prague, Czech Republic, 2012.
17. Crawford, P.B.; Story, M.; Wang, M.C.; Ritchie, L.D.; Sabry, Z.I. Ethnic issues in the epidemiology of childhood obesity. *Pediatr. Clin. N. Am.* **2001**, *48*, 855–878. [CrossRef]

18. Satia-Abouta, J.; Patterson, R.E.; Kristal, A.R.; Teh, C.; Tu, S.P. Psychosocial predictors of diet and acculturation in Chinese American and Chinese Canadian women. *Ethn. Health* **2002**, *7*, 21–39. [CrossRef] [PubMed]
19. World Health Organization (WHO). *Obesity: Preventing and Managing the Global Epidemic: Report of a WHO Consultation on Obesity, Geneva, 3–5 June 1997*; WHO: Geneva, Switzerland, 1998. Available online: http://apps.who.int/iris/handle/10665/63854 (accessed on 11 January 2018).
20. Strauss, A.; Corbinová, J. Základy kvalitativního výzkumu. In *Postupy a Techniky Metody Zakotvené Teorie*; Albert: Brno, Czech Republic, 1999.
21. Adámková, V. Obezita a nadváha jako celospolečenský problem. In *Prevence Obesity a Nadváhy u Romské Minority v Komunitním Ošetřovatelství*; Tóthová, V., Ed.; NLN, s.r.o.: Praha, Czech Republic, 2016; pp. 16–25.
22. Brewiss, A.A. *Obesity: Cultural and Biocultural Perspectives*; Rutgers University Press: New Brunswick, NJ, USA, 2011.
23. Saxena, S.; Ambler, G.; Cole, T.J.; Majeed, A. Ethnic group differences in overweight and obese children and young people in England: Cross sectional survey. *Arch. Dis. Child.* **2004**, *89*, 30–36. [PubMed]
24. Robertson, A.; Lobstein, T.; Knai, C. Obesity and Socio-Economic Groups in Europe: Evidence Review and Implications for Action. 2007. Available online: http://ec.europa.eu/health/ph_determinants/life_style/nutrition/documents/ev20081028_rep_en.pdf (accessed on 11 January 2017).
25. Higgins, V.; Dale, A. *Ethnic Differences in Overweight and Obese Children in England*; The University of Manchester: Manchester, UK, 2010. Available online: http://www.cmist.manchester.ac.uk/medialibrary/archive-publications/working-papers/2010/2010-07-ethnic-differences.pdf (accessed on 11 January 2017).
26. Karlsen, S.; Morris, S.; Kinra, S.; Vallejo-Torres, L.; Viner, R.M. Ethnic variations in overweight and obesity among children over time: Findings from analyses of the Health Surveys for England 1998–2009. *Pediatr. Obes.* **2013**, *9*, 186–196. [CrossRef] [PubMed]
27. Urban, D.; Kajanová, A. Kouření a konzumace alkoholu u romských komunit v České a Slovenské republice. *Kontakt* **2011**, *13*, 328–335.
28. Oláhová, L. *Nejen Romská Kuchařka*; Fortuna: Praha, Czech Republic, 2000.
29. Šišková, T. *Menšiny a Migranti v České Republice: My a Oni v Multikulturní Společnosti 21. Století*; Portál: Praha, Czech Republic, 2001.
30. Davidová, E. Způsob života a kultura: Změny ve hmotné kultuře Romů—Bydlení, strava. In *Černobílý Život*; Černá, M., Ed.; Gallery: Praha, Czech Republic, 2000; pp. 80–89.
31. Stávková, J.; Derflerová Brázdová, Z. Konzumace ovoce a zeleniny a jiné stravovací zvyklosti Romské populace. *Hygiena* **2014**, *59*, 179–183. [CrossRef]
32. Cachelin, F.M.; Rebeck, R.M.; Chung, G.H.; Pelayo, E. Does ethnicity influence body-size preference? A comparison of body image and body size. *Obes. Res.* **2002**, *10*, 158–166. [CrossRef] [PubMed]

10

Eicosapentaenoic and Docosahexaenoic Acid-Enriched High Fat Diet Delays Skeletal Muscle Degradation in Mice

Nikul K. Soni [1,*], Alastair B. Ross [1], Nathalie Scheers [1], Otto I. Savolainen [1], Intawat Nookaew [2,3], Britt G. Gabrielsson [1] and Ann-Sofie Sandberg [1]

1 Division of Food and Nutrition Science, Department of Biology and Biological Engineering, Chalmers University of Technology, Gothenburg SE-41296, Sweden; alastair.ross@chalmers.se (A.B.R.); nathalie.scheers@chalmers.se (N.S.); otto.savolainen@chalmers.se (O.I.S.); bggabr@gmail.com (B.G.G.); ann-sofie.sandberg@chalmers.se (A.-S.S.)

2 Division of Systems and Synthetic Biology, Department of Biology and Biological Engineering, Chalmers University of Technology, Gothenburg SE-412 96, Sweden; intawat@chalmers.se

3 Department of Biomedical Informatics, College of Medicine, University of Arkansas for Medical Sciences, Little Rock, AR 72204, USA

* Correspondence: soni@chalmers.se

Abstract: Low-grade chronic inflammatory conditions such as ageing, obesity and related metabolic disorders are associated with deterioration of skeletal muscle (SkM). Human studies have shown that marine fatty acids influence SkM function, though the underlying mechanisms of action are unknown. As a model of diet-induced obesity, we fed C57BL/6J mice either a high fat diet (HFD) with purified marine fatty acids eicosapentaenoic acid (EPA) and docosahexaenoic acid (DHA) (HFD-ED), a HFD with corn oil, or normal mouse chow for 8 weeks; and used transcriptomics to identify the molecular effects of EPA and DHA on SkM. Consumption of ED-enriched HFD modulated SkM metabolism through increased gene expression of mitochondrial β-oxidation and slow-fiber type genes compared with HFD-corn oil fed mice. Furthermore, HFD-ED intake increased nuclear localization of nuclear factor of activated T-cells (Nfatc4) protein, which controls fiber-type composition. This data suggests a role for EPA and DHA in mitigating some of the molecular responses due to a HFD in SkM. Overall, the results suggest that increased consumption of the marine fatty acids EPA and DHA may aid in the prevention of molecular processes that lead to muscle deterioration commonly associated with obesity-induced low-grade inflammation.

Keywords: eicosapentaenoic acid (EPA)/Docosahexaenoic acid (DHA); obesity; skeletal-muscle metabolism; mitochondrial β-oxidation; transcriptome

---

1. Introduction

The World Health Organization (WHO) estimates that chronic inflammatory conditions accounts for more than 17 million deaths every year [1]. Obesity is considered one of the main underlying factors for chronic inflammation and has almost doubled since 1980 and now over 1.4 billion adults worldwide are obese. Obesity, once considered a problem only in developed countries, is now also a major problem in low- and middle-income countries. Parallel to the increase in obesity, diseases associated with chronic inflammation such as cardiovascular diseases and type 2 diabetes are also rising [1]. One of the major concerns associated with low-grade inflammation is sarcopenia—loss of muscle mass. Generally, after the age of 50 the muscle mass reduces at a rate of up to 1%–2% annually, while fat mass increases [2,3]. At the same time, muscle strength drops at the rate of 1.5% annually between the age of 50 and 60 years and at the rate of 3% thereafter [4]. Obesity accelerates age-related muscle deterioration [5] exacerbating the risk for type 2 diabetes (T2D) by approximately 30% [6]. The negative feedback loop defined as the combination of excess weight-gain and reduced muscle mass, strength and performance is known as sarcopenic obesity [7]. Further suggestions of a role for inflammation in sarcopenia includes an association between increased TNF-α [8] and Il-6 [9] and decreased muscle mass and strength.

Skeletal muscle (SkM) constitutes about 40% of total body mass in adult lean men and is an adaptable tissue in response to changes in lifestyle such as diet and physical training [10,11]. SkM is one of the major sites of glucose metabolism, accounting for about 30% of postprandial glucose disposal [12]. This makes SkM a crucial organ for maintaining healthy glucose concentrations in the body, with loss of muscle mass also associated with increased type 2 diabetes risk. Changes to diet may impact on SkM and use of fish oil rich in the fatty acids eicosapentaenoic acid (EPA) and docosahexaenoic acid (DHA) have been proposed to improve SkM metabolism [13]. An intervention with marine fatty acids improved muscle mass and function in older adults [13] and animal studies suggest a role for marine fatty acids in SkM anabolism and increased protein synthesis [14,15]. In addition, marine fatty acids have anti-inflammatory activity in animals and humans [16], which may reduce the loss of inflammation-mediated SkM mass in older adults. Supplementation with EPA and DHA, the two main marine fatty acids, could be the basis for a simple, safe and low-cost solution for preventing and mitigating negative changes to SkM metabolism. For such a strategy to be credible, it is crucial to understand the underlying signaling mechanisms mediated by EPA and DHA on SkM.

Our previous intervention studies showed that mice fed high fat diets (HFDs) supplemented with herring improve muscle mass compared with mice fed HFD supplemented with beef [17,18]. In several randomized control trials in humans, marine fatty acids improve muscle volume, a surrogate marker for improved muscle performance [13,19,20]. In order to build on these results and determine if EPA and DHA, or other components in fatty fish, are responsible for improving muscle metabolism and to determine what the underlying mechanisms could be, we conducted a follow-up trial on earlier work with fatty fish [17,18]. Here we have used transcriptomics to explore how replacing a commonly used source of dietary fat, corn oil with purified EPA and DHA interacts with gastrocnemicus skeletal muscle (gSkM) gene expression, in order to investigate how EPA and DHA can affect muscle deterioration.

2. Materials and Methods

2.1. Animal Experiment

Six-week old male C57BL/6 J mice (Harlan BV, The Netherlands) were grouped 5–6 mice/cage, and were housed in a temperature and humidity-controlled environment with 12 h light/dark cycle for three weeks to acclimatize to the facility. At nine weeks of age, mice were switched from a normal mouse chow to one of three intervention diets: high fat diet with EPA and DHA (HFD-ED), a high fat diet with corn oil (HFD-corn oil) or the same mouse chow as during the acclimatization period (control group). Mice were maintained on these diets for 8-weeks (see Diets for details). After 8-weeks the animals were anesthetized by intraperitoneal injection of sodium pentobarbital (>60 mg/kg) and blood was collected from the heart followed by cervical dislocation. Plasma was obtained by centrifugation at 4 °C of EDTA whole blood (10 min; 10,000× g). The tissues were weighed and snap-frozen in liquid nitrogen immediately after dissection. Both, tissues and plasma were stored at −80 °C until further analysis. The animal experiments were approved by the Animal Ethics Committee at the University of Gothenburg (Dnr: 253-2009) [21].

2.2. Diets

The mice were fed a standard control chow during the 3-weeks acclimatization period. The mice did not differ in body weight at the start of the study (Table 1) and the body weights were measured weekly during the study. We removed two mice from the control group due to unsocial behavior, thus there were $n = 9$ mice in control and $n = 12$ mice in either HFD group. HFD were used to induce obesity in the mice. The two HFD used in the study differed only in their fatty acid composition. The reference

HFD was prepared with 5 weight/weight (*w*/*w*)% corn oil, while the treatment HFD was prepared with 2 *w*/*w*% purified EPA and DHA (EPAX AS Lysaker, Norway) plus 3 *w*/*w*% corn oil. The control diet provided 24 energy% (E%) as protein, 12 E% as fat and 65 E% as carbohydrates, whereas the two HFD contained 25 E% as protein, 32 E% as fat and 44 E% as carbohydrates (Table 2). The diets were prepared by Lantmännen AB (Kimstad, Sweden). Access to water and diet was ad libitum and the diets were changed three times per week throughout the study.

Table 1. Changes in Body Weight Composition and Plasma Lipid Composition.

Parameter	Control	HFD-ED	HFD-Corn oil
Total number of animals; *n*	9	12	12
Initial body weight (g)	27.5 ± 0.8	28.6 ± 0.8	24.3 ± 0.5
Final body weight (g)	31.4 ± 1	33.8 ± 0.8	36.2 ± 0.9
Change in body weight (g)	3.9 ± 0.5 [a]	5.2 ± 0.3 [a]	8.6 ± 0.5 [b]
plasma cholesterol (mmol/L)	5.6 ± 0.4	5.5 ± 0.4	5.2 ± 0.6
plasma triglyceride (mmol/L)	0.9 ± 0.1 [a,b]	1.1 ± 0.1 [a]	0.7 ± 0.1 [b]

The data are shown as mean ± SEM; different letters show significant different tested by ANOVA followed by Tukey's multiple comparison test. To calculate the changes in body weight (g), initial body weight values from individual animals was subtracted from the final body weight measurement.

Table 2. Diet Compositions Namely Control, HFD-ED and HFD-Corn Oil (CO) [21].

Ingredient (g/100 g Diet)		Control	HFD-ED	HFD-CO
Protein	Casein	22.2	25.6	25.6
Carbohydrates	Sucrose	5.0	10.0	10.0
	Corn starch	56.0	34.8	34.8
	Cellulose	5.0	5.8	5.8
Fat	Total	5.0	15.0	15.0
	Corn oil	2.5	3.0	5.0
	Coconut oil	2.5	10.0	10.0
	EPAX oils [a]	0	2.0	0
Minerals [b]		2.0	2.5	2.5
Miconutrients [c]		3.0	3.0	3.0
Choline bitartrate		1.6	2.0	2.0
Cholesterol		0	1.0	1.0
Methionine		0.2	0.3	0.3
Energy content (kJ/100 g)		1599	1752	1752
Protein E%		24	25	25
Carbohydrate E%		65	44	44
Fat E%		12	32	32
Fatty acid composition [d] (mg/g diet)	C10:0	0.20	1.47	1.33
	C12:0	2.37	7.58	7.72
	C14:0	1.54	4.58	4.78
	C16:0	1.90	3.44	3.59
	C18:0	0.68	2.26	2.49
	SFA	6.70	19.33	19.91
	C18:1*n*9	2.82	4.80	5.26
	MUFA	2.82	4.80	5.26
	C18:2*n*6	3.62	5.03	7.36
	C18:3*n*6	0.12	0.22	0.26
	n-6 PUFA	3.74	5.26	7.62
	C20:5*n*3 (EPA)	0.00	2.03	0.01
	C22:6*n*3 (DHA)	0.00	4.58	0.01
	n-3 PUFA	0.00	6.61	0.02

[a] EPAX 1050. EPAX 6015. [b] $CaCO_3$ (57.7%); KCl (19.9%); KH_2PO_4 (11.9%); $MgSO_4$ (10.4%). [c] Corn starch (98.22%); $Ca(IO_3)_2$ (0.0007%); $CoCO_3$ (0.064%); CuO (0.02%); $FeSO_4$ (0.5%); MnO_2 (0.035%); Na_2MoO_4 (0.001%); $NaSeO_3$ (0.0007%); ZnO (0.1%); Vitamin A (0.013%); B_2 (Riboflavin-5-phosphate sodium; 0.027%); B_3 (0.1%); B_5 (Ca Pantothenate; 0.057%); B_6 (0.023%); B_7 (0.0007%); B_9 (0.007%); B_{12} (0.00008%); D_3 (0.007%); E (0.25%); K (0.003%). [d] Analyses were performed in triplicate and data was obtained by Gas chromatography mass spectroscopy.

2.3. Muscle Composition

Gastrocnemicus skeletal muscles were dissected and weighed directly after sacrifice. Plasma total triglyceride and cholesterol was measured enzymatically with Konelab Autoanalyser version 2.0 at the Department of Clinical Chemistry, Sahlgrenska University Hospital, Gothenburg, Sweden. Clinical chemistry procedures have been previously described in detail [21].

2.4. RNA Isolation and Quality Assurance

Four mice, representative from each diet group on the basis of body weight, plasma triglyceride and plasma cholesterol levels were selected for RNA isolation and microarray analysis (Supplemental Table S1). Total RNA from gSkM was purified using the RNeasy® Plus Universal Mini kit (Qiagen Nordic, Sollentuna, Sweden). RNA samples were quantified spectrophotometrically (NanoDrop 2000c UV-Vis Spectrophotometer, Thermo Scientific, Wilmington, NC, USA) and the quality of the RNA was controlled by the ratio of 28S and 18S rRNA (RNA 6000 Nano LabChip for Agilent 2100 Bioanalyzer (Agilent Technologies, Santa Clara, CA, USA).

2.5. Western Blot Analysis

Nuclear and cytosolic extracts were prepared using NE-PER Nuclear and Cytoplasmic Extraction Reagents kit (78833, Thermo Fisher Scientific). Western blot analysis was performed as described earlier [22]. Briefly, the protein concentration was measured in duplicate using the Pierce BCA Protein Assay kit (Thermo Fisher Scientific) for equal protein loading to the SDS-PAGE. After transfer of the proteins to the membranes, the membranes were stained with 0.5% Ponceau S (Merck Chemicals, Darmstadt, Germany) to visualize the protein transfer. For the detection of specific proteins, the following primary antibodies were used: Rb-anti-m acetyl-CoA carboxylase (Acc; 3662; Cell Signaling Technology), Rb-anti-m phospho-acetyl-CoA carboxylase (P-Acc; Ser79, 3661; Cell Signaling Technology), Rb-anti-m troponin c1 (Tnnc1; sc-20642, Santa Cruz Biotechnology), Rb-anti-m Nuclear factor of activated T-cells (Nfatc4; sc-13036, Santa Cruz Biotechnology). The secondary antibodies were: HRP-conjugated Horse-anti-m IgG (7076; Cell Signaling Technology), Goat-anti-m IgG (sc-2020; Santa Cruz Biotechnology) and Rb-anti-m IgG (7074; Cell Signaling Technology). As loading control for each western blot, either glyceraldehyde 3-phosphate dehydrogenase (anti-Gapdh; sc-47724; Santa Cruz Biotechnology), or lamin (anti-lamin A/C, sc-6215; Santa Cruz Biotechnology) was used. Western blots for the protein Acc, P-Acc and Tnnc1 are in supplemental Figure S1.

2.6. Microarray—Data Acquisition and Analysis

RNA was labeled and hybridized to MouseWG-6_V2.0 Expression BeadChip (R3_11278593_A; Illumina, CA, USA) that contains 45,281 transcripts, at the SCIBLU Genomics core facility (Swegene Centre for Integrative Biology at Lund University, Sweden). The content of this BeadChip is derived from the National Center for Biotechnology Information Reference Sequence (NCBI RefSeq) database (Build 36, Release 22) [23], supplemented with probes from the Mouse Exonic Evidence Based Oligonucleotide (MEEBO) [24] set, as well as example protein-coding sequences from RIKEN FANTOM2 database [25]. The raw and normalized data is available in SOFT format at the Gene Expression Omnibus database under Accession Number GSE76361.

The Illumina bead array files were imported to GenomeStudio Gene Expression (GSGX) software 1.9.0. The un-normalized expression data (fluorescence intensities) were extracted for the mean intensity of arrays. R Studio software (Version 3.2.3, © 2015 RStudio, Inc., Boston, MA, USA) was used for microarray data analysis. The data was quantile normalized and variance-stabilizing transformation (VST) was performed using the default setting of *lumiExpresso* function from the lumi package [26]. The top 100 differentially expressed genes regulated by HFD-ED compared with HFD-corn oil are provided in supplemental Table S2. The Empirical Bayes method from the limma package was then applied to the signals to calculate moderated *t*- and *F*-statistics, log odds and differential expression for comparisons between the diets from skeletal muscle tissue [27]. The Generally Applicable Gene-Set/Pathway Analysis (GAGE) Bioconductor package was used for gene-set enrichment analysis (GSEA) for functional inference [28]. Before implementing the gage function, canonical signaling and metabolic pathways from the KEGG mouse database was prepared for better-defined results. For the microarray data, false discovery rate (FDR) adjusted p-values were calculated and FDR adjusted p-value < 0.05 was considered significant. The Pathview package was used to visualize the data, where the *pathview* function downloads KEGG graph data and renders a pathway map, based on experimental results [29].

2.7. Fatty Acid Analysis

Approximately 100 mg gSkM tissue was weighed, freeze-dried and extracted using the Folch total lipid extraction method [30]. Briefly, 5 mL chloroform–methanol (2:1 v/v) was added to the samples followed by sonication at 40 Hz for 30 min at RT (Branson 8510, Branson Ultrasonics Corp, CT, USA). One mL of physiological saline (0.9% NaCl) was mixed with the samples followed by brief vortexing and centrifugation for 5 min at 3000 rpm (1700$\times$ g), to separate the two phases. The organic lower phase was collected and the remaining aqueous phase was re-extracted with 1.5 mL chloroform. The two extracted phases were combined and evaporated under N_2 and re-dissolved in 1 mL isopropanol. All solvents were from Sigma-Aldrich, Sweden.

Solid phase extraction (SPE) method was used to separate lipid classes [31]. Internal phospholipid (C17:0) and triglyceride (C19:0) standards (Nu-Chek prep, Inc., Elysian, MN, USA) were added to the samples. Hexane conditioned aminopropyl SPE columns were loaded with 1 mL of extracted SkM lipid samples. Neutral lipids, free fatty acid and phospholipids were eluted with chloroform–isopropanol (2:1), diethylether-2% acetone and methanol, respectively and evaporated under N_2. Dried SPE fractions were methylated by overnight incubation with 1 mL 10% acetyl chloride in methanol and 1 mL toluene. After methylation, 0.3 mL water and 4 mL petroleum ether was added to the samples and the resulting two phases were separated by 3 min centrifugation at 3000$\times$ g. The upper phase was then removed, evaporated under N_2 and re-dissolved in 250 μL isooctane [32].

The fatty acid methyl esters (FAMEs) were analyzed by gas chromatography mass spectrometry (Focus GC, ISQ, Thermo Fischer Scientific, USA) using a ZB-WAX column (30 $\times$ 0.25 mm I.D., 0.25 μm) (Phenomenex, UK). One μl of sample was injected in splitless mode. The injector temperature was 240 and helium was used as the carrier gas with the flow of 1 mL/min. Oven temperature was as follows: 50 °C 1.5 min, ramped to 180 °C at 25 °C/min where held for 1 min, ramped to 220 °C at 10 °C/min, held for 1 min and ramped to 250 °C at 15 °C/min and held for 3 min. The transfer line was kept at 250 °C and ion source at 200 °C. Electron impact ionization (70 eV) was used and the FAMEs were detected by scanning a mass range from 50 to 650 m/z. An external FAME standard mix GLC 463 (Nu-Chek prep, Inc., Elysian, MN, USA) was used for identification of peaks in gSkM samples. Fatty acids were quantified against internal standards, summed and expressed as mg/g dry gSkM biomass and as a percentage of total lipid fractions.

2.8. Statistical Analysis of Western Blot and Fatty Acid Analyses

Differences in SkM western blot and fatty acid analyses were tested using ANOVA with Tukey's honest significant difference (Tukey-HSD) post-hoc test. Statistical significance between the protein groups was calculated with an unpaired 2-tailed Student's t-test. A p-value < 0.05 was considered statistically significant. Statistical calculations were performed using Microsoft® Excel® for Mac 2011 version 14.5.8 and R software (Version 3.2.3) under RStudio interface. All data are presented as mean $\pm$ SEM.

3. Results

3.1. *Effect of EPA and DHA vs Corn Oil on gSkM Weight and Transcriptome*

Delayed weight gain was observed in HFD-ED compared with HFD-corn oil fed animals (Table 1). Moreover, relative adiposity was lower in HFD-ED compared with HFD-corn oil fed mice [21]. Principle component analysis of the gSkM transcriptome did not detect any outliers in the data (Supplemental Figure S2a) indicating good analytical reproducibility. To visualize the global effects of different diets on gSkM, differential expression of the genes was performed on the following comparisons: HFD-ED versus control diet, HFD-corn oil versus control diet and HFD-ED versus HFD-corn oil. Venn diagrams show the number of differentially expressed genes (DEGs) corrected for multiple testing by Benjamini and Hochberg at p-value < 0.001 (supplemental Figure S2b). The total number of DEGs was 365, 129 and 383 for the comparison HFD-ED versus control diet, HFD-corn oil versus control diet and HFD-ED versus HFD-corn oil, respectively. Differential gene expression analysis found that the different fat composition of the two HFDs affected gene expression in gSkM differently when compared to the control group (Supplemental Figure S3).

3.2. *gSkM Fatty Acid Composition*

Neutral lipids: The total amount of neutral lipids was significantly higher in the mice fed HFD-corn oil compared to mice fed the other two study diets (Table 3). The concentration of fatty acid C12:0 was higher in HFD-corn oil fed animals compared with both HFD-ED and control diets (Table 3). C14:0 was higher in HFD-corn oil fed animals compared with control diet but there was no difference compared with HFD-ED fed animals. Fatty acids C16:0, C18:1 and C18:2 n-6 (linoleic acid) were higher in HFD-corn oil fed animals compared with mice fed HFD-ED or control diets, whereas no difference was observed between the control and HFD-ED fed animals. C22:6 n-3 (DHA) was higher in the HFD-ED fed animals compared to the control diet.

Free fatty acids: Free fatty acids (FFA) mainly comprised of saturated and monounsaturated fatty acids including C16:0, C19:0, C16:1 and C18:1 (Table 3). Apart from C12:0, which was higher in HFD-ED fed animals, the remaining FFAs were higher in HFD-corn oil fed animals compared with the other two diets. The concentration of C20:3 n-3 was higher in the HFD-corn oil fed animals compared with HFD-ED and the concentration did not differ compared with control diet. As expected, C22:6 n-3 concentrations were higher in the HFD-ED fed animals compared with HFD-corn oil. The total amount of FFAs in gSkM did not differ between the different groups.

Phospholipids: The concentration of C14:0 was significantly higher in the HFD-ED fed animals compared with the other two diets (Table 3). The amount of C18:1 was significantly lower in the HFD-ED fed animals compared with HFD-corn oil fed animals. The amount of C20:4 n-6 (arachidonic acid) was lower in HFD-ED fed animals compared with either HFD-corn oil or control diet fed animals. The amount of n-3 PUFA C20:5 n-3 (EPA) did not differ for any of the diets, with only very low concentrations measured, whereas the concentrations of C22:5 n-3 (DPA) and C22:6 n-3 (DHA) were significantly higher in the animals fed HFD-ED compared with animals fed HFD-corn oil but the expected increase in EPA was not found. The total phospholipid content was significantly lower in the HFD-ED fed animals compared with control diet fed animals but did not differ from that found in gSkM from the animals fed HFD-corn oil.

Table 3. The Fatty Acid Profiles of Different Lipid Fractions in Gastrocnemicus Skeletal Muscle.

Lipid Fraction	mg/g	mg/g	mg/g	% value	% value	% value
Neutral lipids	**Control**	**HFD-ED**	**HFD-Corn oil**	**Control**	**HFD-ED**	**HFD-Corn oil**
C12:0	0.12 ± 0.06 [a]	1.51 ± 0.42 [b]	2.87 ± 0.41 [c]	0.44 ± 0.18 [a]	3.93 ± 0.21 [b]	4.02 ± 0.33 [b]
C14:0	1.18 ± 0.24 [a]	3.15 ± 0.76	4.81 ± 0.49 [b]	4.35 ± 0.48 [a]	8.19 ± 0.52 [b]	6.74 ± 0.23 [c]
C16:0	8.11 ± 2.31 [a]	9.75 ± 2.28 [a]	19.01 ± 2.11 [b]	29.93 ± 1.78	25.35 ± 1.51	26.63 ± 2.34

Table 3. *Cont.*

Lipid Fraction	mg/g	mg/g	mg/g	% value	% value	% value
Neutral lipids	**Control**	**HFD-ED**	**HFD-Corn oil**	**Control**	**HFD-ED**	**HFD-Corn oil**
C18:0	0.55 ± 0.05	0.65 ± 0.05	0.68 ± 0.04	2.03 ± 0.48 ^{a}	1.69 ± 0.4 ^{a}	0.95 ± 0.09 ^{b}
C18:1	13.11 ± 3.05 ^{a}	14.86 ± 3.45 ^{a}	29.2 ± 2.19 ^{b}	48.38 ± 0.81 ^{a}	38.64 ± 1.06 ^{b}	40.91 ± 1.6 ^{b}
C18:2 *n6*	3.75 ± 0.78 ^{a}	7.29 ± 1.89 ^{a}	14.55 ± 1.25 ^{b}	13.84 ± 0.67 ^{a}	18.95 ± 0.9 ^{b}	20.38 ± 0.73 ^{b}
C18:3 *n3*	0.07 ± 0.04	0.07 ± 0.03	0.09 ± 0.02	0.26 ± 0.08	0.18 ± 0.04	0.13 ± 0.03
C20:3 *n6*	0.02 ± 0.01	0.01 ± 0 ^{a}	0.03 ± 0 ^{b}	0.07 ± 0.06	0.03 ± 0	0.04 ± 0
C22:5 *n3*	0.03 ± 0.01	0.06 ± 0.01	0 ± 0	0.11 ± 0.09	0.16 ± 0.01 ^{a}	0 ± 0 ^{b}
C22:6 *n3*	0.14 ± 0.02 ^{a}	1.1 ± 0.09 ^{b}	0.14 ± 0.02 ^{a}	0.52 ± 0.25 ^{a}	2.86 ± 0.68 ^{b}	0.2 ± 0.04 ^{a}
Total neutral lipids	27.1 ± 6.48 ^{a}	38.46 ± 8.89 ^{a}	71.38 ± 6.13 ^{b}			
Free fatty acids	**Control**	**HFD-ED**	**HFD-Corn oil**	**Control**	**HFD-ED**	**HFD-Corn oil**
C12:0	0.13 ± 0.04	0.16 ± 0.04 ^{a}	0.04 ± 0.01 ^{b}	6.6 ± 2.11	8.21 ± 2.26 ^{a}	1.61 ± 0.43 ^{b}
C16:0	0.52 ± 0.07 ^{a}	0.64 ± 0.02	0.78 ± 0.04 ^{b}	26.4 ± 3.14 ^{a}	32.82 ± 1.34 ^{b}	31.33 ± 2.03 ^{b}
C16:1	0.12 ± 0.03	0.09 ± 0.03	0.15 ± 0.05	6.09 ± 1.17	4.62 ± 1.3	6.02 ± 1.58
C18:1	1.07 ± 0.09	0.89 ± 0.07 ^{a}	1.29 ± 0.12 ^{b}	54.31 ± 4.03 ^{a}	45.64 ± 1.96 ^{b}	51.81 ± 1.68
C18:2 *n6*	0 ± 0 ^{a}	0 ± 0 ^{a}	0.11 ± 0.02 ^{b}	0 ± 0 ^{a}	0 ± 0 ^{a}	4.42 ± 0.46 ^{b}
C18:3 *n3*	0.09 ± 0	0.07 ± 0.01	0.07 ± 0.01	4.57 ± 0.64 ^{a}	3.59 ± 0.51	2.81 ± 0.27 ^{b}
C20:3 *n3*	0.04 ± 0 ^{a}	0 ± 0 ^{b}	0.04 ± 0.01 ^{a}	2.03 ± 0.27 ^{a}	0 ± 0 ^{b}	1.61 ± 0.24 ^{c}
C22:6 *n3*	0 ± 0 ^{a}	0.09 ± 0.03 ^{b}	0 ± 0 ^{a}	0 ± 0 ^{a}	4.62 ± 1.25 ^{b}	0 ± 0.14 ^{a}
Total free fatty acids	1.97 ± 0.17	1.95 ± 0.12	2.49 ± 0.21			
Phospholipids	**Control**	**HFD-ED**	**HFD-Corn oil**	**Control**	**HFD-ED**	**HFD-Corn oil**
C14:0	0.33 ± 0.02 ^{a}	0.83 ± 0.04 ^{b}	0.64 ± 0.07	2.17 ± 0.14 ^{a}	6.14 ± 0.28 ^{b}	4.7 ± 0.49 ^{c}
C16:0	5.06 ± 0.06 ^{a}	4.93 ± 0.09	4.73 ± 0.06 ^{b}	33.29 ± 0.76 ^{a}	36.49 ± 0.55 ^{b}	34.75 ± 1.37
C18:0	1.97 ± 0.33	2.65 ± 0.18	2.01 ± 0.26	12.96 ± 2.38	19.62 ± 1.41	14.77 ± 2.02
C18:1	3.67 ± 0.68 ^{a}	0.39 ± 0.26 ^{b}	2.07 ± 0.44 ^{a}	24.14 ± 3.71 ^{a}	2.89 ± 1.81 ^{b}	15.21 ± 3.12 ^{a}
C18:2 *n6*	1.73 ± 0.06 ^{a}	0.58 ± 0.09 ^{b}	2.13 ± 0.05 ^{c}	11.38 ± 0.28 ^{a}	4.29 ± 0.61 ^{b}	15.65 ± 0.6 ^{c}
C20:3 *n6*	0.05 ± 0 ^{a}	0 ± 0 ^{b}	0.06 ± 0.01 ^{a}	0.33 ± 0 ^{a}	0 ± 0 ^{b}	0.44 ± 0.04 ^{a}
C20:4 *n6*	0.57 ± 0.01 ^{a}	0.1 ± 0 ^{b}	0.55 ± 0.01 ^{a}	3.75 ± 0.12 ^{a}	0.74 ± 0.01 ^{b}	4.04 ± 0.28 ^{a}
C20:5 *n3*	0 ± 0	0.04 ± 0	0.02 ± 0.02	0 ± 0	0.3 ± 0.01	0.15 ± 0.15
C22:3 *n6*	0.54 ± 0.02 ^{a}	0.07 ± 0 ^{b}	0.26 ± 0.03 ^{c}	3.55 ± 0.18 ^{a}	0.52 ± 0.01 ^{b}	1.91 ± 0.23 ^{c}
C22:5 *n3*	0.05 ± 0 ^{a}	0.11 ± 0 ^{b}	0.06 ± 0.01 ^{a}	0.33 ± 0.02 ^{a}	0.81 ± 0.02 ^{b}	0.44 ± 0.05 ^{c}
C22:6 *n3*	1.23 ± 0.03 ^{a}	3.45 ± 0.06 ^{b}	1.07 ± 0.1 ^{a}	8.09 ± 0.3 ^{a}	25.54 ± 0.53 ^{b}	7.86 ± 0.73 ^{a}
Total phospholipids	15.2 ± 0.47 ^{a}	13.15 ± 0.34 ^{b}	13.61 ± 0.45 ^{b}			
Total Fat content	44.26 ± 6.99	53.56 ± 9	87.47 ± 6.45			

The fatty acid profiles from the mice fed, either control, HFD-corn oil or HFD-ED are shown as mean ± SEM and as a proportion of total fatty acid fraction; different letters show statistical difference tested by ANOVA followed by Tukey's multiple comparison test. For details see methods section.

3.3. Increased Mitochondrial B—Oxidation and Oxidative Phosphorylation in the Gskm of Mice Fed HFD-ED

Energy metabolism is a biochemical process to generate energy from nutrients via aerobic or anaerobic pathways. KEGG pathway analysis suggested that HFD-ED intake led to an increased regulation of energy metabolism relating to lipid metabolism, Krebs cycle and oxidative phosphorylation, leading to increased capacity for ATP production in gSkM compared with HFD-corn oil fed animals.

Eight gene transcripts were upregulated by HFD-ED compared with the HFD-corn oil fed mice (Figure 1a). Functionally, the enzymes in the β-oxidation pathway facilitate the breakdown of fatty acids to form acetyl-CoA, which enters the Krebs cycle. The upregulated gene products, which are responsible for transporting fatty acids into the mitochondria, were two carnitine palmitoyltransferases (*Cpt1a* and *Cpt2*). In addition, RNA transcription of genes responsible for the subsequent degradation of fatty acids within the mitochondrial matrix producing acetyl-CoA including short/medium chain acyl-CoA dehydrogenase (*Acadm*), long chain acyl-CoA dehydrogenase (*Acadl*), very long chain acyl-CoA dehydrogenase (*Acadvl*), acetyl-CoA acyl transferase 2 (*Acaa2*), enoyl-CoA delta isomerase 1 (*Eci1*) and aldehyde dehydrogenese (*Aldh2*), were upregulated by the HFD-ED diet.

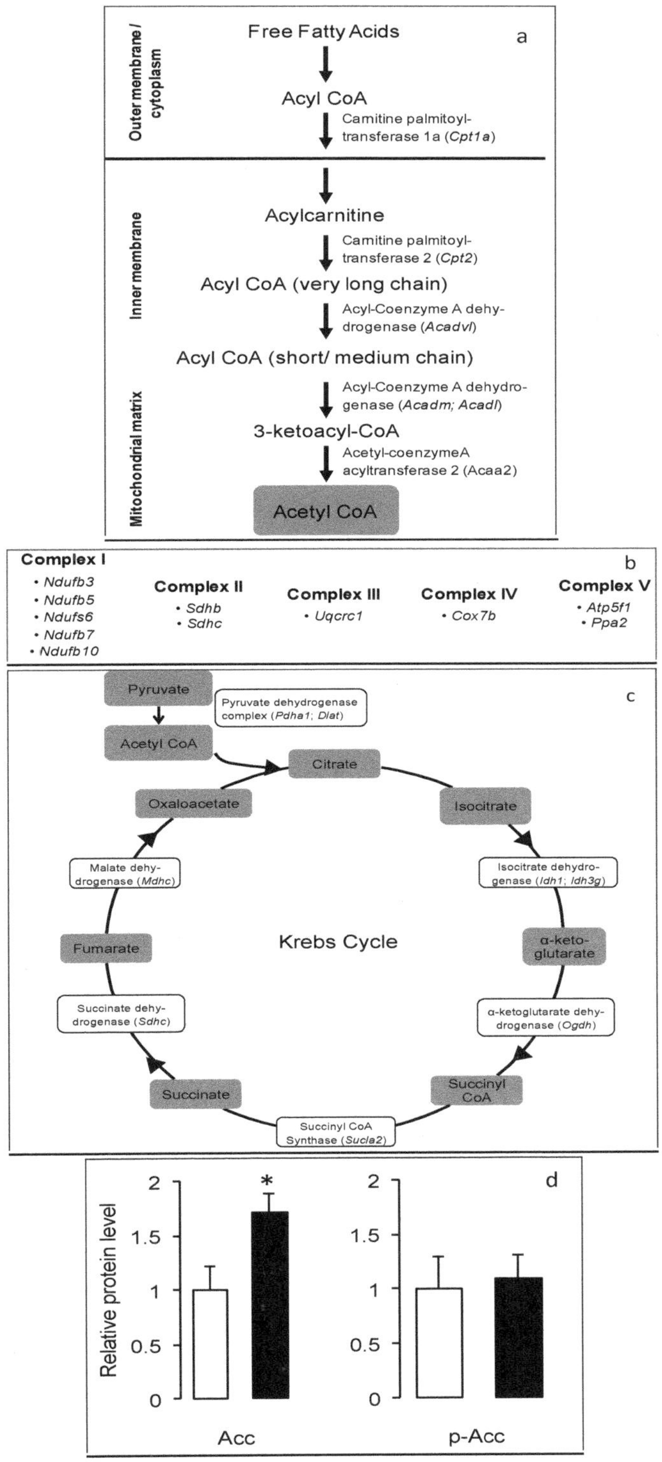

Figure 1. Pathway analysis of the gSkM transcriptome for the comparison of HFD-ED and HFD-corn oil fed mice. The illustration is based on the Kegg pathway database (http://www.genome.jp/kegg/pathway.html). (**a**) Fatty acid β-oxidation: Genes highlighted in red are upregulated in gSkM of mice fed HFD-ED compared with HFD-corn oil; (**b**) Electron transport chain: Genes highlighted in red are upregulated in gSkM of mice fed HFD-ED compared with HFD-corn oil; (**c**) Krebs Cycle: Genes highlighted in red are upregulated in gSkM of mice fed HFD-ED compared with HFD-corn oil; (**d**) Relative Acc protein levels in HFD-ED (white bars) fed mice was lower than HFD-corn oil (black bars) and there was no difference in the phosphorylation of Acc (p-Acc) protein after 8-weeks diet intervention. * Different at $p < 0.05$.

Pathway analyses showed a significant increase in the oxidative phosphorylation pathway in gSkM from the HFD-ED fed mice compared with HFD-corn oil animals (Figure 1b). Several genes involved in electron transport complex I-V were upregulated by HFD-ED fed mice compared with HFD-corn oil. Genes from the NADH dehydrogenase family that constitutes complex I (*Ndufa11, Ndufb3, Ndufb5, Ndufb7, Ndufb10* and *Ndufs6*); two succinate dehydrogenases (*Sdhb* and *Sdhc*) from complex II; ubiquinol-cytochrome c reductase core protein 1, cytochrome c oxidase subunit VIIb-Muscle and ATP synthase H+ transporting mitochondrial F0 complex subunit B1 (*Uqcrc1, Cox7b* and *Atp5f1*) constituting complex-III, IV and complex-V respectively, were upregulated.

HFD-ED upregulated the Krebs cycle in mice gSkM compared with HFD-corn oil (Figure 1c). The mitochondrial event consumes Acetyl-CoA producing NADH, $FADH_2$, GTP and the by-product CO_2. NADH and $FADH_2$ are in turn used by oxidative phosphorylation to generate ATP. Genes for key proteins in this metabolic pathway that were upregulated by EPA and DHA include pyruvate dehydrogenase E1 alpha 1 (*Pdha1*) and dihydrolipoamide S-acetyl transferase (*Dlat*), which converts pyruvate to Acetyl-CoA. HFD-ED upregulated several Krebs cycle genes including two kinds of isocitrate dehydrogenases (*Idh1* and *Idh3g*), oxoglutarate dehydrogenase (*Ogdh*), Succinate-CoA ligase GDP forming alpha subunit 2 (*Sucla2*), succinate dehydrogenase subunit a (*Sdha*) and malate dehydrogenase 2 (*Mdh2*), when compared with HFD-corn oil. There was no difference in the gene expression of *Acacb* (Acetyl-CoA carboxylase beta) but the total protein content of total acetyl-CoA carboxylase (Acc) was markedly lower in the gSkM of HFD-ED fed mice (Figure 1d). However, the phosphorylation levels of Acc did not differ in between the two HFDs (Figure 1d). This suggests increased internalization of fatty acids in mitochondria for potential β-oxidation in gSkM of HFD-ED fed mice rather than synthesis of fatty acids, as seems to be ongoing in HFD-corn oil animals.

3.4. Increased Expression of Muscle Contraction Pathway Genes in the Gskm of Mice Fed HFD-ED

Skeletal muscle fibers require stimulation from the neuromuscular junctions acting on the cholinergic nicotine receptor on the muscle cells to initiate contraction. These efferent cholinergic nerves are crucial for voluntary control of skeletal muscles. Gene expression of the cholinergic receptor nicotinic α polypeptide 1 (*Chrna1*), insulin growth factor receptor (*Igfr*) and two L-type voltage dependent Ca-channel genes (*Cacna1s* and *Cacnb2*), two calcium ATPases (*Atp1a1* and *Atp2a2*, a.k.a *Serca* 1 and 2, respectively), were upregulated by HFD-ED compared with HFD-corn oil fed mice (Figure 2a).

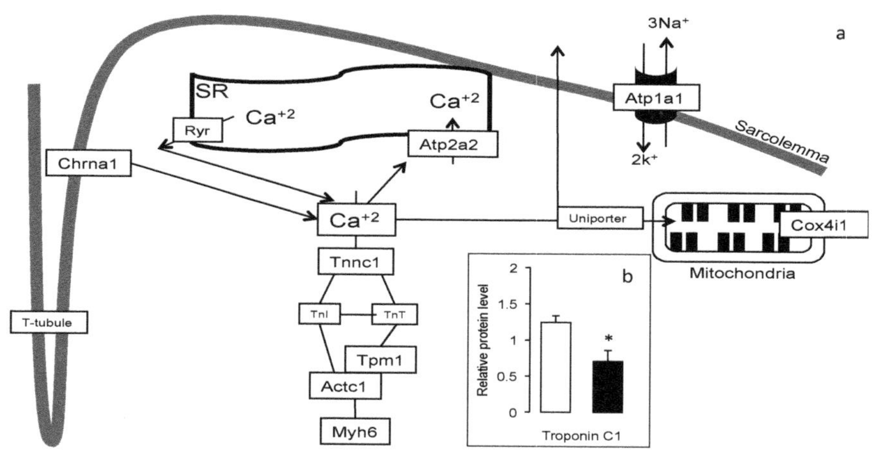

Figure 2. Pathway analysis of the gSkM transcriptome for the comparison HFD-ED versus HFD-corn oil fed mice. The illustration is based on the Kegg pathway database (http://www.genome.jp/kegg/pathway.html). (**a**) Nerve-Muscle contraction: Genes highlighted in red are upregulated in gSkM of mice fed HFD-ED compared with HFD-corn oil; (**b**) Relative Troponin C1 protein level in HFD-corn oil (black bars) fed mice was lower than HFD-ED (white bars). * Different at $p < 0.05$.

3.5. Increased Slow-Fiber-Specific Gene Expression Program in the Gskm of Mice Fed HFD-ED

The calcium mediated calcineurin-Nfat signaling cascade has been suggested to upregulate slow-fiber type gene expression. Differential gene expression of gSkM from the mice fed HFD-ED compared with HFD-corn oil suggested upregulation of several Nfat (*Nfatc1; Nfatc2; Nfatc4*) isoforms. The slow-fiber type genes troponin C1, cardiac/slow skeletal (*Tnnc1*), tropomyosin 1 alpha (*Tpm1*) and actin alpha 1 (*Actc1*) complex genes and crossbridge myosin heavy polypeptide isoforms (*Myh1, Myh2, Myh3, Myh6, Myh7, Myh8*) were upregulated in gSkM of HFD-ED fed mice compared with HFD-corn oil animals. Protein levels of *Tnnc1,* a biomarker for slow muscle fiber type, were higher in gSkM of HFD-ED fed mice compared with HFD-corn oil animals (Figure 2b). Furthermore, the gene product forming complex with *Nfatc2* and *Nfact4,* namely myogenin (*Myog*) and GATA Binding Protein 5 (*Gata5*) regulating the transcription of slow-fiber type gene expression was upregulated in the HFD-ED gSkM compared with HFD-corn oil. Nuclear localization of Nfat protein is essential for regulation of the slow-fiber-type gene expression. In the gSkM of HFD-ED fed mice, nuclear protein Nfat levels were significantly higher than HFD-corn oil fed animals (Figure 3). The master regulator of the calcineurin-Nfat signaling cascade, the regulator of calcineurin-2, *Rcan2,* was upregulated and its inhibitor glycogen synthase kinase 3β (*Gsk3*β) was downregulated in mice fed HFD-ED, compared with HFD-corn oil animals. Another transcriptional activator, suggested to be a direct target of marine fatty acids, peroxisome proliferator-activated receptor-γ coactivator 1α (*Ppargc1*α) was upregulated in gSkM of HFD-ED compared with HFD-corn oil fed mice.

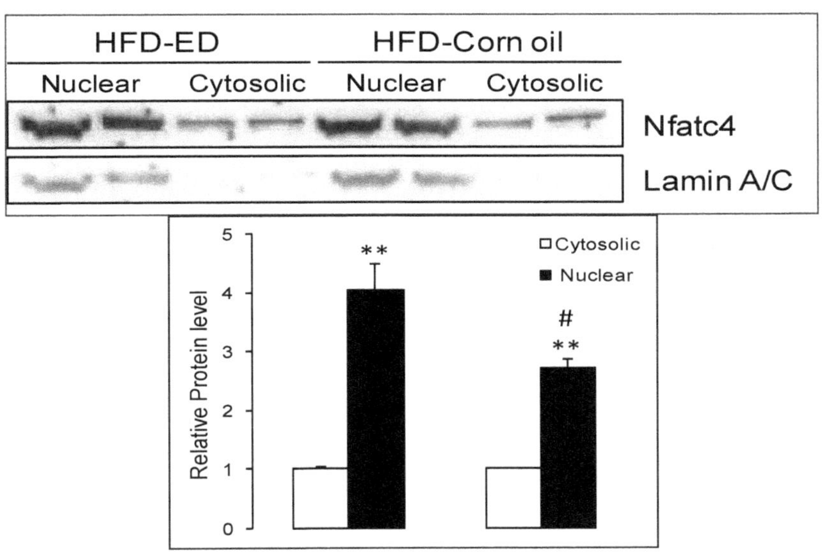

Figure 3. Representative Western blot is shown with LaminA/C loading control. Nuclear (black bars) and cytosolic (white bars) protein extract from the gSkM of HFD-ED (left-panel) and HFD-corn oil (right-panel) were analyzed by Western blot using antibodies for total anti-Nfatc4 antibody and the cytosolic protein levels in the HFD-ED was kept to 1. Different at ** $p < 0.05$ and # $p < 0.01$.

4. Discussion

In this study, we have shown that HFD-ED improves muscle metabolism and promotes a switch to slow-fiber type compared to HFD-corn oil. HFD-ED improves metabolism of fatty acids in gSkM by upregulating expression of genes coding for proteins involved in fatty acid β-oxidation, the Krebs cycle and oxidative phosphorylation. Lipid analysis shows that the HFD-ED fed animals had lower total fatty acid content compared to HFD-corn oil and control diet fed animals. Reduced ectopic fat accumulation in HFD-ED compared with HFD-corn oil fed animals suggests a physiological effect of EPA and DHA on muscle metabolic health. Higher expression of the genes involved in muscle contraction was found in gSkM of HFD-ED fed animals compared with HFD-corn oil fed animals. Western blot analysis showed reduced Acc protein levels in gSkM of HFD-ED fed animals compared with HFD-corn oil, confirming gene expression results. Acc is an inhibitor of fatty acid β-oxidation in mitochondria and the lower levels shows increase in mitochondrial fatty acid β-oxidation. In addition, increased Tnnc1 levels suggest increased muscle contraction in gSkM of HFD-ED fed animals compared with HFD-corn oil. Moreover, increased nuclear protein levels of the Nfatc4 isoform strongly suggests up-regulation of slow-fiber-type gene expression in gSkM of HFD-ED fed animals compared with HFD-corn oil fed animals (Figure 4).

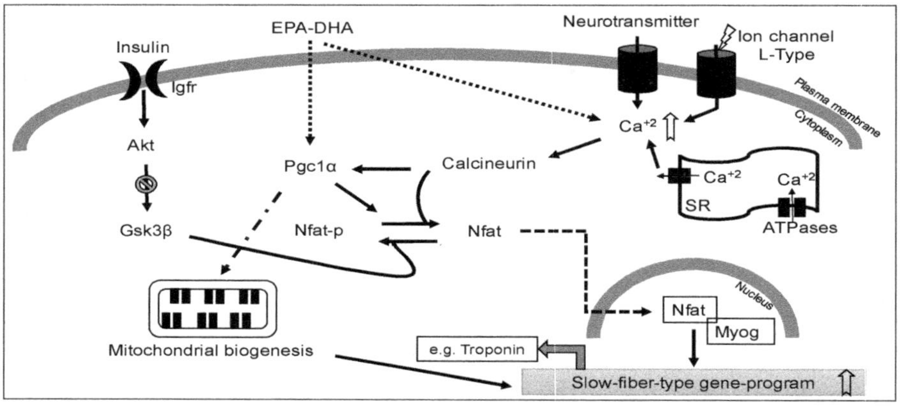

Figure 4. Schematic representation of the role of ED—enriched HFD on the gSkM transcriptome and modulation of ageing and/or obesity-induced sarcopenia in C57Bl/6J mice. Briefly, ED enriched HFD downregulates glucose synthase kinase 3 beta (*Gsk3β*) that phosphorylates nuclear factor of activated T cells (*Nfatc4*) and excludes it from entering into the nucleus. It also increases cytosolic calcium concentrations that in turn regulate calcineurin that then dephosphorylates Nfat allowing its localization in the nucleus. Upon localization, *Nfat* forms complex with myogenin (*Myog*) to turn on slow-fiber-type specific gene-program for e.g., Troponin C1. *Pgc1α*, a known master regulator of mitochondrial biogenesis was also seen upregulated by ED enriched HFD that could act upon multiple targets, one of which regulating dephosphorylation of *Nfatc4* isoforms and its further nuclear localization.

The gSkM neutral lipid and free fatty acid profiles reflect the higher amount of DHA in the feed of HFD-ED fed mice, though EPA was not detected in either fraction, in line with our previous findings in liver; that EPA was present in very low amounts, not in proportion to EPA in the diet [21]. There was no substantial proportional difference in gSkM fatty acid composition between the two HFD groups, even though HFD-corn oil fed mice had nearly twice the amount of total neutral lipids. This suggests that ED does not specifically upregulate any of the reactions related to β-oxidation and rather, leads to stimulation of β-oxidation in general, resulting in reduced total neutral lipids in SkM. Although there were several differences in the amount and proportion of free fatty acids and phospholipids, these differences were not quantitatively important aside from the increase DPA and DHA in mice fed HFD-ED but lower EPA in phospholipids fractions [33]. Notably C18:1 was substantially higher in HFD-corn oil fed mice compared with HFD-ED fed mice and this result was reversed for DHA. This could have implications for membrane fluidity within SkM and this may play a role in the observed transcriptome changes.

Previously we found that HFD-ED induced β-oxidation reduced liver fat compared to HFD-corn oil [21], similarly, reduced SkM fat can be due to the increase in β-oxidation and the lower amount of neutral lipids in HFD-ED fed mice. Reduced SkM mitochondrial fatty acid β-oxidation has been proposed as a key feature leading to insulin resistance [34,35] and high fat diets led to downregulation of the group of genes involved in oxidative phosphorylation in human SkM biopsies [36–38]. In the gSkM of the HFD-ED fed mice, the expression of rate limiting enzymes in fatty acid β-oxidation in mitochondria, *Cpt1* and *Cpt2* were upregulated compared with HFD-corn oil fed mice. Notably, the protein level of Acc was significantly reduced in gSkM of HFD-ED fed mice compared with HFD-corn oil. Acc regulates fatty acid metabolism by synthesizing malonyl-CoA (building blocks for new fatty acids) but suppresses mitochondrial β-oxidation by inhibiting fatty acid transporter *Cpt1*. Therefore, lower protein levels of Acc suggests entry of fatty acid into mitochondria via *Cpt1* transporter for mitochondrial β-oxidation in gSkM of HFD-ED fed mice compared with HFD-corn oil. A SkM specific isoform of *Acc* (*Acc2*) knockout mice were protected against fat-induced peripheral insulin resistance [39] whereas overexpression of *Cpt1* is sufficient to reduce insulin resistance [40]. Impairments in mitochondrial oxidative capacity in skeletal muscle have been seen in relation to a decrease in energy expenditure [35,41,42]. Thus, increased mitochondrial oxidative capacity in the gSkM of HFD-ED fed animals, supported by increased levels by *Cpt1* and decreased total protein levels of Acc may contribute to increased energy expenditure. Further work on a possible stimulation of energy expenditure by EPA and DHA, possibly via diet-induced thermogenesis is required.

Ageing and obesity may contribute to the decrease in the contractibility of skeletal muscle. Muscle contraction is regulated by intracellular calcium concentration via the thin filament regulatory proteins troponin and tropomyosin. In the absence of calcium, actin-myosin interaction and subsequently muscle contraction is inhibited. In the gSkM of HFD-ED, two ATPases, namely Na^+/K^+-ATPase transporting α2 polypeptide (*Atp1a2*; sodium pump) and ATPase Ca^{+2} transporting skeletal muscle slow switch 2 (*Atp2a2*; *Serca2a*) were upregulated compared with HFD-corn oil. A tissue specific knockout study shows that the sodium pump (*Atp1a2*) is required to prevent fatigue, and systematic analysis of Serca isoforms in calcium transport showed their importance for restoring muscle contractibility [43,44]. Protein levels of the oxidative fiber biomarker Troponin C1 were higher in gSkM of HFD-ED fed mice compared with HFD-corn oil, indicative of increased muscle contraction via control of intracellular calcium in mice fed HFD-ED. Together, these results suggest that HFD-ED contributes to increased calcium release into the sarcoplasm, compared with HFD-corn oil fed mice.

Calcineurin has been proposed to play a major role in the upregulation of slow-fiber-specific gene expression [45–47]. Earlier, it was found that inhibition of calcineurin by cyclosporin-A could result in an increased number of fast fibers in rat skeletal muscle [45]. Activated calcineurin phosphatase capacity is required for dephosphorylation of Nfat proteins, which then localize to the nucleus to initiate slow-fiber-specific gene expression [45,47]. Our data shows that the gSkM of HFD-ED fed animals has markedly higher nuclear levels of Nfat (Nfatc4 isoform) compared with HFD-corn oil, which could contribute to upregulation of the slow-fiber-specific gene expression upon nuclear localization. An earlier study showed abundant myogenin mRNA in slow oxidative muscles and this relationship followed phenotype transition caused by cross-innervation [48]. In HFD-ED fed mice, myogenin (P_{adj}-value = 0.06) tends to be higher compared with HFD-corn oil fed animals suggesting upregulation of genes for the slower muscle fiber phenotype. We also found that EPA and DHA increased gene expression of *Ppargc1α*, a master regulator of mitochondrial biogenesis leading to red type I fiber, also suggests genetic programing towards stimulating slower muscle fiber [49–52]. It is known that the products of peroxisomal β-oxidation are also targeted towards mitochondria for oxidation in skeletal muscle and therefore assist in complete lipid disposal [53]. Further support for an effect on muscle fiber type comes from stimulation of insulin growth factor 1 (*Igf*-1), which regulates the *Akt* pathway. Activation of *Akt* phosphorylates *Gsk3*β thereby inactivating it. *Gsk3*β phosphorylates *Nfat* and excluding its entry into the nucleus and subsequent DNA binding [54], which would down-regulate slow-fiber gene expression. In our study, *Gsk3*β was downregulated in the gSkM of HFD-ED compared with HFD-corn oil animals, indicating little Nfat phosphorylation and thus, conditions that would favor production of slow-fiber type. Resistance training, testosterone treatment, growth hormone, or dehydroepiandrosterone interventions have shown favorable effects in retaining muscle mass and function [19,55–58]. However, long-term use of growth hormone treatment can be harmful due to associated side effects, making this a poor choice for intervention against muscle loss. Our findings suggest a mechanistic basis for the human results and supports the case for further research on either

ED or fish oil supplements as potential molecules for the long-term prevention of sarcopenia. In this study we were unable to determine if muscle fiber type regulation is due to the effects of increased β-oxidation, or a direct effect of EPA or DHA on gene transcription.

Although the effects of EPA and DHA on gSkM gene expression are conclusive, due to the limited sample amount we have been unable to validate many of the possible physiological effects found from transcriptome analysis. Ideally, future work should study these effects across a wider range of SkM and perform histology to confirm the hypothesis on fiber-type regulation. Similarly, our results suggest an effect on many parameters related to energy metabolism, supported in part by finding a lower fat content in the gSkM of HFD-ED fed mice compared with HFD-corn oil. Future work will need to see if this effect extends to improved glucose disposal which could extend the findings to possible relevance for T2D. A role for regulation of calcium concentrations for signaling should also be tested using muscle cell models. Future work will also need to test if these pathways are still relatively upregulated with lower proportions of n-3 fatty acids and at lower amounts, to test if they are relevant at normal amounts of dietary fat.

These results clearly demonstrate the wide-ranging impact a difference in dietary fatty acid composition can have on SkM gene-transcription. It is unclear if ED regulates all of these gene targets simultaneously, or if some are a result of downstream interactions with initial ED targets. Given the clear sequential effects on energy metabolism from β-oxidation to oxidative phosphorylation, it appears likely that the observed upregulation of these processes is directly related to increased circulating EPA and DHA. Further studies on cell and rodent models of ageing and functional analysis of SkM are required to confirm these effects and the likely regulatory nodes for these mechanisms.

5. Conclusions

The skeletal muscle transcriptome from mice fed HFDs differing in fat composition for 8 weeks, showed marked differences in expression of genes coding for metabolic proteins. Our results suggest muscle-protective effects of EPA and DHA against catabolic degradation, possibly via stimulation of pathways that increase mitochondrial β-oxidation capacity and control calcium release for muscle contraction. These shifts in gene expression, even against a background of HFD are clearly favorable for hindering molecular progression towards muscle loss. With the limited availability of clinical treatments for preventing muscle loss, increased intake of fatty fish that are abundant in EPA and DHA, or supplementation with marine fatty acids could provide a safe and economic alternative to pharmaceutical interventions.

Supplementary Materials

Figure S1: Protein lysate from the gSkM of HFD-ED and HFD-corn oil were analyzed by Western blot using antibodies for total Acc, p-Acc (Ser79) and total anti-Troponin C1. Gapdh was used as a loading control for the Western blot, Figure S2:(a) Principle Component Analysis (PCA) plot based on the normalized gene expression from the gSkM tissue fed control, HFD-ED and HFD-corn oil is plotted for assessing the quality of the datasets. No animals or any related data was excluded from further assessment. (b) Venn diagrams showing the number of differentially expressed genes (FDR adjusted p-value < 0.001) in each diet-comparison for gSkM tissue. HFD-ED compared with control diet and HFD-corn oil fed mice shows most transcriptional response to the diet. Key: ED = HFD-ED; CO = HFD-corn oil and CD = control diet, Figure S3: (a) Fatty acid β-oxidation pathway rendered by the pathview function from the Kegg pathway database. Genes highlighted in red are upregulated for the comparison HFD-ED vs. HFD-corn oil. (b) Krebs cycle pathway rendered by the pathview function from the Kegg pathway database. Genes highlighted in red are upregulated for the comparison HFD-ED vs. HFD-corn oil. (c) Oxidative phosphorylation pathway rendered by the pathview function from the Kegg pathway database. Genes highlighted in red are upregulated for the comparison HFD-ED vs. HFD-corn oil, Table S1: Table for the selection criteria for animals for microarray analysis. Animals marked in green were selected for microarray analysis, Table S2: The top 100 differentially regulated genes regulated by HFD-ED compared to HFD-corn oil fed mice, based on adjusted p-value.

Acknowledgments: The study was supported by grants from Stiftelsen Olle Engkvist, Byggmästare; The Swedish Research Council for Environment, Agricultural Sciences and Spatial Planning (222-2011-1322); the Region of Västra Götaland (VGR; RUN 612-0959-11) and the Swedish Research Council (VR project number 2013-4504). IN gracefully acknowledge Swedish Research Council (VR-2013-4504). We would like to acknowledge SCIBLU, Lund University for the labelling of RNA and hybridization to the Illumina microarrays chips, and CBI, University of Gothenburg, for the assistance with the animal experiments. We also acknowledge Chalmers Mass Spectrometry Infrastructure (CMSI), Chalmers University of Technology for their help with fatty acid profiling. We also gratefully acknowledge the kind gifts of the EPAX oils from EPAX AS, Norway (now FMC Corporation, USA).

Author Contributions: B.G., I.N., and A.S. designed the study. B.G. performed the animal experiments; B.G. and N.So. conducted the RNA isolation and microarray data collection. I.N. coordinated microarray experiment and analysis. N.So. and O.I.S. performed fatty acid analysis. N.So. performed statistical analyses and wrote the manuscript. A.B.R. and N.Sc. aided in the interpretation of the data and gave their input during the preparation of manuscript. All authors reviewed and approved the final version of manuscript.

References and Notes

1. World Health Organization. *Obesity and Overweight Fact Sheet N°311*; World Health Organization Media Centre: Geneva, Switzerland, 2015.
2. Lauretani, F.; Russo, C.R.; Bandinelli, S.; Bartali, B.; Cavazzini, C.; Di Iorio, A.; Corsi, A.M.; Rantanen, T.; Guralnik, J.M.; Ferrucci, L. Age-associated changes in skeletal muscles and their effect on mobility: An operational diagnosis of sarcopenia. *J. Appl. Physiol.* **2003**, *95*, 1851–1860. [CrossRef] [PubMed]
3. Candow, D.G.; Chilibeck, P.D. Differences in size, strength, and power of upper and lower body muscle groups in young and older men. *J. Gerontol.* **2005**, *60*, 148–156. [CrossRef]
4. Von Haehling, S.; Morley, J.E.; Anker, S.D. An overview of sarcopenia: Facts and numbers on prevalence and clinical impact. *J. Cachexia Sarcopenia Muscle* **2010**, *1*, 129–133. [CrossRef] [PubMed]
5. Rosenberg, I.H. Sarcopenia: Origins and clinical relevance. *J. Nutr.* **1997**, *127*, 990S–991S. [CrossRef] [PubMed]
6. Schmidt, M.; Johannesdottir, S.A.; Lemeshow, S.; Lash, T.L.; Ulrichsen, S.P.; Botker, H.E.; Sorensen, H.T. Obesity in young men, and individual and combined risks of type 2 diabetes, cardiovascular morbidity and death before 55 years of age: A danish 33-year follow-up study. *BMJ Open* **2013**, *3*. [CrossRef] [PubMed]
7. Roubenoff, R. Sarcopenic obesity: The confluence of two epidemics. *Obes. Res.* **2004**, *12*, 887–888. [CrossRef] [PubMed]
8. Schaap, L.A.; Pluijm, S.M.; Deeg, D.J.; Harris, T.B.; Kritchevsky, S.B.; Newman, A.B.; Colbert, L.H.; Pahor, M.; Rubin, S.M.; Tylavsky, F.A.; et al. Higher inflammatory marker levels in older persons: Associations with 5-year change in muscle mass and muscle strength. *J. Gerontol.* **2009**, *64*, 1183–1189. [CrossRef] [PubMed]
9. Visser, M.; Pahor, M.; Taaffe, D.R.; Goodpaster, B.H.; Simonsick, E.M.; Newman, A.B.; Nevitt, M.; Harris, T.B. Relationship of interleukin-6 and tumor necrosis factor-alpha with muscle mass and muscle strength in elderly men and women: The health abc study. *J. Gerontol.* **2002**, *57*, M326–M332. [CrossRef]
10. Zhao, X.; Wang, Z.; Zhang, J.; Hua, J.; He, W.; Zhu, S. Estimation of total body skeletal muscle mass in chinese adults: Prediction model by dual-energy X-ray absorptiometry. *PLoS ONE* **2013**, *8*. [CrossRef] [PubMed]
11. Kim, J.; Wang, Z.; Heymsfield, S.B.; Baumgartner, R.N.; Gallagher, D. Total-body skeletal muscle mass: Estimation by a new dual-energy X-ray absorptiometry method. *Am. J. Clin. Nutr.* **2002**, *76*, 378–383.
12. Meyer, C.; Dostou, J.M.; Welle, S.L.; Gerich, J.E. Role of human liver, kidney, and skeletal muscle in postprandial glucose homeostasis. *Am. J. Physiol. Endocrinol. Metab.* **2002**, *282*, 419–427. [CrossRef] [PubMed]
13. Smith, G.I.; Julliand, S.; Reeds, D.N.; Sinacore, D.R.; Klein, S.; Mittendorfer, B. Fish oil-derived *n*-3 pufa therapy increases muscle mass and function in healthy older adults. *Am. J. Clin. Nutr.* **2015**, *102*, 115–122. [CrossRef] [PubMed]
14. Alexander, J.W.; Saito, H.; Trocki, O.; Ogle, C.K. The importance of lipid type in the diet after burn injury. *Ann. Surg.* **1986**, *204*, 1–8. [CrossRef] [PubMed]
15. Gingras, A.A.; White, P.J.; Chouinard, P.Y.; Julien, P.; Davis, T.A.; Dombrowski, L.; Couture, Y.; Dubreuil, P.; Myre, A.; Bergeron, K.; et al. Long-chain omega-3 fatty acids regulate bovine whole-body protein metabolism by promoting muscle insulin signalling to the akt-mtor-s6k1 pathway and insulin sensitivity. *J. Physiol.* **2007**, *579*, 269–284. [CrossRef] [PubMed]
16. Fetterman, J.W., Jr.; Zdanowicz, M.M. Therapeutic potential of *n*-3 polyunsaturated fatty acids in disease. *Am. J Health Syst. Pharm.* **2009**, *66*, 1169–1179. [CrossRef] [PubMed]

17. Gabrielsson, B.G.; Wikstrom, J.; Jakubowicz, R.; Marmon, S.K.; Carlsson, N.G.; Jansson, N.; Gan, L.M.; Undeland, I.; Lonn, M.; Holmang, A.; et al. Dietary herring improves plasma lipid profiles and reduces atherosclerosis in obese low-density lipoprotein receptor-deficient mice. *Int. J. Mol. Med.* **2012**, *29*, 331–337. [CrossRef] [PubMed]
18. Nookaew, I.; Gabrielsson, B.G.; Holmang, A.; Sandberg, A.S.; Nielsen, J. Identifying molecular effects of diet through systems biology: Influence of herring diet on sterol metabolism and protein turnover in mice. *PLoS ONE* **2010**, *5*. [CrossRef] [PubMed]
19. Rodacki, C.L.; Rodacki, A.L.; Pereira, G.; Naliwaiko, K.; Coelho, I.; Pequito, D.; Fernandes, L.C. Fish-oil supplementation enhances the effects of strength training in elderly women. *Am. J. Clin. Nutr.* **2012**, *95*, 428–436. [CrossRef] [PubMed]
20. Smith, G.I.; Atherton, P.; Reeds, D.N.; Mohammed, B.S.; Rankin, D.; Rennie, M.J.; Mittendorfer, B. Dietary omega-3 fatty acid supplementation increases the rate of muscle protein synthesis in older adults: A randomized controlled trial. *Am. J. Clin. Nutr.* **2011**, *93*, 402–412. [CrossRef] [PubMed]
21. Soni, N.K.; Nookaew, I.; Sandberg, A.S.; Gabrielsson, B.G. Eicosapentaenoic and docosahexaenoic acid-enriched high fat diet delays the development of fatty liver in mice. *Lipids Health Dis.* **2015**, *14*. [CrossRef] [PubMed]
22. Amrutkar, M.; Cansby, E.; Nunez-Duran, E.; Piraz zi, C.; Stahlman, M.; Stenfeldt, E.; Smith, U.; Boren, J.; Mahlapuu, M. Protein kinase stk25 regulates hepatic lipid partitioning and progression of liver steatosis and nash. *FASEB J.* **2015**, *29*, 1564–1576. [CrossRef] [PubMed]
23. For More Information about ncbi refseq, Please Go to http://ftp.Ncbi.Nih.Gov/refseq/release/.
24. For More Information about meebo, Please Go to http://www.Arrays.Ucsf.Edu/archive/meebo.Html.
25. Functional Annotation of Mouse. Available online: http://fantom2.Gsc.Riken.Jp/ (accessed on 25 August 2016).
26. Du, P.; Kibbe, W.A.; Lin, S.M. Lumi: A pipeline for processing illumina microarray. *Bioinformatics* **2008**, *24*, 1547–1548. [CrossRef] [PubMed]
27. Ritchie, M.E.; Phipson, B.; Wu, D.; Hu, Y.; Law, C.W.; Shi, W.; Smyth, G.K. Limma powers differential expression analyses for RNA-sequencing and microarray studies. *Nucl. Acids Res.* **2015**, *43*. [CrossRef]
28. Luo, W.; Friedman, M.S.; Shedden, K.; Hankenson, K.D.; Woolf, P.J. Gage: Generally applicable gene set enrichment for pathway analysis. *BMC Bioinformatics* **2009**, *10*, 1–17. [CrossRef] [PubMed]
29. Luo, W.; Brouwer, C. Pathview: An R/Bioconductor package for pathway-based data integration and visualization. *Bioinformatics* **2013**, *29*. [CrossRef] [PubMed]
30. Folch, J.; Lees, M.; Stanley, G.H.S. A simple method for the isolation and purification of total lipids from animal tissues. *J. Biol. Chem.* **1957**, *226*, 497–509. [PubMed]
31. Kaluzny, M.A.; Duncan, L.A.; Merritt, M.V.; Epps, D.E. Rapid separation of lipid classes in high yield and purity using bonded phase columns. *J. Lipid Res.* **1985**, *26*, 135–140. [PubMed]
32. Lepage, G.; Roy, C.C. Improved recovery of fatty acid through direct transesterification without prior extraction or purification. *J. Lipid. Res.* **1984**, *25*, 1391–1396. [PubMed]
33. Tuazon, M.A.; Henderson, G.C. Fatty acid profile of skeletal muscle phospholipid is altered in mdx mice and is predictive of disease markers. *Metable* **2012**, *61*, 801–811. [CrossRef] [PubMed]
34. Lowell, B.B.; Shulman, G.I. Mitochondrial dysfunction and type 2 diabetes. *Science* **2005**, *307*, 384–387. [CrossRef] [PubMed]
35. Petersen, K.F.; Dufour, S.; Befroy, D.; Garcia, R.; Shulman, G.I. Impaired mitochondrial activity in the insulin-resistant offspring of patients with type 2 diabetes. *N. Engl. J. Med.* **2004**, *350*, 664–671. [CrossRef] [PubMed]
36. Patti, M.E.; Butte, A.J.; Crunkhorn, S.; Cusi, K.; Berria, R.; Kashyap, S.; Miyazaki, Y.; Kohane, I.; Costello, M.; Saccone, R.; et al. Coordinated reduction of genes of oxidative metabolism in humans with insulin resistance and diabetes: Potential role of pgc1 and nrf1. *Proc. Natl. Acad. Sci. USA* **2003**, *100*, 8466–8471. [CrossRef] [PubMed]
37. Sparks, L.M.; Xie, H.; Koza, R.A.; Mynatt, R.; Hulver, M.W.; Bray, G.A.; Smith, S.R. A high-fat diet coordinately downregulates genes required for mitochondrial oxidative phosphorylation in skeletal muscle. *Diabetes* **2005**, *54*, 1926–1933. [CrossRef] [PubMed]
38. Mootha, V.K.; Lindgren, C.M.; Eriksson, K.F.; Subramanian, A.; Sihag, S.; Lehar, J.; Puigserver, P.; Carlsson, E.; Ridderstrale, M.; Laurila, E.; et al. Pgc-1alpha-responsive genes involved in oxidative phosphorylation are coordinately downregulated in human diabetes. *Nat. Genet.* **2003**, *34*, 267–273. [CrossRef] [PubMed]

39. Choi, C.S.; Savage, D.B.; Abu-Elheiga, L.; Liu, Z.X.; Kim, S.; Kulkarni, A.; Distefano, A.; Hwang, Y.J.; Reznick, R.M.; Codella, R.; et al. Continuous fat oxidation in acetyl-coa carboxylase 2 knockout mice increases total energy expenditure, reduces fat mass, and improves insulin sensitivity. *Proc. Natl. Acad. Sci. USA* **2007**, *104*, 16480–16485. [CrossRef] [PubMed]
40. Bruce, C.R.; Hoy, A.J.; Turner, N.; Watt, M.J.; Allen, T.L.; Carpenter, K.; Cooney, G.J.; Febbraio, M.A.; Kraegen, E.W. Overexpression of carnitine palmitoyltransferase-1 in skeletal muscle is sufficient to enhance fatty acid oxidation and improve high-fat diet-induced insulin resistance. *Diabetes* **2009**, *58*, 550–558. [CrossRef] [PubMed]
41. Schwerzmann, K.; Hoppeler, H.; Kayar, S.R.; Weibel, E.R. Oxidative capacity of muscle and mitochondria: Correlation of physiological, biochemical, and morphometric characteristics. *Proc. Natl. Acad. Sci. USA* **1989**, *86*, 1583–1587. [CrossRef] [PubMed]
42. Petersen, K.F.; Befroy, D.; Dufour, S.; Dziura, J.; Ariyan, C.; Rothman, D.L.; DiPietro, L.; Cline, G.W.; Shulman, G.I. Mitochondrial dysfunction in the elderly: Possible role in insulin resistance. *Science* **2003**, *300*, 1140–1142. [CrossRef] [PubMed]
43. Periasamy, M.; Kalyanasundaram, A. Serca pump isoforms: Their role in calcium transport and disease. *Muscle Nerve* **2007**, *35*, 430–442. [CrossRef] [PubMed]
44. Radzyukevich, T.L.; Neumann, J.C.; Rindler, T.N.; Oshiro, N.; Goldhamer, D.J.; Lingrel, J.B.; Heiny, J.A. Tissue-specific role of the na,k-atpase alpha2 isozyme in skeletal muscle. *J. Biol. Chem.* **2013**, *288*, 1226–1237. [CrossRef] [PubMed]
45. Dunn, S.E.; Burns, J.L.; Michel, R.N. Calcineurin is required for skeletal muscle hypertrophy. *J. Biol. Chem.* **1999**, *274*, 21908–21912. [CrossRef] [PubMed]
46. Dunn, S.E.; Chin, E.R.; Michel, R.N. Matching of calcineurin activity to upstream effectors is critical for skeletal muscle fiber growth. *J. Cell. Biol.* **2000**, *151*, 663–672. [CrossRef] [PubMed]
47. Dunn, S.E.; Simard, A.R.; Bassel-Duby, R.; Williams, R.S.; Michel, R.N. Nerve activity-dependent modulation of calcineurin signaling in adult fast and slow skeletal muscle fibers. *J. Biol. Chem.* **2001**, *276*, 45243–45254. [CrossRef] [PubMed]
48. Hughes, S.M.; Taylor, J.M.; Tapscott, S.J.; Gurley, C.M.; Carter, W.J.; Peterson, C.A. Selective accumulation of myod and myogenin mrnas in fast and slow adult skeletal muscle is controlled by innervation and hormones. *Development* **1993**, *118*, 1137–1147.
49. Lin, J.; Wu, H.; Tarr, P.T.; Zhang, C.Y.; Wu, Z.; Boss, O.; Michael, L.F.; Puigserver, P.; Isotani, E.; Olson, E.N.; et al. Transcriptional co-activator pgc-1 alpha drives the formation of slow-twitch muscle fibres. *Nature* **2002**, *418*, 797–801. [CrossRef] [PubMed]
50. Vega, R.B.; Huss, J.M.; Kelly, D.P. The coactivator pgc-1 cooperates with peroxisome proliferator-activated receptor alpha in transcriptional control of nuclear genes encoding mitochondrial fatty acid oxidation enzymes. *Mol. Cell Biol.* **2000**, *20*, 1868–1876. [CrossRef] [PubMed]
51. Wu, Z.; Puigserver, P.; Andersson, U.; Zhang, C.; Adelmant, G.; Mootha, V.; Troy, A.; Cinti, S.; Lowell, B.; Scarpulla, R.C.; et al. Mechanisms controlling mitochondrial biogenesis and respiration through the thermogenic coactivator PGC-1. *Cell* **1999**, *98*, 115–124. [CrossRef]
52. Puigserver, P.; Wu, Z.; Park, C.W.; Graves, R.; Wright, M.; Spiegelman, B.M. A cold-inducible coactivator of nuclear receptors linked to adaptive thermogenesis. *Cell* **1998**, *92*, 829–839. [CrossRef]
53. Noland, R.C.; Woodlief, T.L.; Whitfield, B.R.; Manning, S.M.; Evans, J.R.; Dudek, R.W.; Lust, R.M.; Cortright, R.N. Peroxisomal-mitochondrial oxidation in a rodent model of obesity-associated insulin resistance. *Am. J. Physiol. Endocrinol. Metab.* **2007**, *293*, E986–E1001. [CrossRef] [PubMed]
54. Neal, J.W.; Clipstone, N.A. Glycogen synthase kinase-3 inhibits the DNA binding activity of NFATc. *J. Biol. Chem.* **2001**, *276*, 3666–3673. [CrossRef] [PubMed]
55. Baker, W.L.; Karan, S.; Kenny, A.M. Effect of dehydroepiandrosterone on muscle strength and physical function in older adults: A systematic review. *J. Am. Geriatr. Soc.* **2011**, *59*, 997–1002. [CrossRef] [PubMed]
56. Emmelot-Vonk, M.H.; Verhaar, H.J.; Pour, H.R.N.; Aleman, A.; Lock, T.M.; Bosch, J.L.; Grobbee, D.E.; van der Schouw, Y.T. Effect of testosterone supplementation on functional mobility, cognition, and other parameters in older men: A randomized controlled trial. *J. Am. Med. Assoc.* **2008**, *299*, 39–52. [CrossRef] [PubMed]

57. Giannoulis, M.G.; Sonksen, P.H.; Umpleby, M.; Breen, L.; Pentecost, C.; Whyte, M.; McMillan, C.V.; Bradley, C.; Martin, F.C. The effects of growth hormone and/or testosterone in healthy elderly men: A randomized controlled trial. *J. Clin. Endocrinol. Metab.* **2006**, *91*, 477–484. [CrossRef] [PubMed]
58. Kirwan, J.P.; Solomon, T.P.; Wojta, D.M.; Staten, M.A.; Holloszy, J.O. Effects of 7 days of exercise training on insulin sensitivity and responsiveness in type 2 diabetes mellitus. *Am. J. Physiol. Endocrinol. Metab.* **2009**, *297*, E151–E156. [CrossRef] [PubMed]

11

An Exploratory Study Examining Obesity Risk in Non-Obese Mothers of Young Children Using a Socioecological Approach

Jennifer Martin-Biggers [1], Virginia Quick [1,*], Kim Spaccarotella [2] and Carol Byrd-Bredbenner [1]

[1] Department of Nutritional Sciences, Rutgers University, 26 Nichol Avenue, New Brunswick, NJ 08901, USA; jmartinbiggers@rutgers.edu (J.M.-B.); bredbenner@sebs.rutgers.edu (C.B.-B.)

[2] Department of Biological Sciences, Kean University, 1000 Morris Avenue, Union, NJ 07082, USA; kspaccar@kean.edu

* Correspondence: vquick@njaes.rutgers.edu

Abstract: This cross-sectional, exploratory study aimed to (1) develop an obesity risk score using a comprehensive set of variables assessing mothers' intrapersonal weight-related characteristics and those of their homes' interpersonal and physical environments, and (2) determine how weight-related characteristics differ by obesity risk level. U.S. mothers (N = 550) of preschool-aged children completed an online survey that assessed maternal self-report weight status, sociodemographics, health-related characteristics, and maternal intrapersonal and their homes' interpersonal and physical environment weight-related characteristics. Binomial logistic regression analysis identified variables significantly associated with obesity. Scores for all obesity risk variables were summed to create a weighted obesity risk score for non-obese participants (n = 386). Analysis of variance and Tukey post-hoc tests determined how non-obese mothers' sociodemographic, health-related, and intrapersonal and their homes' interpersonal and physical environment characteristics differed among obesity risk score tertiles. Results revealed that eight variables explained 53 percent of maternal obesity risk, including African American race, lower education level, more children in household, poorer maternal health, higher weight teasing history, higher body dissatisfaction, primary relative with obesity, and greater concern about children's overweight risk. Non-obese mothers in the highest obesity risk tertile had greater food insecurity risk, lower family affluence, worse sleep quality, less fruit/vegetable availability, and reported less frequent modeling of healthy behaviors and more family conflict. In conclusion, eight characteristics that explained more than half of the risk for obesity in non-obese mothers of young children, may help healthcare professionals identify mothers at increased risk of obesity and offer preventive care early.

Keywords: obesity risk; mothers; women; young children; socioecological

---

1. Introduction

Recent data from the National Health and Nutrition Examination Survey (NHANES) indicate that nearly 34.9 percent of U.S. adults are obese [1]. It is no longer debated that obesity and its comorbidities are significantly impacting Americans both in financial and quality of life costs. A systematic review of 33 studies found that the overall estimated medical costs of obesity accounted for approximately 10 percent of all medical spending in the United States [2]. The physical health consequences of obesity are numerous and include effects on the pulmonary, orthopedic, neurological, gastroenterological, endocrine, and cardiovascular systems, as well as causing systemic inflammation, thereby greatly impacting quality of life [3–6].

The increase in obesity rates in the U.S. likely reflects changes in environmental factors and lifestyle choices related to increased energy intake and inadequate energy expenditure, rather than genetic changes because of the slow rate at which population-wide genetic changes occur [7–9]. Changes in lifestyles and the environment that have occurred in tandem with the increase in obesity include ready availability of food and shifting dietary patterns, which have led to an increase in calorie intake [10,11], combined with a decline in energy expenditure associated with a sedentary lifestyle [12]. Macro-level factors have a more indirect (yet important) role in influencing behaviors and include social norms, agriculture policies, economic policies, advertising, and more. Factors that are more directly influenced by an individual include his or her physical and social environments and personal factors (e.g., home environment, skills, behaviors).

In recent years, health behavior change experts have recognized the influence of factors in the physical environment, as well as in the social environment, on obesity and health outcomes [13]. This ecological approach to public health issues posits that an individual's motivation and skills alone are not adequate to facilitate behavior change; environments also need to support and facilitate the practice of healthful behaviors [14–16]. Reciprocal determinism, a construct of the Social Cognitive Theory, describes how a person's characteristics and behaviors, as well as the physical and social environment where behaviors occur, mutually affect each other [17]. Environments not supportive of weight-management behaviors make it difficult to engage in practices that prevent unhealthy weight gain. Research has increasingly provided evidence that environmental factors significantly influence diet, physical activity, and obesity in adults [15,18,19] and children [16,20–22], yet their relative contribution to obesity risk remains unknown.

The home environment deserves in-depth study given its potential influence on health behaviors [23]. An understanding of factors in the home environment associated with obesity could assist healthcare providers, researchers, parents, and caregivers in creating home environments that support healthy weights for the whole family. Mothers tend to be food gatekeepers in the home and, thus, are well suited to providing an appraisal of their homes' social (interpersonal) and physical environment characteristics [23,24]. Mothers also are children's role models and often the household food decision-maker, thus mothers' own intrapersonal cognitions, behaviors, and weight status play a role in weight-related decisions affecting the entire family [23,24]. Moreover, behaviors directly affecting weight are developed during childhood and track into adulthood [25–28], thereby making it vital to identify factors affecting maternal obesity risk and address them in obesity prevention interventions. A deeper understanding of the full interplay of intrapersonal and interpersonal characteristics and behaviors along with environments could provide a more complete picture of the aspects of the home environment that may place mothers of young children at risk for weight gain. A method for assessing risk for weight gain could enable health care providers and researchers to tailor and design more effective nutrition education.

Health experts acknowledge that lifestyles and the environment play a role in obesity risk [29]; however, few studies have considered these factors when examining obesity risk and none could be located that examined a comprehensive array of factors. Thus, the aims of this exploratory study were to (1) develop an obesity risk score using a comprehensive set of variables assessing mothers' own intrapersonal weight-related characteristics as well as the weight-related characteristics of their homes' interpersonal and physical environments, and (2) determine how these weight-related characteristics differ among levels of obesity risk.

2. Materials and Methods

This research was approved by the Institutional Review Board at Rutgers University. All participants gave informed consent.

2.1. *Sample*

Survey Sampling International (SSI), a global research company whose services include survey sample participant recruitment (www.surveysampling.com), was utilized. SSI panel members received invitations to participate in an online survey that would help researchers create "a program to help parents to build healthier kids". The goal was to recruit mothers of children in the target age range who had most of the food decision-making authority in their households to adequately capture the most representative responses. To meet eligibility requirements, panel members had to be female, between 18- and 45-years-old, have one or more children 2- to 5-years-old, and be the household's primary food gatekeeper (i.e., made most or all food purchasing and preparation decisions). As an incentive to complete the cross-sectional online survey, participating mothers accrued points from SSI that were redeemable for gifts. A total sample size of 384 was estimated based on a 95% confidence interval, and total population of women in the U.S. that are 20–45 years old using 2010 U.S. Census data [30].

2.2. *Instrument*

Development and content of the online Home Obesogenicity Measure of EnvironmentS (HOMES) survey is described in detail elsewhere [31–33]. In summary, development began with a comprehensive literature review to identify salient weight-related demographic, environmental, behavioral, and psychographic characteristics. Self-report scales assessing these characteristics, preferably those previously used and validated with a diverse sample of U.S. adults, also were identified. When multiple scales for assessing a characteristic were found, each was reviewed to determine which was most relevant to the study sample, easy to administer and score, and had good reliability and validity. If an instrument assessing a characteristic of interest or fitting the needs of the study could not be located in the literature, items were developed *de novo*. For scales with items substantially modified from their original form or developed *de novo*, standard processes for developing and refining scales were applied [34]. That is, experts (n = 5) in subject matter areas appropriate to the scale content (e.g., nutrition, physical activity, psychology, child development, obesogenic environment), psychometrics, and survey design iteratively reviewed and refined them to ensure scale clarity and content validity [34,35]. The items then underwent cognitive testing with participants who were similar to the study population to assess whether the items were interpreted as intended [35] and to determine ways to reduce participant burden and increase understandability and acceptability [36].

After refinement, the scales were consolidated into a single survey that was posted online (using Qualtrics®). The survey was pilot-tested with 48 participants whose characteristics were the same as those of the target audience for the final study (but were not participants in the final sample) to gauge completion time, identify further refinements needed to improve clarity and ease of completion, ensure protocols for scoring of scales were accurate, and conduct preliminary psychometric analyses. The survey was administered online for ease of data collection and convenience to participants, to help reduce the potential for social desirability bias that can occur during in-person administration, and to increase researcher ability to reach individuals who would be otherwise difficult to access (i.e., distance from researchers or limited time to meet in-person) [37,38].

The HOMES survey included an array of measures that focused on mother's intrapersonal weight-related characteristics and their homes' interpersonal and physical environment characteristics and yielded 79 variables. Table 1 lists the variables in the HOMES survey considered in the creation of the obesity risk score, including number of items, possible score range, and Cronbach's alpha (when applicable).

Table 1. Description of Sociodemographic, Intrapersonal, Interpersonal and Home Environment Characteristics of Participants (N = 550).

Measure	# Items	Possible Score Range	Scale Type	Cronbach's α	Mean ± SD or N (%)
Sociodemographic Characteristics					
Race/Ethnicity	1	n/a	categorical response	*	
White					396 (72.0)
Black or African American					52 (9.5)
Hispanic					25 (4.5)
Multi-racial					43 (7.8)
Asian					31 (5.6)
Other					3 (0.6)
Education Level	1	n/a	categorical response	*	
High School or less					99 (18.0)
Some college or technical/Associate's degree					245 (44.5)
Bachelor's degree or higher					206 (37.5)
Maternal Employment	1	n/a	categorical response	*	
Do not work					303 (55.1)
Part-time (less than 30 h/week)					103 (18.7)
Full-time (30 or more h/week)					143 (26.0)
Number of Children in Household	1	0 to more than 6	Total #	*	2.20 ± 1.01
Family Affluence Score [39,40]	3	0 to 7	varies per item [A]	*	5.61 ± 1.56
Food Insecurity Risk [41]	2	1 to 4	4-point agreement rating [B]	0.84	2.04 ± 1.91
Weight Status					
Mother's BMI	1	n/a	Self-reported height/weight	*	27.69 ± 7.90
Child's BMI percentile (n = 339)	1	n/a	Self-reported height/weight/sex/age	*	63.93 ± 34.93
Health-Related Assessments					
General Health Rating [42,43]	1	1 to 5	5-point excellence rating [C]	*	3.52 ± 0.87
Health-related Quality of Life (# of unhealthy days) [42,43]	1	0 to 30	days/month	*	2.89 ± 4.56
Depression Severity [44]	2	1 to 4	4-point occurrence rating [D]	0.81	1.05 ± 1.44
Age at Birth of First Child (years)	1	n/a	years	*	24.46 ± 5.39
Perception of Weight Teasing History [45]	3	1 to 5	5-point frequency rating [E]	0.95	1.84 ± 1.15
Body Dissatisfaction [46]	1	1 to 4	4-point frequency rating [F]	*	2.58 ± 1.10
Primary Relative with History of Obesity (% yes)	1	0 or 1	yes/no	*	207 (37.6)
Primary Relative with History of Diabetes (% yes)	1	0 or 1	yes/no	*	140 (25.5)

Table 1. *Cont.*

Measure	# Items	Possible Score Range	Scale Type	Cronbach's α	Mean ± SD or *N* (%)
Intrapersonal Characteristics					
Maternal Weight-Related Behaviors					
Physical Activity Level [47–49]	3	0 to 42	8-point exercise scale [G]	*	15.44 ± 9.98
Screentime	1	0 to 1440	minutes/day	*	273.52 ± 253.99
Sleep Duration	1	0 to 24	hours/day	*	7.11 ± 1.84
Sleep Quality [50,51]	1	1 to 5	5-point rating [H]	*	3.24 ± 0.89
Fruit and Vegetable Intake [52–54]	10	0 to 12.17	6-point servings [I] eaten per day scale	*	4.56 ± 2.22
% Calories from Total Fat [52–54]	17	0 to 100	5-point servings eaten scale [J]	*	37.4 ± 5.91
Milk [55,56]	1	0 to 8	9-point servings drank per day scale [K]	*	3.95 ± 3.08
Sugar-Sweetened Beverage [55,56]	4	0 to 4.6	9-point servings drank per day scale [K]	*	0.89 ± 0.88
Maternal Eating Styles					
Disinhibited Eating [57,58]	3	1 to 4	4-point agreement rating [B]	0.81	1.96 ± 0.76
Emotional Eating [57,58]	3	1 to 4	4-point agreement rating [B]	0.75	2.07 ± 0.88
Dietary Restraint Eating [57,58]	4	1 to 4	4-point agreement rating [B]	0.74	2.42 ± 0.74
Adventurous Eating [59–61]	2	1 to 4	4-point agreement rating [B]	0.72	3.16 ± 0.68
Maternal Self-Perceptions					
Personal Organization [62]	4	1 to 5	5-point agreement rating [L]	0.69	3.68 ± 0.82
Need for Cognition [63,64]	1	1 to 5	5-point agreement rating [L]	*	3.49 ± 0.98
Parenting Self-Efficacy [65,66]	1	1 to 5	5-point agreement rating [L]	*	4.1 ± 0.81
Stress Management [67]	2	1 to 4	4-point agreement rating [D]	0.84	3.94 ± 0.76
Stress Management Self-Efficacy	2	1 to 4	4-point agreement rating [D]	0.79	2.63 ± 1.01
Child Weight Cognitions		1 to 5			
Belief that Chubby Kids are Healthy	2	1 to 5	5-point agreement rating [L]	0.65	2.70 ± 0.74
Concern for Child's Overweight Risk [68]	3	1 to 5	5-point agreement rating [L]	0.91	1.91 ± 1.03
Health Behavior Values [31,69–72]					
Importance of Physical Activity for Self	3	1 to 5	5-point agreement rating [L]	0.82	3.49 ± 0.97
Importance of Physical Activity for Child	3	1 to 5	5-point agreement rating [L]	0.68	3.83 ± 0.87
Encourages/Facilitates Child Physical Activity	5	1 to 5	5-point agreement rating [L]	0.88	4.23 ± 0.66
Importance of Modeling Physical Activity to Child	2	1 to 5	5-point agreement rating [L]	0.79	4.13 ± 0.82
Engages in Physical Activity with Child Frequently	2	0 to 7	8-point frequency scale [M]	*	3.67 ± 1.85
Models Physical Activity to Child Frequently	2	0 to 7	8-point frequency scale [M]	*	3.08 ± 1.22
Models Sedentary Behaviors Infrequently	2	0 to 7	8-point frequency scale [M]	*	2.79 ± 2.18
Models Healthy Eating to Child	4	1 to 5	5-point agreement rating [L]	0.56	3.51 ± 0.73
Belief that TV Positively Affects Child Learning	2	1 to 5	5-point agreement rating [L]	0.85	3.89 ± 0.76
Talks Often with Child about TV	2	1 to 5	5-point agreement rating [L]	0.50	3.24 ± 0.97
Limits Child Exposure to TV Commercials and Inappropriate Programs Shows	2	1 to 5	5-point agreement rating [L]	0.50	3.67 ± 0.93
Limits Child to Educational TV	1	1 to 5	5-point agreement rating [L]	*	3.52 ± 1.09

Table 1. *Cont.*

Measure	# Items	Possible Score Range	Scale Type	Cronbach's α	Mean ± SD or *N* (%)
Home Interpersonal Characteristics					
Child Feeding Practices [68–71,73–75]					
Restricts Child Food Intake	2	1 to 5	5-point agreement rating [L]	0.63	3.84 ± 0.86
Pressures Child to Eat	3	1 to 5	5-point agreement rating [L]	0.69	2.17 ± 0.96
Maternal Control Over Child Food Access and Choices	7	1 to 5	5-point agreement rating [L]	0.65	3.33 ± 0.52
Non-Acceptance of Food Waste	2	1 to 5	5-point agreement rating [L]	0.61	3.05 ± 0.97
Instrumental Feeding Practices (uses food to reward children for eating a healthy food)	3	1 to 5	5-point agreement rating [L]	0.73	2.63 ± 0.91
Non-Food Rewards (uses non-food (e.g., extra playtime) to reward children for eating a healthy food)	2	1 to 5	5-point agreement rating [L]	0.65	2.90 ± 0.95
Allows Child to Independently Access Nutrient Dense Foods	5	0 to 5	yes/no	*	1.82 ± 1.74
Allows Child to Independently Access Low Nutrient Density Foods	6	0 to 6	yes/no	*	0.68 ± 1.32
Nutrient Dense Foods Stored in Locations Visible to Child	5	0 to 5	yes/no	*	2.44 ± 1.71
Low Nutrient Dense Foods Stored in Locations Visible to Child	6	0 to 6	yes/no	*	0.82 ± 1.35
Family Meal Patterns [70,76–80]					
Family Meal Frequency	3	0 to 21	0–7 days for breakfast, lunch, dinner; score is sum of 3 meals	*	13.64 ± 5.05
Importance of Family Meals	3	1 to 5	5-point agreement rating [L]	0.70	4.52 ± 0.64
Positive Family Meal Atmosphere	3	1 to 5	5-point agreement rating [L]	0.70	4.12 ± 0.85
Fast Food Eaten at Family Meals	1	0 to 7	days/week	*	0.93 ± 1.18
TV on During Family Meals	1	0 to 7	days/week	*	2.24 ± 2.48
Family Meals Eaten at Kitchen or Dining Table	1	0 to 7	days/week	*	4.69 ± 2.51
Family Meals Eaten in the Car	1	0 to 7	days/week	*	0.43 ± 1.16
Family Meal Planning	2	1 to 5	5-point agreement rating [L]	0.70	3.40 ± 0.88
Time and Energy for Family Meals	2	1 to 5	5-point agreement rating [L]	0.78	4.34 ± 0.85
Family Functioning and Maternal Engagement					
Family Support for Healthy Behaviors [81–83]	4	1 to 5	5-point agreement rating [L]	0.81	4.40 ± 0.73
Family Conflict and Lack of Cohesion [84–86]	5	1 to 5	5-point agreement rating [L]	0.84	1.83 ± 0.70
Household Disorganization [87,88]	3	1 to 5	5-point agreement rating [L]	0.76	2.47 ± 0.92
Verbal Engagement with Children	1	1 to 5	5-point agreement rating [L]	*	4.17 ± 0.93
Physical Engagement with Children	1	1 to 5	5-point agreement rating [L]	*	4.74 ± 0.51

Table 1. *Cont.*

Measure	# Items	Possible Score Range	Scale Type	Cronbach's α	Mean ± SD or *N* (%)
Home Physical Environment Characteristics					
Physical Activity [69–72,82,89]					
Physical Activity Availability	12	1 to 5	5-point agreement rating [L]	0.72	3.78 ± 0.67
Physical Activity Accessibility †	2	1 to 5	5-point agreement rating [L]	0.90	4.21 ± 1.14
Media Devices in the Home	6	0 to more than 10	Total devices [N]	*	11.57 ± 4.21
Media Devices in Child's Bedroom	7	0 to 7	Total # of media device types [O]	*	1.39 ± 1.62
Daily Screentime Child Allowed	1	0 to 1440	minutes/day	*	495.14 ± 714.22
Food Availability					
Household Fruit and Vegetable Availability (serving/person/day) [52,90]	10	0 to 19.94	9-point servings scale [P]	*	6.41 ± 2.53
Household Fatty/Salty Snack Availability (serving/person/day) [52,90]	4	0 to 32	9-point servings scale [P]	*	8.37 ± 7.22
Household Sugar-Sweetened Beverage Availability (serving/person/day) [55,56]	4	0 to 4.57	9-point servings scale [P]	*	1.87 ± 1.79
Household Breakfast Cereal Availability (serving/person/day) [52,90]	1	0 to 8	9-point servings scale [P]	*	5.35 ± 2.72

Note: n/a = not applicable. * Cronbach's alpha is not appropriate for the scale type or because the scale has <2 items. † n = 524. [A] Family affluence assessed by three questions asking the total number of cars, vans, or trucks the family owns (0 = none, 1 = 1 vehicle, 2 = 2 or more vehicles), # of times family traveled on vacation in past year (0 = never, 1 = 1 time, 2 = 2 times, 3 = 3 or more times), and whether participant had their own bedroom (1 = yes, 0 = no); items are summed. [B] 4-point Agreement Rating: definitely false, mostly false, mostly true, definitely true; scored 1 to 4, respectively. Items averaged with higher scores indicating greater expression of the trait. [C] 5-point Excellence Rating: poor, fair, good, very good, excellent; scored 1 to 5 respectively; higher score indicates better health. [D] 4-point Occurrence Rating: not at all, several days, more than half the days, nearly every day; scored 1 to 4, respectively; scale scores equals average of items with higher scores indicating greater expression of the behavior. [E] 5-point Frequency Rating: never, rarely, sometimes, often, very often; scored 1 to 5 respectively; scale score equals average of item scores with higher scores indicating greater weight teasing history. [F] 4-point Frequency Rating: not at all, slightly, moderately, a lot; scored 1 to 4 respectively; higher scores indicate greater body dissatisfaction. [G] 8-point Exercise Days/week: 0, 1, 2, 3, 4, 5, 6, and 7; days/week weighted by exercise intensity (weights of 1, 2, 3 for walking, moderate, and vigorous activity, respectively) and summed to create scale score; higher scale score indicates greater activity level. [H] 5-point rating scale: very good, good, okay, bad, and very bad; scored 1 to 5 respectively with higher scores indicate poorer sleep quality. [I] 6-point Fruit/Vegetable Servings Rating: <1 serving/week, 1 serving /week, 2 to 3 servings/week, 4 to 6 servings/week, 1 serving/day, 2 or more servings/day; scored 0 to 5 respectively; scale scoring algorithm is protected by copyright and described in detail elsewhere. Possible score range = 0 to 12.17. [J] 5-point Fatty Food Servings Rating: 1 time/month or less, 2 to 3 times/month, 1 to 2 times/week, 3 to 4 times/week, 5 or more times/week; scored 0 to 4 respectively; scale scoring algorithm is protected by copyright and described in detail elsewhere. [K] 9-point Beverage Servings Rating: <1 time/week, 1 day/week, 2 days/week, 3 days/week, 4 days/week, 5 days/week, 6 days/week, 7 days/week, >1 time/day; scored 0 to 8 respectively. Possible score ranges for Sugar-Sweetened Beverages = 0 to 4.6; Milk = 0 to 8. [L] 5-point Agreement Rating: strongly disagree, disagree, neither agree nor disagree, agree, strongly agree; scored 1 to 5 respectively; scale score equals average of item scores with higher scale score indicating greater expression of the trait. [M] 8-point Modeling Days/week: 0 (almost never), 1, 2, 3, 4, 5, 6, and 7; days averaged to create scale score with higher score indicating more frequent modeling. [N] 11-point Media Device Count: 1 = 1 to 10 = 10, 11 = more than 10; scale score equals sum of items; higher score indicates greater number of media devices. Possible score range = 0 to 66. [O] Sum of 7 media devices found in child's bedroom (i.e., TV, DVD player, Computer/Laptop, Smarphone/Tablet/LeapPad, video game devices (Nintendo DS, XBoxKinect), and Internet access). [P] 9-point Household Servings Rating: <1 time/week, 1 day/week, 2 days/week, 3 days/week, 4 days/week, 5 days/week, 6 days/week, 7 days/week, >1 time/day; scored 0 to 8 respectively. Possible score ranges for fruits/vegetables (0 to 19.94), salty/fatty snacks (0 to 32), sugar-sweetened beverages (0 to 4.57), and breakfast cereal (0 to 8) servings/household/member/day.

2.3. Sociodemographics and Health-Related Characteristics

Variables addressing maternal sociodemographic data included race/ethnicity, education level, number of children in the household, family affluence [39,40], maternal employment, and food insecurity risk [41]. There were eight variables examining health-related characteristics (e.g., general health status [42,43], health-related quality of life [42,43], depression severity [44], age at birth of first child, perception of weight teasing history [45], body dissatisfaction [46], primary relative with obesity and/or obesity.

2.3.1. Weight Status

Self-reported heights and weights of participants were used to calculate body mass index (BMI) (weight (kg)/(height (m^2)). Participants also reported their children's height, weight, sex, and age which were used to calculated their children's BMI percentile [91].

2.3.2. Intrapersonal Characteristics

Mothers' personal weight-related behaviors (e.g., physical activity level and screentime [47–49], sleep quality and duration [50,51], fruit/vegetable intake [52–54], percent calories from fat [52–54], milk intake [55,56], sugar-sweetened beverage intake [55,56]) accounted for eight variables. Scales evaluating maternal eating styles (e.g., disinhibited eating [57,58], emotional eating [57,58], dietary restraint eating [57,58], adventurous eating [59–61]) generated four variables. Five variables were produced from measures of mothers' self-perceptions (i.e., personal organization [62], need for cognition [63,64], parenting self-efficacy [65,66], stress management [67], stress management self-efficacy). Cognitions related to children's weight (i.e., belief that chubby kids are healthy, concern about own children's overweight risk [68]) were assessed with two scales. The value of engaging in healthy behaviors for self and child (i.e., importance placed on physical activity, encouragement and facilitation of children's physical activity, importance of modeling physical activity to children, frequency of engaging in active play with children, parent modeling of healthy eating, parenting cognitions and behaviors associated with children's television viewing) [31,69–72] was examined with 12 measures, each generating a variable.

2.3.3. Home Interpersonal Characteristics

Assessments of mothers' child feeding behaviors (e.g., food restriction, pressuring, rewarding) [68–71,73–75] yielded 10 variables. Family meal patterns (e.g., frequency and location of meals) [70,76–80] resulted in nine variables. Scales assessing family functioning and engagement (e.g., family support for healthy behaviors [81–83], family conflict and lack of cohesion [84–86], household organization [87,88]) included five variables.

2.3.4. Home Physical Environment

Appraisal of the home physical environment's accessibility to and availability of physical activity and sedentary activity opportunities (e.g., physical activity supports, media devices in the home, children's TV accessibility) [69–72,82,89] contributed five variables. Measures of household food availability (e.g., fruit/vegetables, sugar-sweetened beverages) [52,55,56,90] generated 4 variables.

2.4. Data Analysis

Internal consistencies of all measures, when applicable, were calculated using Cronbach's alpha. Descriptive statistics of all variables in the total sample were evaluated in four steps before further development of the obesity risk score. First, Spearman rank order correlations of all variables, except mothers' and children's weight status, were examined for multicollinearity. In the correlation matrix, race/ethnicity was categorized into two dichotomous variables (i.e., white or non-white, black or non-black) and education level was dichotomized into low (some college or less) or high (baccalaureate degree or higher). Variables that were intercorrelated (i.e., $r > 0.50$) were reviewed to select a single variable from among them to use in further analyses. The criterion for selecting a single variable from among those that were intercorrelated was that the variable under consideration had to be significantly correlated ($p < 0.05$) with maternal BMI. If none of the intercorrelated variables met this criterion, none were considered in further analyses. If more than one variable met this criterion, the variable with the highest correlation (absolute value) with maternal BMI was selected. In the second step of data analysis, binomial logistic regression was conducted to identify variables significantly associated with obesity. Variables remaining after the first step of the data analysis served as independent variables. The dependent variable was maternal weight status of obese (i.e., BMI ≥ 30) vs. non-obese (i.e., BMI ≤ 30). In step three of data analysis, the significant obesity risk variables identified in step two were again entered into the binomial logistic regression analysis to determine the best model fit and confirm results. In step four, data for non-obese mothers' were extracted from the data set and median scores were calculated for all variables found to be significantly associated with obesity.

To create the weighted obesity risk score, each non-obese mother was assigned a score for each obesity risk variable found in the regression model, as stated above, to be significantly associated with obesity. If a participant's score for an obesity risk variable was above the median for continuous variables or mothers had the characteristic for dichotomous variables, the score assigned for the variable was the beta coefficient value generated by the binomial logistic regression (reflecting an increased risk for obesity); if a particiapant's score was below the median for continuous variables or mothers did not have the characteristic for dichotomous variables, thereby indicating reduced obesity risk, a score of 0 was awarded for that variable. Scores for all obesity risk variables were then summed to yield a participant's total weighted obesity risk score.

To determine how non-obese mothers differed by obesity risk level, they were assigned to groups based on their obesity risk score tertile (i.e., low, moderate, and high risk). ANOVA and Tukey post-hoc tests were conducted to determine how maternal sociodemographic, health-related, and intrapersonal and their homes' interpersonal and physical environment characteristics differed among and between obesity risk score tertiles. For variables that were statically significant ($p < 0.05$), effect sizes were estimated by examining partial Eta squared, Analyses were performed with SPSS software version 24.0 (IBM corporation, Chicago, IL, USA). Given the number of variables investigated, significance level for main effects was set at 0.01 to reduce the risk of type 1 errors while maintaining sufficient power. Significance level for post-hoc procedures was set at $p < 0.05$.

3. Results

Out of 910 participants who responded to the online survey, only 550 participants were eligible and completed the survey (i.e., 188 did not complete the survey, 96 did not meet inclusion criteria, and 76 had implausible responses (e.g., multiple items had the same answers)) with a survey response rate of 60%. Most participants (n = 550; mean age 32.25 $\pm$ 5.81 SD years) were white (72%) with some post-secondary education (82%). Nearly all measures had good to excellent internal consistency as determined by Cronbach's alpha (see Table 1). Spearman rank order correlation coefficients of the study variables revealed that several variables were multicollinear. Table 2 lists each group of multicollinear variables and the variable selected from each group based on the criteria previously described in the Data Analysis section.

Table 2. Selection Rationale for Single Variable from Multicollinear Variable Groups.

Multicollinear Variable Group	Variable Most Highly and Significantly Correlated with BMI Was Retained in Further Analysis
Depression Severity, Health-related Quality of Life, and Stress Management	Health-Related Quality of Life
Disinhibited Eating and Emotional Eating	Emotional Eating
Importance of Physical Activity for Self with (1) Maternal Physical Activity Level and (2) Importance of Modeling Physical Activity to Child	Importance of Physical Activity for Self
Encourages/Facilitates Child Physical Activity with (1) Importance of Physical Activity for Child and (2) Importance of Modeling Physical Activity to Child	Encourages/Facilitate Child Physical Activity (Note: Importance of Modeling Physical Activity to Child had a higher correlation with BMI; however, it could not be selected because it is intercorrelated with Importance of Physical Activity for Self; see above)
Models Physical Activity to Child Frequently with (1) Maternal Physical Activity Level and (2) Mother: Child Co-Physical Activity	Models Physical Activity to Child Frequently
Instrumental Feeding Practices and Non-Food Rewards	Instrumental Feeding Practices
Allows Child to Independently Access Nutrient Dense Foods and Nutrient Dense Foods Stored in Locations Visible to Child	Neither variable was significantly correlated with BMI (none included)
Allows Child to Independently Access Low Nutrient Density Foods and Low Nutrient Dense Foods Stored in Locations Visible to Child	Low Nutrient Dense Foods Stored in Locations Visible to Child
Family Meals Eaten at Kitchen or Dining Table and TV on During Family Meals	Family Meals Eaten at Kitchen or Dining Table
Positive Family Meal Atmosphere and Household Disorganization	Neither variable was significantly correlated with BMI (none included)
Importance of Family Meals and Time and Energy for Family Meals	Importance of Family Meals
Household Fruit and Vegetable Availability with (1) Fruit and Vegetable Intake and (2) Household Sugar-sweetened Beverage Availability	Household Fruit and Vegetable Availability

Of the original 79 variables examined, scores for the 62 variables that were not highly intercorrelated were retained for further analysis. Binomial logistic regression on the dichotomous dependent variable of non-obese (n = 386) vs obese (n = 164) weight status revealed that all of the variables combined explained 64 percent of maternal obesity risk, with 12 of the variables being significantly associated with obesity risk. The 12 significant obesity risk variables were retained and again subjected to binomial logistic regression resulting in a final model with 8 variables explaining 53 percent of maternal risk for obesity (Table 3). Three of the obesity risk variables were dichotomous variables (i.e., being black or African American, having lower education level, having a primary relative with a history of obesity) and five were continuous variables (i.e., larger number of children in household, poorer general health rating, higher perceived weight teasing history, greater body dissatisfaction, more concern about their children's overweight risk). Using the variable scoring procedure described in the Data Analysis section, the weighted obesity risk score averaged 1.66 $\pm$ 0.98 SD and ranged from 0 to 5.49.

Table 3. Binomial Logistic Regression of Variables Associated with Maternal Obesity (n = 550).

Dependent Variable: Maternal Obesity †					
Independent Variables	**B** ‡	**SE** #	**Odds Ratio**	**95% CI**	***p*-value**
Race (black or African American)	1.25	0.41	3.48	(1.56, 7.70)	0.002
Education Level (some college or less)	0.61	0.26	1.83	(1.09, 3.07)	0.021
Number of Children in Household	0.32	0.12	1.38	(1.08, 1.75)	0.010
General Health Rating [a]	0.89	0.17	2.43	(1.73, 3.41)	<0.001
Perception of Weight Teasing History	0.52	0.11	1.69	(1.35, 2.11)	<0.001
Body Dissatisfaction	0.91	0.14	2.29	(1.91, 3.25)	<0.001
Primary Relative with History of Obesity	0.71	0.25	2.04	(1.25, 3.23)	0.004
Concern for Child's Overweight Risk	0.28	0.13	1.32	(1.03, 1.69)	0.026
R					
Cox and Snell R Square	0.374				
Nagelkerke R Square	0.531				
Tests of Model Coefficients	**DF** *	χ^2	***p*-value**		
	8	257.92	<0.001		

‡ Beta coefficient. * DF = Degrees of Freedom. # Standard Error. † Maternal obesity defined at body mass index ≥ 30.
[a] Higher scores indicate poorer perceptions of health status.

ANOVA and Tukey post-hoc tests comparing obesity risk scores by tertiles, as shown in Table 4, revealed significant differences ($p < 0.001$) among low-, moderate-, and high risk groups with a large effect size (i.e., $\eta^2 = 0.833$) for the obesity risk score, as estimated by partial Eta squared. A review of the characteristics related to sociodemographic variables, weight status, and health showed that non-obese mothers in the low obesity risk tertile had significantly higher family affluence ($p < 0.001$), lower food security risk ($p = 0.006$), and higher BMIs ($p < 0.001$) than those in the high obesity risk tertile. Additionally, the high obesity risk tertile reported significantly more days of "not good" health in the past month ($p < 0.001$), younger age at birth of first child ($p = 0.007$), and higher depression severity ($p < 0.001$) compared with those in lower obesity risk tertiles. There were no significant child BMI percentile differences among obesity risk tertiles although there was an increasing trend.

An examination of maternal intrapersonal characteristics showed that those in the high obesity risk tertile were significantly more likely to report worse sleep quality ($p < 0.001$), greater emotional eating ($p < 0.001$), perceive themselves as having less personal organization ($p < 0.001$), lower confidence in parenting ($p = 0.004$), and poorer stress management skills ($p < 0.001$) than those in the lower obesity risk tertiles. Compared to the high obesity risk tertile, mothers in the low obesity risk tertile were significantly more likely to value the importance of physical activity for self ($p < 0.001$) and child ($p = 0.006$), value the importance of modeling physical activity ($p = 0.01$), frequently model physical activity ($p < 0.001$) and less frequently model sedentary activity ($p = 0.007$), model healthy eating ($p = 0.003$), and place more child limits on children's TV program choices ($p = 0.01$). None of the other intrapersonal characteristics differed significantly among obesity risk tertile groups.

The only interpersonal characteristics that differed significantly among obesity risk tertile groups were the frequency of family meals eaten at the kitchen or dining table and family conflict and lack of cohesion. That is, mothers in the high obesity risk tertile reported eating significantly ($p = 0.006$) fewer family meals at a kitchen or dining table and had more family conflict and less cohesion ($p = 0.005$) compared with those in the low obesity risk tertile.

Household fruit and vegetable availability was the only home physical environment characteristic that differed significantly among obesity risk tertiles. That is, mothers in the low obesity risk tertile had greater household availability of fruits and vegetables ($p = 0.013$) than those in the high obesity risk tertile. Estimated effect sizes, as determined by partial Eta squared, for the significantly different intrapersonal, interpersonal, and home environment characteristics were low.

Table 4. ANOVA of Sociodemographic, Intrapersonal, Interpersonal and Home Environment Characteristics among Obesity Risk Score Tertiles of Non-Obese Participants.

	Obesity Risk Score Tertiles of Non-Obese Participants (N = 386)				
	Low Risk (n = 120)	Moderate Risk (n = 135)	High Risk (n = 131)		
Weighted Score Cut-offs	0 to 1.12	1.13 to 2.07	≥2.08	ANOVA *	
	Mean ± SD or N (%)	Mean ± SD or N (%)	Mean ± SD or N (%)	F or χ^2	p-value
Obesity risk score (possible score range 0–5.49)	0.58 ± 0.36 †[a]	1.52 ± 0.27 [b]	2.78 ± 0.53 [c]	953.53	<0.001
Sociodemographic Characteristics					
Maternal Employment				5.03	0.284
Do not work	56 (46.7)	73 (54.1)	78 (59.5)		
Part-time (less than 30 h/week)	24 (20.0)	28 (20.7)	21 (16.0)		
Full-time (30 or more h/week)	40 (33.3)	34 (25.2)	32 (24.4)		
Number of Children in Household	2.07 ± 0.97	2.21 ± 1.02	2.22 ± 0.96	0.94	0.392
Family Affluence Score	6.09 ± 1.49 [a]	5.63 ± 1.61 [b]	5.49 ± 1.53 [b]	5.16	0.006
Food Insecurity Risk	1.38 ± 1.76 [a]	1.78 ± 1.80	2.27 ± 1.82 [b]	7.81	<0.001
Weight Status					
Mother's BMI	22.15 ± 2.64 [a]	22.93 ± 3.03 [a]	25.19 ± 3.05 [b]	37.36	<0.001
Child's BMI percentile (n = 339)	59.85 ± 34.58	62.07 ± 34.76	65.45 ± 35.45	0.89	0.413
Health-Related Assessments					
Health-Related Quality of Life (# of unhealthy days)	0.94 ± 1.57 [a]	1.61 ± 2.51 [a]	4.16 ± 5.49 [b]	27.97	<0.001
Depression Severity	0.57 ± 1.02 [a]	0.85 ± 1.41 [a]	1.33 ± 1.48 [b]	10.68	<0.001
Age at Birth of First Child (years)	25.92 ± 4.72 [a]	24.30 ± 5.12 [a]	23.92 ± 5.59 [b]	5.08	0.007
Primary Relative with History of Diabetes (% yes)	23 (19.2)	21 (15.6)	38 (29.0)	7.64	0.022
Intrapersonal Characteristics					
Maternal Weight-Related Behaviors					
Physical Activity Level	17.43 ± 9.78	15.93 ± 9.49	14.65 ± 10.50	2.46	0.087
Screentime (minutes/day)	216.25 ± 214.87	270.78 ± 249.99	277.67 ± 251.36	2.43	0.089
Sleep Duration (hours/day)	7.49 ± 1.97	7.22 ± 1.85	6.87 ± 1.89	3.31	0.038
Sleep Quality	3.58 ± 0.87 [a]	3.46 ± 0.82 [a]	3.03 ± 0.83 [b]	15.00	<0.001
Fruit and Vegetable (servings/day)	4.98 ± 2.37	4.84 ± 2.30	4.24 ± 2.29	3.65	0.027
% Calories from Total Fat	36.83 ± 5.36	37.61 ± 6.55	36.98 ± 5.87	0.64	0.530
Milk (servings/day)	4.18 ± 3.19	4.31 ± 2.95	3.33 ± 3.11	3.79	0.023
Sugar-Sweetened Beverage (servings/day)	0.70 ± 0.78	0.95 ± 1.06	0.93 ± 0.86	2.83	0.060
Maternal Eating Styles					
Disinhibited Eating	1.77 ± 0.77	1.95 ± 0.76	2.00 ± 0.73	2.25	0.040
Emotional Eating	1.73 ± 0.74 [a]	1.87 ± 0.80 [a]	2.19 ± 0.88 [b]	10.95	<0.001
Dietary Restraint Eating	2.31 ± 0.79	2.47 ± 0.79	2.49 ± 0.69	2.27	0.105

Table 4. *Cont.*

	Obesity Risk Score Tertiles of Non-Obese Participants (N = 386)				
	Low Risk (n = 120)	Moderate Risk (n = 135)	High Risk (n = 131)		
Weighted Score Cut-offs	0 to 1.12	1.13 to 2.07	≥2.08	ANOVA *	
	Mean ± SD or N (%)	Mean ± SD or N (%)	Mean ± SD or N (%)	F or χ^2	p-value
Adventurous Eating	3.21 ± 0.69	3.16 ± 0.66	3.12 ± 0.67	0.52	0.597
Maternal Self-Perceptions					
Personal Organization (self-effectiveness)	3.91 ± 0.75 [a]	3.79 ± 0.79 [a]	3.49 ± 0.83 [b]	9.31	<0.001
Need for Cognition	3.66 ± 1.01	3.47 ± 0.94	3.37 ± 0.98	2.76	0.065
Parenting Self-Efficacy	4.23 ± 0.71 [a]	4.23 ± 0.75 [a]	3.95 ± 0.82 [b]	5.71	0.004
Stress Management	4.19 ± 0.54 [a]	4.02 ± 0.71 [a]	3.79 ± 0.83 [b]	10.41	<0.001
Stress Management Self-Efficacy	2.88 ± 1.01	2.51 ± 1.05	2.64 ± 0.99	1.43	0.242
Child Weight Cognitions					
Belief that Chubby Kids are Healthy	2.72 ± 0.75	2.79 ± 0.68	2.61 ± 0.72	1.95	0.143
Health Behavior Values					
Importance of Physical Activity for Self	3.90 ± 0.92 [a]	3.75 ± 0.81 [a]	3.34 ± 0.92 [b]	13.94	<0.001
Importance of Physical Activity for Child	4.03 ± 0.78 [a]	3.85 ± 0.85	3.69 ± 0.87 [b]	5.12	0.006
Encourages/Facilitates Child Physical Activity	4.37 ± 0.67	4.29 ± 0.61	4.16 ± 0.64	3.44	0.033
Importance of Modeling Physical Activity to Child	4.35 ± 0.82 [a]	4.26 ± 0.71	4.07 ± 0.76 [b]	4.61	0.010
Engages in Physical Activity with Child Frequently	3.92 ± 1.90	3.61 ± 1.91	3.44 ± 1.80	2.11	0.123
Models Physical Activity to Child Frequently	3.55 ± 1.10 [a]	3.13 ± 1.21 [b]	2.93 ± 1.18 [b]	9.14	<0.001
Models Sedentary Behaviors Infrequently	3.54 ± 2.11 [a]	2.84 ± 2.08 [b]	2.75 ± 2.27 [b]	5.00	0.007
Models Healthy Eating to Child	3.72 ± 0.75 [a]	3.62 ± 0.63	3.43 ± 0.69 [b]	5.74	0.003
Belief that TV Positively Affects Child Learning	3.91 ± 0.68	3.91 ± 0.8	3.78 ± 0.78	1.30	0.274
Talks Often with Child about TV	3.38 ± 1.01	3.27 ± 0.94	3.26 ± 0.94	0.60	0.548
Limits Child Exposure to TV Commercials and Inappropriate Programs Shows	3.77 ± 0.90	3.71 ± 0.86	3.66 ± 0.93	0.48	0.621
Limits Child to Educational TV	3.68 ± 1.03 [a]	3.64 ± 1.02 [a]	3.31 ± 1.09 [b]	4.66	0.010
Home Interpersonal Characteristics					
Child Feeding Practices					
Restricts Child Food Intake	3.85 ± 0.88	3.91 ± 0.84	3.83 ± 0.83	0.31	0.737
Pressures Child to Eat	2.22 ± 1.04	2.18 ± 0.95	2.15 ± 0.89	0.18	0.837
Maternal Control Over Child Food Access and Choices	3.44 ± 0.49	3.38 ± 0.55	3.30 ± 0.48	2.40	0.092
Non-Acceptance of Food Waste	3.12 ± 0.96	3.26 ± 0.94	3.05 ± 0.89	1.75	0.175
Instrumental Feeding Practices (uses food to reward children for eating a healthy food)	2.74 ± 0.97	2.77 ± 0.93	2.55 ± 0.87	2.01	0.136
Non-Food Rewards (uses non-food [e.g., extra playtime] to reward children for eating a healthy food)	2.93 ± 1.00	2.95 ± 0.98	2.89 ± 0.86	0.16	0.854
Allows Child to Independently Access Nutrient Dense Foods	1.74 ± 1.74	1.96 ± 1.68	1.73 ± 1.78	0.75	0.475
Allows Child to Independently Access Low Nutrient Density Foods	0.48 ± 1.04	0.78 ± 1.43	0.70 ± 1.40	1.81	0.166
Nutrient Dense Foods Stored in Locations Visible to Child	2.30 ± 1.72	2.42 ± 1.71	2.61 ± 1.78	1.03	0.360
Low Nutrient Dense Foods Stored in Locations Visible to Child	0.58 ± 1.21	0.79 ± 1.39	0.94 ± 1.36	2.26	0.106

Table 4. *Cont.*

	Obesity Risk Score Tertiles of Non-Obese Participants (N = 386)				
	Low Risk (n = 120)	Moderate Risk (n = 135)	High Risk (n = 131)		
Weighted Score Cut-offs	0 to 1.12	1.13 to 2.07	≥2.08	ANOVA *	
	Mean ± SD or N (%)	Mean ± SD or N (%)	Mean ± SD or N (%)	F or χ^2	p-value
Family Meal Patterns					
Family Meal Frequency (per week)	14.25 ± 5.00	13.92 ± 4.49	12.97 ± 5.09	2.39	0.093
Importance of Family Meals	4.64 ± 0.57	4.53 ± 0.64	4.42 ± 0.65	3.69	0.026
Positive Family Meal Atmosphere	4.18 ± 0.86	4.09 ± 0.88	4.08 ± 0.79	0.57	0.569
Fast Food Eaten at Family Meals					
TV on During Family Meals (days/week)	1.53 ± 2.17	2.22 ± 2.53	2.24 ± 2.43	3.55	0.030
Family Meals Eaten at Kitchen or Dining Table (days/week)	5.38 ± 2.23 [a]	4.82 ± 2.48	4.42 ± 2.42 [b]	5.13	0.006
Family Meals Eaten in the Car	0.51 ± 1.29	0.54 ± 1.39	0.35 ± 0.90	0.92	0.401
Family Meal Planning	3.53 ± 0.93	3.46 ± 0.9	3.4 ± 0.80	0.70	0.496
Time and Energy for Family Meals	4.46 ± 0.78	4.33 ± 0.85	4.22 ± 0.92	2.57	0.078
Family Functioning and Maternal Engagement					
Family Support for Healthy Behaviors	4.54 ± 0.74	4.34 ± 0.86	4.37 ± 0.65	2.56	0.079
Family Conflict and Lack of Cohesion	1.65 ± 0.62 [a]	1.76 ± 0.64	1.91 ± 0.66 [b]	5.29	0.005
Household Disorganization	2.32 ± 0.96	2.48 ± 0.92	2.55 ± 0.87	2.03	0.133
Verbal Engagement with Children	4.33 ± 0.84	4.15 ± 0.91	4.05 ± 1.01	2.91	0.056
Physical Engagement with Children	4.81 ± 0.44	4.67 ± 0.6	4.73 ± 0.51	2.11	0.122
Home Physical Environment Characteristics					
Physical Activity					
Physical Activity Availability	3.90 ± 0.68	3.82 ± 0.62	3.78 ± 0.64	1.12	0.327
Physical Activity Accessibility	4.42 ± 0.98	4.39 ± 1.16	4.12 ± 1.15	2.84	0.060
Media Devices in the Home (total number)	11.53 ± 4.29	11.09 ± 4.19	11.5 ± 3.71	0.49	0.613
Media Devices in Child's Bedroom (total number)	1.05 ± 1.55	1.37 ± 1.70	1.63 ± 1.75	3.71	0.025
Daily Screentime Child Allowed (minutes/day)	342.00 ± 413.14	433.78 ± 642.76	509.54 ± 710.46	2.39	0.093
Food Availability					
Household Fruit and Vegetable Availability (serving/person/day)	6.96 ± 2.41 [a]	6.80 ± 2.62	6.09 ± 2.44 [b]	4.40	0.013
Household Fatty/Salty Snack Availability (serving/person/day)	9.21 ± 7.81	8.67 ± 7.73	8.07 ± 6.81	0.73	0.481
Household Sugar-Sweetened Beverage Availability (serving/person/day)	1.70 ± 2.02	2.21 ± 2.02	1.72 ± 1.51	3.15	0.044
Household Breakfast Cereal Availability (servings/person/day)	5.67 ± 2.78	5.39 ± 2.70	5.49 ± 2.52	0.36	0.698

* Analysis of Variance (ANOVA) for continuous variables and Chi-square analysis for categorical variables examined characteristic differences among the Obesity Risk Score Tertile groups (low risk, moderate risk, and high risk). Tukey post-hoc tests were conducted for characteristics that were statistically significant ($p < 0.01$) in the ANOVA to determine significant between group differences. † Differing superscript lowercase letters in the same row indicate significant ($p < 0.05$) between group differences as determined by Tukey post-hoc tests.

4. Discussion

This study developed an obesity risk score for non-obese mothers of young children using a comprehensive array of sociodemographic and weight-related intrapersonal, interpersonal, and home environmental characteristics. The eight characteristics comprising the obesity risk score may help health professionals identify non-obese mothers with young children at increased risk for obesity and provide early obesity prevention intervention.

The eight independent variables identified in this study explained over half of maternal risk for obesity have been shown in other studies to be strongly associated with obesity. That is, women of African American race are more likely to be overweight or obese than other racial and ethnic groups [1]; lower education attainment is associated with overweight and obesity [1,83]; obese adults have more chronic disease [92,93] and report poorer health [94]; obese women are more likely to report being teased growing up [95,96]; and body shape dissatisfaction is associated with overweight and obesity [97,98]. The study reported here also provides insight into variables that are associated with obesity which are not changeable through nutrition and health promotion programs (e.g., race, family history, affluence), and those which are, yet are rarely targeted in nutrition education interventions (e.g., family conflict, body dissatisfaction).

Examining non-obese mothers by high, moderate, and low obesity risk tertiles provided an efficient means for exploring how risk level was associated with interpersonal, intrapersonal, and environmental characteristics. Several sociodemographic variables, health-related assessments, and intrapersonal, and interpersonal characteristics were associated with high obesity risk score among non-obese mothers whereas home physical environment factors tended to not be associated with obesity risk. Trends in sociodemographic and health-related characteristics noted among participants at high risk for obesity (e.g., food insecurity, lower family affluence, more unhealthy days in past month, and greater depression severity) mirror national data [1,83]. For instance, mothers in the high obesity risk group reported less family affluence and greater depression severity, which is consistent with literature indicating obesity rates are higher among adult women with low socio-economic status [99] and obese women are more likely to suffer from depression (although this association may be bi-directional) [100,101].

High obesity risk mothers did not significantly differ from lower obesity risk moms in their physical activity and screentime behaviors possibly because at risk, but not obese, women are not yet hindered by their weight interfering with their activity level. These findings suggest that activity level may not be a significant risk factor for maternal obesity but is associated with obesity weight status, raising the question of reverse causality. That is, are obese mothers inactive and more sedentary [102] because their weight inhibits physical activity instead of inactivity causing weight gain; or, are there other factors contributing to these relationships, such as the environmental supports for physical activity? Environments that promote access to and availability of physical activity are associated with more physical activity behaviors [103–107]. However, a recent systematic review has found inconsistent results in the associations between the built physical environment and obesity in adults [108], perhaps due to the great variation in metrics used and differing contexts of prior studies [108].

There is growing interest in the associations of sleep duration and quality with weight [109]. In the present study, poor sleep quality was significantly more prevalent in high obesity risk mothers. Although non-significant, the number of total hours slept each night linearly decreased as obesity risk increased, with those in the high obesity risk group receiving less than the recommended total sleep hours per night for adults of 7 to 9 h [110]. These findings suggest the need for continued investigation of the mechanisms of how sleep may be related to weight gain, and indicate the importance of including sleep management in weight-management interventions.

A linear trend showed that high obesity risk mothers were less active with their children and allowed children to have more minutes of screentime daily than lower obesity risk mothers. This finding is similar to reports of associations between maternal characteristics, child activity, and sedentary behaviors [111,112], and further highlights the importance of maternal modeling, encouraging, and facilitating physical activity for their children [69]. Not surprisingly, low obesity risk mothers engaged in significantly more modeling of both physical activity and less sedentary behaviors. Additionally, mothers at low obesity risk were less likely to model unhealthy emotional eating behaviors for their children. Parents and caregivers act as powerful socialization agents and serve as models of eating that children learn to emulate [113]. Future work should explore how low obesity risk mothers' modeling of healthy behaviors affects the health and weight status of their children.

Home food availability, parental diet, and family eating habits are associated with diet quality of children [114,115]. In this study, high obesity risk moms had less household availability of fruits and vegetables and ate fewer family meals at a kitchen or dining room table which may have influenced their child's diet quality and weight status. Although non-significant, there was a positive linear trend in child BMI percentile and maternal obesity risk score. Studies on weight-resilience (i.e., maintaining a healthy weight despite living in an obesogenic environment) suggest that homes with healthy weight children and teens are more likely to have healthier food options available and limit access to unhealthy foods [116,117]. In the study reported here, only a non-significant linear trend occurred, with mothers at low obesity risk limiting children's access to low nutrient dense foods and storing nutrient dense foods in a manner that was clearly visible to children. Thus, future interventions should consider targeting family nutrition education that encourages positive changes in the home food supply and healthful dietary practices in the home.

This study found a non-significant decreasing trend in the relationships among obesity risk tertiles and family meal frequency. Other studies have found cross-sectional associations of family meal frequency were inversely associated with obesity in adolescents, but longitudinal analyses have not corroborated those results [118–120]. The results of this study contribute to the mixed associations among family meals and weight status [121]. It may be that characteristics of the family meal environment are confounding potential associations. For example, non-obese mothers at high risk for obesity reported significantly more family conflict and lack of cohesion. Having poor family functioning (i.e., more conflict and less cohesion) during mealtimes may lead to less frequent family meals, especially when there is a negative meal atmosphere [122–124]. Further research examining the influences of family dynamics with family meal frequency and weight-related behaviors are warranted [122,125].

The relationships between home food availability and maternal dietary intake are not clear. For instance, sugar-sweetened beverage intake was relatively lower among low obesity risk mothers yet household availability of sugar-sweetened beverages was similar in households across maternal obesity risk tertiles. Mothers at low obesity risk ate relatively more fruits and vegetables and had significantly greater household availability of fruits and vegetables than those of higher obesity risk. Whether foods were eaten from household food stores or outside the home was not investigated; the incongruence of beverage intake and household availability may indicate these beverages were consumed at home as well as outside the home, whereas the relative consistency between fruit and vegetable intake and household food supplies may indicate these foods are typically eaten at home. Further research is needed to understand where food and beverages are typically consumed and the impact of consumption location on household food supplies, overall family dietary intakes, and obesity risk.

A major strength of this study was the use of a socioecological framework to guide the comprehensive selection of constructs obesity risk in mothers of young children. A systematic method [34] was used to examine the potential scales for application to the study population (i.e., mothers and young children of varying races/ethnicities and educational attainment). Use of reliable and valid scales is vital to ensure the most accurate responses. In this survey, previously validated and refined tools were used when possible, and nearly all had good to high internal consistency with the study sample. Despite the strengths of this study, it is important to note its limitations. Inference of causality of observed associations cannot be made due to the cross-sectional study design. In addition, the study sample only included mothers of preschool-aged children in the U.S. with greater educational attainment than the national average, so findings may not be generalizable to mothers with lower education levels or mothers with children of different ages or those residing in other countries. This study also did not evaluate characteristics and behaviors of other family or friends or environments outside of the home environment. Although the estimated effect size for the obesity risk score was high, the significantly different intrapersonal, interpersonal, and home environment characteristics that occurred across obesity risk tertiles had low effect sizes. Lastly, data collected from participants were self-reported and may be subject to both reporting error and bias. However, heights and weights self-reported by adults are highly correlated with measured heights and weights [126] and online data collection offers privacy and relative anonymity that may improve veracity when answering questions [127–129].

5. Conclusions

In conclusion, this exploratory study identified eight characteristics that, together, explain more than half of the risk of obesity in non-obese mothers of young children. These eight characteristics may help healthcare professionals identify mothers at increased risk of obesity and offer preventive care early and more specifically tailor care (e.g., psychological assistance for those with body dissatisfaction). Many of the eight characteristics are not usually assessed in clinical practice, but are simple to assess and may yield valuable obesity risk information to healthcare providers. In addition, nutrition communication and health promotion professionals can apply the findings by targeting intervention efforts to those at increased risk and expanding intervention content to address topics not typically addressed in obesity prevention programs, such as strategies for managing family conflicts and changing the home food environment. Further research with larger, more diverse samples who are longitudinally assessed is needed to confirm the results of this study. Additional research to clarify the contribution of early identification of those at high risk for obesity and inclusion of new topics in obesity prevention programs also is warranted.

Author Contributions: C.B.-B. and J.M.-B. conceived and designed the study. J.M.-B. and C.B.-B. collected data. J.M.-B., V.Q., and C.B.-B. analyzed the data. J.M.-B., V.Q., K.S., and C.B.-B. were involved in manuscript preparation and revision and approved the final manuscript.

Acknowledgments: This study was funded by USDA NIFA #2011-68001-30170. An earlier draft of parts of this manuscript were from J. Martin-Biggers (2016) Home Environment Characteristics Associated with Obesity Risk In Preschool-Aged Children and Their Mothers, doctoral dissertation, Rutgers, The State University of New Jersey, New Brunswick, NJ.

References

1. Ogden, C.; Carroll, M.; Kit, B.; Flegal, K. Prevalence of childhood and adult obesity in the United States, 2011–2012. *JAMA* **2014**, *311*, 806–814. [CrossRef] [PubMed]
2. Tsai, A.; Williamson, D.; Glick, H. Direct medical cost of overweight and obesity in the United States: A qunatitative systematic review. *Obes. Rev.* **2012**, *12*, 50–61. [CrossRef] [PubMed]
3. Pi-Sunyer, F.X. The Obesity Epidemic: Pathophysiology and Consequences of Obesity. *Obesity* **2002**, *10* (Suppl. 12), 97S–104S. [CrossRef] [PubMed]
4. Organization, W.H. *Obesity: Preventing and Managing the Global Epidemic*; World Health Organization: Geneva, Switzerland, 2000.
5. Lobstein, T.; Baur, L.; Uauy, R. Obesity in children and young people: A crisis in public health. *Obes. Rev.* **2004**, *5*, 4–85. [CrossRef] [PubMed]
6. Hassan, M.K.; Joshi, A.V.; Madhavan, S.S.; Amonkar, M.M. Obesity and health-related quality of life: A cross-sectional analysis of the US population. *Int. J. Obes. Relat. Metab. Disord.* **2003**, *27*, 1227–1232. [CrossRef] [PubMed]

7. Brinkley, J.; Eales, J.; Jekanowski, M. The relation between dietary change and rising US obesity. *Int. J. Obes. Relat. Metab. Disord.* **2000**, *24*, 1032–1039. [CrossRef]
8. Golan, M.; Crow, S. Parents are key players in the prevention and treatment of weight-related problems. *Nutr. Rev.* **2004**, *62*, 39–50. [CrossRef] [PubMed]
9. Hill, J.; Wyatt, H.; Reed, G.; Peters, J. Obesity and the environment: Where do we go from here? *Science* **2003**, *203*, 853–856.
10. Wang, Y.C.; Bleich, S.N.; Gortmaker, S.L. Increasing caloric contribution from sugar-sweetened beverages and 100% fruit juices among US children and adolescents, 1988–2004. *Pediatrics* **2008**, *121*, e1604–e1614. [PubMed]
11. Wang, Y.C.; Orleans, C.T.; Gortmaker, S.L. Reaching the healthy people goals for reducing childhood obesity: Closing the energy gap. *Am. J. Prev. Med.* **2012**, *42*, 437–444. [PubMed]
12. *Diet, Nutrition and the Prevention of Chronic Diseases*; World Health Organization Technical Report Series 916, backcover; World Health Organization: Geneva, Switzerland, 2003; Volume i–viii, pp. 1–149.
13. Richard, L.; Gauvin, L.; Raine, K. Ecological Models Revisited: Their Uses and Evolution in Health Promotion Over Two Decades. *Annu. Rev. Public Health* **2011**, *32*, 307–326. [CrossRef] [PubMed]
14. Sallis, J.; Owen, N. *Ecological Models of Health Behavior*, 5th ed.; Jossey-Bass: San Francisco, CA, USA, 2015.
15. Giskes, K.; van Lenthe, F.; Avendano-Pabon, M.; Brug, J. A systematic review of environmental factors and obesogenic dietary intakes among adults: Are we getting closer to understanding obesogenic environments? *Obes. Rev.* **2011**, *12*, e95–e106. [CrossRef] [PubMed]
16. Van der Horst, K.; Oenema, A.; Ferreira, I.; Wendel-Vos, W.; Giskes, K.; van Lenthe, F.; Brug, J. A systematic review of environmental correlates of obesity-related dietary behaviors in youth. *Health Educ. Res.* **2007**, *22*, 203–226. [CrossRef] [PubMed]
17. Kelder, S.; Hoelscher, D.; Perry, C. How individuals, environments, and health behavior interact; Social Cognitive Theory. In *Health Behavior: Theory, Research, and Practice*, 5th ed.; Glanz, K., Rimer, B., Viswanath, K., Eds.; Jossey-Bass: San Francisco, CA, USA, 2015; pp. 159–182.
18. Saelens, B.; Sallis, J.; Frank, L. Environmental correlates of walking and cycling: Findings from the transportation, urban design, and planning literatures. *Ann. Behav. Med.* **2003**, *25*, 80–91. [CrossRef] [PubMed]
19. Humpel, N.; Owen, N.; Leslie, E. Environmental factors associated with adults' participation in physical activity: A review. *Am. J. Prev. Med.* **2002**, *22*, 188–199. [CrossRef]
20. Berge, J.M.; Larson, N.; Bauer, K.W.; Neumark-Sztainer, D. Are parents of young children practicing healthy nutrition and physical activity behaviors? *Pediatrics* **2011**, *127*, 881–887. [CrossRef] [PubMed]
21. Evans, A.E.; Dave, J.; Tanner, A.; Duhe, S.; Condrasky, M.; Wilson, D.; Griffin, S.; Palmer, M.; Evans, M. Changing the home nutrition environment: Effects of a nutrition and media literacy pilot intervention. *Fam. Community Health* **2006**, *29*, 43–54. [CrossRef] [PubMed]
22. *Children's Food Environment State Indicator Report*; Centers for Disease Control and Prevention: Atlanta, GA, USA, 2011.
23. Vaughn, A.; Ward, D.; Fisher, J.; Faith, M.; Hughes, S.; Kremers, S.; Musher-Eizenman, D.; O'Connor, T.; Patrick, H.; Power, T. Fundamental constructs in food parenting practices: A content map to guide future research. *Nutr. Rev.* **2016**, *74*, 98–117. [CrossRef] [PubMed]
24. Reid, M.; Worsley, A.; Mavondo, F. The obesogenic household: Factors influencing dietary gatekeeper satisfaction with family diet. *Psychol. Mark.* **2015**, *32*, 544–557. [CrossRef]
25. Mamun, A.; O'Callaghan, M.; Callaway, L.; Williams, G.; Najman, J.; Lawlor, D. Associations of Gestational Weight Gain with Offspring Body Mass Index and Blood Pressure at 21 Years of Age Evidence from a Birth Cohort Study. *Circulation* **2009**, *119*, 1720–1727. [CrossRef] [PubMed]
26. Lagström, H.; Hakanen, M.; Niinikoski, H.; Viikari, J.; Rönnemaa, T.; Saarinen, M.; Pahkala, K.; Simell, O. Growth Patterns and Obesity Development in Overweight or Normal-Weight 13-Year-Old Adolescents: The STRIP Study. *Pediatrics* **2008**, *122*, e876–e883. [CrossRef] [PubMed]
27. Shibli, R.; Rubin, L.; Akons, H.; Shaoul, R. Morbidity of overweight (85th percentile) in the first 2 years of life. *Pediatrics* **2008**, *122*, 267–272. [CrossRef] [PubMed]
28. Ogata, B.; Hayes, D. Position of the Academy of Nutrition and Dietetics: Nutrition guidance for healthy children ages 2 to 11 years. *J. Acad. Nutr. Diet.* **2014**, *114*, 1257–1276. [CrossRef] [PubMed]

29. Centers for Disease Control and Prevention Adult Obesity Causes & Consequences. Available online: https://www.cdc.gov/obesity/adult/causes.html (accessed on 1 November 2017).
30. U.S. Census Bureau Age and Sex Composition: 2010. Available online: https://www.census.gov/prod/cen2010/briefs/c2010br-03.pdf (accessed on 1 May 2017).
31. Martin-Biggers, J. Home Environment Characteristics Associated with Obesity Risk in Preschool-Aged Children and THEIR mothers. Ph.D. Dissertation, Rutgers, The State University of New Jersey, New Brunswick, NJ, USA, 2016.
32. Martin-Biggers, J.; Cheng, C.; Spaccarotella, K.; Byrd-Bredbenner, C. The Physical Activity Environment in Homes and Neighborhoods. In *Recent Advances in Obesity in Children*; Avid Science Publications: Berlin, Germany, 2016; Available online: www.avidscience.com/wp-content/uploads/2016/05/OIC-15-04_May-06-2016.pdf (accessed on 1 November 2017).
33. Martin-Biggers, J.M.; Worobey, J.; Byrd-Bredbenner, C. Interpersonal Characteristics in the Home Environment Associated with Childhood Obesity. In *Recent Advances in Obesity in Children*; Avid Science Publications: Berlin, Germany, 2016; Chapter 3.
34. Redding, C.A.; Maddock, J.E.; Rossi, J.S. The sequential approach to measurement of health behavior constructs: Issues in selecting and developing measures. *Calif. J. Health Promot.* **2006**, *4*, 83–101.
35. Linn, R.; Gronlund, N. *Measuring and Assessment in Teaching*, 8th ed.; Prentice-Hall: Englewood Cliffs, NJ, USA, 2000.
36. Carbone, E.T.; Campbell, M.K.; Honess-Morreale, L. Use of cognitive interview techniques in the development of nutrition surveys and interactive nutrition messages for low-income populations. *J. Am. Diet. Assoc.* **2002**, *102*, 690–696. [CrossRef]
37. Wright, K.B. Researching Internet-Based Populations: Advantages and Disadvantages of Online Survey Research, Online Questionnaire Authoring Software Packages, and Web Survey Services. *J. Comput.-Med. Commun.* **2005**, *10*. [CrossRef]
38. Masse, L. Innovations in Measurement of Parenting Constructs, Parenting Meausurement: Current Status and Consensus Reports. In Proceedings of the International Society for Behavioral Nutrition and Physical Activity, Houston, TX, USA, 20 May 2012.
39. Hartley, J.; Levin, K.; Currie, C. A new version of the HBSC Family Affluence Scale—FAS III: Scottish qualitative findings from the international FAS developments study. *Child Indic. Res.* **2016**, *9*, 233–245. [CrossRef] [PubMed]
40. Currie, C.; Mollcho, M.; Boyce, W.; Holstein, B.; Torsheim, T.; Richter, M. Researching health inequalities in adolescents: The development of the health behavior in school-aged children (HBSC) family affluence scale. *Soc. Sci. Med.* **2008**, *66*, 1429–1436. [CrossRef] [PubMed]
41. Hager, E.; Quigg, A.; Black, M.; Coleman, S.; Heeren, T.; Rose-Jacobs, R.; Cook, J.; Ettinger de Cuba, S.; Casey, P.; Chilton, M.; et al. Development and validity of a 2-Item screen to identify families at risk for food insecurity. *Pediatrics* **2010**, *126*, e26–e32. [CrossRef] [PubMed]
42. Centers for Disease Control and Prevention HRQOL Concepts. Why Is Quality of Life Important? Available online: www.cdc.gov/hrqol/concept.htm (accessed on 9 May 2016).
43. Centers for Disease Control and Prevention CDC HRQOL-14 Healthy Days Measure. Available online: www.cdc.gov/hrqol/hrqol14_measure.htm (accessed on 9 May 2016).
44. Kroenke, K.; Spitzer, R.L.; Williams, J.B.W. The Patient Health Questionnaire-2: Validity of a two-item depression screener. *Med. Care* **2003**, *41*, 1284–1292. [CrossRef] [PubMed]
45. Thompson, J.; Cattarin, J.; Fowler, B.; Fisher, E. The Perception of Teasing Scale (POTS): A revision and extension of the Physical Appearance Related Teasing Scale (PARTS). *J. Personal. Assess.* **1995**, *65*, 146–157. [CrossRef] [PubMed]
46. Fairburn, C.; Beglin, S. Assessment of eating disorders: Interview or self-report questionnaire? *Int. J. Eat. Disord.* **1994**, *16*, 363–370. [PubMed]
47. Quick, V.; Byrd-Bredbenner, C.; Shoff, S.; White, A.; Lohse, B.; Horacek, T.; Kattlemann, K.; Phillips, B.; Hoerr, S.; Greene, G. A streamlined, enhanced self-report physical activity measure for young adults. *Int. J. Health Promot. Educ.* **2016**. [CrossRef]
48. Lee, P.; Macfarlane, D.; Lam, T.; Stewart, S. Validity of the international physical activity questionnaire short form (IPAQ-SF): A systematic review. *Int. J. Behav. Nutr. Phys. Act.* **2011**, *8*, 115. [CrossRef] [PubMed]

49. Craig, C.L.; Marshall, A.L.; Sjorstrom, M.; Bauman, A.E.; Booth, M.L.; Ainsworth, B.E.; Pratt, M.; Ekelund, U.L.; Yngve, A.; Sallis, J.F.; et al. International Physical Activity Questionnaire: 12-country reliability and validity. *Med. Sci. Sports Exerc.* **2003**, *35*, 1381–1395. [CrossRef] [PubMed]
50. Buysse, D.; Reynolds, C.; Monk, T.; Berman, S.; Kupfer, D. The Pittsburgh Sleep Quality Index: A new instrument for psychiatric practice and research. *Psychiatr. Res.* **1989**, *28*, 193–213. [CrossRef]
51. Carpenter, J.; Andrykowski, M. Psychometric evaluation of the Pittsburgh Sleep Quality Index. *J. Psychosom. Res.* **1998**, *45*, 5–13. [CrossRef]
52. Block, G.; Gillespie, C.; Rosenbaum, E.H.; Jenson, C. A rapid food screener to assess fat and fruit and vegetable intake. *Am. J. Prev. Med.* **2000**, *18*, 284–288. [CrossRef]
53. Block, G.; Hartman, A.; Naughton, D. A reduced dietary questionnaire: Development and validation. *Epidemiology* **1990**, *1*, 58–64. [CrossRef] [PubMed]
54. Block, G.; Thompson, F.; Hartman, A.; Larkin, F.; Guire, K. Comparison of two dietary questionnaires validated against multiple dietary records collected during a 1-year period. *J. Am. Diet. Assoc.* **1992**, *92*, 686–693. [PubMed]
55. Nelson, M.; Lytle, L. Development and evaluation of a brief screener to estimate fast-food and beverage consumption among adolescents. *J. Am. Diet. Assoc.* **2009**, *109*, 730–734. [CrossRef] [PubMed]
56. West, D.; Bursac, Z.; Quimby, D.; Prewit, T.; Spatz, T.; Nash, C.; Mays, G.; Eddings, K. Self-reported sugar-sweetened beverage intake among college students. *Obesity* **2006**, *14*, 1825–1831. [CrossRef] [PubMed]
57. Stunkard, A.; Messick, S. The three-factor eating questionnaire to measure dietary restraint, disinhibition and hunger. *J. Psychosom. Res.* **1985**, *29*, 71–83. [CrossRef]
58. Karlsson, J.; Persson, L.-O.; Sjostrom, L.; Sullivan, M. Psychometric properties and factor structure of the Three-Factor Eating (TFEQ) in obese men and women. Results from the Swedish Obese Subjects (SOS) study. *Int. J. Obes.* **2000**, *24*, 1715–1725. [CrossRef]
59. Pliner, P.; Hobden, K. Development of a scale to measure the trait of food neophobia in humans. *Appetite* **1992**, *19*, 105–120. [CrossRef]
60. Ullrich, N.V.; Touger-Decker, R.; O'Sullivan-Maillet, J.; Tepper, B.J. PROP taster status and self-perceived food adventurousness influence food preferences. *J. Am. Diet. Assoc.* **2004**, *104*, 543–550. [CrossRef] [PubMed]
61. Pliner, P.; Loewen, E. Temperament and food neophobia in children and their mothers. *Appetite* **1997**, *28*, 239–254. [CrossRef] [PubMed]
62. Matheny, A.; Wachs, T.; Ludwig, J.; Phillips, K. Bringing order out of chaos: Psychometric characteristics of the confusion, hubbub, and order scale. *J. Appl. Dev. Psychol.* **1995**, *16*, 429–444. [CrossRef]
63. Cacioppo, J.; Petty, R. The need for cognition. *J. Personal. Soc. Psychol.* **1982**, *42*, 116–131. [CrossRef]
64. Cacioppo, J.; Petty, R.; Kao, C.F. The efficient assessment of need for cognition. *J. Personal. Assess.* **1984**, *48*, 306–307. [CrossRef] [PubMed]
65. Johnston, C.; Mash, E. A measure of parenting satisfaction and efficacy. *J. Clin. Child Psychol.* **1989**, *18*, 167–175. [CrossRef]
66. Gibaud-Wallston, J.; Wandersmann, L. *Development and Utility of the Parenting Sense of Competence Scale*; John F. Kennedy Center for Research on Education and Human Development: Washington, DC, USA, 1978.
67. Cohen, S.; Kamarck, T.; Mermelstein, R. A global measure of perceived stress. *J. Health Soc. Behav.* **1983**, *24*, 385–396. [CrossRef] [PubMed]
68. Birch, L.; Fisher, J.; Grimm-Thomas, K.; Markey, C.; Sawyer, R.; Johnson, S. Confirmatory factor analysis of the Child Feeding Questionnaire: A measure of parental attitudes, belief and practices about child feeding and obesity proneness. *Appetite* **2001**, *36*, 202–210. [CrossRef] [PubMed]
69. Gattshall, M.; Shoup, J.; Marshall, J.; Crane, L.; Estabrooks, P. Validation of a survey instrument to assess home environments for physical activity and healthy eating in overweight children. *Int. J. Behav. Nutr. Phys. Act.* **2008**, *5*, 3. [CrossRef] [PubMed]
70. Spurrier, N.; Magarey, A.; Golley, R.; Curnow, F.; Sawyer, M. Relationships between the home environment and physical activity and dietary patterns of preschool children: A cross-sectional study. *Int. J. Behav. Nutr. Phys. Act.* **2008**, *5*, 31. [CrossRef] [PubMed]
71. Bryant, M.; Ward, D.; Hales, D.; Vaughn, A.; Tabak, R.; Stevens, J. Reliability and validity of the Healthy Home Survey: A tool to measure factors within homes hypothesized to relate to overweight in children. *Int. J. Behav. Nutr. Phys. Act.* **2008**, *5*, 23. [CrossRef] [PubMed]

72. Earls, F.; Brooks-Gunn, J.; Raudenbush, S.; Sampson, R. *Project on human development in Chicago neighborhoods (PHDCN): Home and life interview, wave 2, 1997–2000. Instruments for ICPSR 13630*; Inter-University Consortium for Political and Social Research: Ann Arbor, MI, USA, undated.
73. Hughes, S.; Cross, M.; Hennessy, E.; Tovar, A.; Economos, C.; Power, T. Caregiver's Feeding Styles Questionnaire. Establishing cutoff points. *Appetite* **2012**, *58*, 393–395. [CrossRef] [PubMed]
74. Wardle, J.; Sanderson, S.; Guthrie, C.A.; Rapoport, L.; Plomin, R. Parental feeding style and the inter-generational transmission of obesity risk. *Obes. Res.* **2002**, *10*, 453–462. [CrossRef] [PubMed]
75. Ogden, J.; Reynolds, R.; Smith, A. Expanding the concept of parental control: A role for overt and covert control in children's snacking behaviour? *Appetite* **2006**, *47*, 100–106. [CrossRef] [PubMed]
76. Neumark-Sztainer, D.; Story, M.; Hannan, P.; Perry, C.; Irving, L. Weight-related concerns and behaviors among overweight and nonoverweight adolescents implications for preventing weight-related disorders. *Arch. Pediatr. Adol. Med.* **2002**, *156*, 171–178. [CrossRef]
77. Neumark-Sztainer, D.; Larson, N.; Fulkerson, J.; Eisenberg, M.; Story, M. Family meals and adolescents: What have we learned from Project EAT (Eating Among Teens)? *Public Health Nutr.* **2010**, *13*, 1113–1121. [CrossRef] [PubMed]
78. Koszewski, W.; Behrends, D.; Nichols, M.; Sehi, N.; Jones, G. Patterns of family meals and food and nutrition intake in limited resource families. *Fam. Consum. Sci. Res. J.* **2011**, *39*, 431–441. [CrossRef]
79. Neumark-Sztainer, D.; Wall, M.; Story, M.; Perry, C. Correlates of unhealthy weight-control behaviors among adolescents: Implications for prevention programs. *Health Psychol.* **2003**, *22*, 88–98. [CrossRef] [PubMed]
80. Storfer-Isser, A. *Association of Maternal Employment with Attitudes, Subjective Norms, and Perceived Behavioral Control Regarding Meal Preparation Among Mothers of 4–5 Years Old Children*; Bowling Green State University: Bowling Green, OH, USA, 2013.
81. Trost, S.G.; Sallis, J.F.; Pate, R.R.; Freedson, P.S.; Taylor, W.C.; Dowda, M. Evaluating a model of parental influence on youth physical activity. *Am. J. Prev. Med.* **2003**, *25*, 277–282. [CrossRef]
82. Sallis, J.F.; Prochaska, J.J.; Taylor, W.C.; Hill, J.O.; Geraci, J.C. Correlates of physical activity in a national sample of girls and boys in Grades 4 through 12. *Health Psychol.* **1999**, *18*, 410–415. [CrossRef] [PubMed]
83. Ball, K.; Crawford, D. An investigation of psychological, social and environmental correlates of obesity and weight gain in young women. *Int. J. Obes.* **2006**, *30*, 1240–1249. [CrossRef] [PubMed]
84. Moos RH, M.B. *Family Environment Scale Manual: Development, Applications, Research*, 3rd ed.; Consulting Psychologists Press: Palo Alto, CA, USA, 1994.
85. Saucier, G.; Wilson, K.; Warka, J. The structure of retrospective accounts of family environments: Related to the structure of personality attributes. *J. Personal. Assess.* **2007**, *88*, 295–308. [CrossRef] [PubMed]
86. Greene, R.; Plank, R. The short-form family environment scale: Testing a different response format. *Psychol. Rep.* **1994**, *74*, 451–464. [CrossRef]
87. Coldwell, J.; Pike, A.; Dunn, J. Household chaos—Links with parenting and child behaviour. *J. Child. Psychol. Psychiatry* **2006**, *47*, 1116–1122. [CrossRef] [PubMed]
88. Matheny, A.W.T., Jr.; Ludwig, J.L.; Phillips, K. Bringing order out of chaos: Psychometric characteristics of the confusion, hubbub, and order scale. *J. Appl. Dev. Psychol.* **1995**, *16*, 319–429. [CrossRef]
89. Crawford, D.; Telford, A.; Salmon, J. Perceptions about the local neighborhood and walking and cycling among children. *Prev. Med.* **2004**, *38*, 39–47.
90. Byrd-Bredbenner, C.; Maurer Abbot, J.; Cussler, E. Nutrient Profile of Household Food Supplies of Families with Young Children. *J. Am. Diet. Assoc.* **2009**, *109*, 2057–2062. [CrossRef] [PubMed]
91. Centers for Disease Control and Prevention CDC Growth Charts: United States. Available online: http://www.cdc.gov/nchs/about/major/nhanes/growthcharts/charts.htm (accessed on 2 June 2004).
92. Chu, S.Y.; Callaghan, W.M.; Kim, S.Y.; Schmid, C.H.; Lau, J.; England, L.J.; Dietz, P.M. Maternal obesity and risk of gestational diabetes mellitus. *Diabetes Care* **2007**, *30*, 2070–2076. [CrossRef] [PubMed]
93. Metzger, B.E.; Coustan, D.R.; Committee, O. Summary and recommendations of the fourth international workshop-conference on gestational diabetes mellitus. *Diabetes Care* **1998**, *21*, B161–B167. [PubMed]
94. Propser, M.-H.; Moczulski, V.; Qureshi, A. Obesity as a predictor of self-rated health. *Am. J. Health Behav.* **2009**, *33*, 319–329.
95. Jackson, T.D.; Grilo, C.M.; Masheb, R.M. Teasing history, onset of obesity, current eating disorder psychopathology, body dissatisfaction, and psychological functioning in binge eating disorder. *Obes. Res.* **2000**, *8*, 451–458. [CrossRef] [PubMed]

96. Quick, V.; McWilliams, R.; Byrd-Bredbenner, C. Fatty, Fatty, Two-By-Four: Weight teasing history and disturbed eating in young adult women. *Am. J. Public Health* **2013**, *103*, 508–515. [CrossRef] [PubMed]
97. Schwartz, M.B.; Brownell, K.D. Obesity and body image. *Body Image* **2004**, *1*, 43–56. [CrossRef]
98. Quick, V.; Eisenberg, M.; Bucchianeri, M.; Neumark-Sztainer, D. Prospective predictors of body dissatifaction in young adults: 10-year longitudinal findings. *Emerg. Adulthood* **2013**, *1*, 271–282. [CrossRef] [PubMed]
99. Newton, S.; Braithwaite, D.; Akinyemiju, T. Socio-economic status over the life course and obesity: Systematic review and meta-analysis. *PLoS ONE* **2017**, *12*, e0177151. [CrossRef] [PubMed]
100. Stunkard, A.J.; Faith, M.S.; Allison, K.C. Depression and obesity. *Biol. Psychiatry* **2003**, *54*, 330–337. [CrossRef]
101. Carey, M.; Small, H.; Yoong, S.; Boyes, A.; Bisquera, A.; Sanson-Fisher, R. Prevalence of comorbid depression and obesity in general practice: A cross-sectional survey. *Br. J. Gen. Pract.* **2014**, *64*, e122–e127. [CrossRef] [PubMed]
102. Thorp, A.; Owen, N.; Neuhas, M.; Dunstan, D. Sedentary behaviors and subsequent health outcomes in adults a systematic review of longitudinal studies, 1996–2011. *Am. J. Prev. Med.* **2011**, *41*, 207–215. [CrossRef] [PubMed]
103. Stronegger, W.; Titze, S.; Oja, P. Perceived characteristics of the neighborhood and its association with physical activiy behavior and self-rated health. *Health Place* **2010**, *16*, 736–743. [CrossRef] [PubMed]
104. Miller, W.D.; Pollack, C.E.; Williams, D.R. Healthy homes and communities: Putting the pieces together. *Am. J. Prev. Med.* **2011**, *40* (Suppl. 1), S48–S57. [CrossRef] [PubMed]
105. Davison, K.; Lawson, C. Do attributes in the physical environment influence children's physical activity? A review of the literature. *Int. J. Behav. Nutr. Phys. Act.* **2006**, *3*, 19. [CrossRef] [PubMed]
106. Kumanyika, S.K.; Parker, L.; Sim, L.J. *Bridging the Evidence Gap in Obesity Prevention: A Framework to Inform Decision Making*; Institute of Medicine of the National Academies: Washington, DC, USA, 2010.
107. Trost, S.G.; Owen, N.; Bauman, A.E.; Sallis, J.F.; Brown, W. Correlates of adults' participation in physical activity: Review and update. *Med. Sci. Sports Exerc.* **2002**, *34*, 1996–2001. [CrossRef] [PubMed]
108. Mackenbach, J.; Rutter, H.; Compernolle, S.; Glonti, K.; Oppert, J.; Charreire, H.; Bourdeaudhuij, I.; Brug, J.; Nijpels, G.; Lakerveld, J. Obesogenic environments: A systematic review of the association between the physical environment and adult weight status, the SPOTLIGHT project. *BMC Public Health* **2014**, *14*, 233. [CrossRef] [PubMed]
109. Golem, D.L.; Martin-Biggers, J.T.; Koenings, M.M.; Davis, K.F.; Byrd-Bredbenner, C. An integrative review of sleep for nutrition professionals. *Adv. Nut. Int. Rev. J.* **2014**, *5*, 742–759. [CrossRef] [PubMed]
110. Hirshkowitz, M.; Whiton, K.; Albert, S.; Alessi, C.; Bruni, O.; DonCarlos, L.; Hazen, N.; Herman, J.; Katz, E.; Kheirandish-Gozal, L.; et al. National Sleep Foundation's sleep time duration recommedations: Methodology and results summary. *Sleep Health* **2015**, *1*, 40–43. [CrossRef] [PubMed]
111. Sallis, J.; Prochaska, J.; Taylor, W. A review of correlates of physical activity of children and adolescents. *Med. Sci. Sports Exerc.* **2000**, *32*, 963–975. [CrossRef] [PubMed]
112. Sonneville, K.; Rifas-Shiman, S.; Kleinman, K.; Gortmaker, S.; Gillman, M.; Taveras, E. Associations of obesogenic behaviors in mothers and obese children participating in a randomized trial. *Obesity* **2012**, *20*, 1449–1454. [CrossRef] [PubMed]
113. Savage, J.; Fisher, J.; Birch, L. Parental influence on eating behavior: Conception to adolescence. *J. Law Med. Ethics* **2007**, *35*, 22–34. [CrossRef] [PubMed]
114. Santiago-Torres, M.; Adams, A.; Carrel, A.; LaRowe, T. Home food availability, parental dietary intake, and familial eating habits influence diet quality of urban Hispanic children. *Child. Obes.* **2014**, *10*, 408–415. [CrossRef] [PubMed]
115. Couch, S.; Glanz, K.; Zhou, C.; Sallis, J.; Saelens, B. Home food environment in relation to children's diet quality and weight status. *J. Acad. Nutr. Diet.* **2014**, *114*, 1569–1579. [CrossRef] [PubMed]
116. Brogan, K.; Idalski Carone, A.; Jen, K.; Ellis, D.; Marshall, S.; Naar-King, S. Factors associated with weight resilience in obesogenic environments in female African-American adolescents. *J. Acad. Nutr. Diet.* **2012**, *112*, 718–724. [CrossRef] [PubMed]
117. Williams, L.; Veitch, J.; Ball, K. What helps children eat well? A qualitative exploration of resilience among disadvantages families. *Health Educ. Res.* **2011**, *26*, 296–307. [CrossRef] [PubMed]
118. Fulkerson, J.A.; Neumark-Sztainer, D.; Hannan, P.J.; Story, M. Family meal frequency and weight status among adolescents: Cross-sectional and 5-year longitudinal associations. *Obesity* **2008**, *16*, 2529–2534. [CrossRef] [PubMed]

119. Sen, B. Frequency of family dinner and adolescent body weight status: Evidence from the national longitudinal survey of youth, 1997. *Obesity* **2006**, *14*, 2266–2276. [CrossRef] [PubMed]
120. Chan, J.C.; Sobal, J. Family meals and body weight. Analysis of multiple family members in family units. *Appetite* **2011**, *57*, 517–524. [CrossRef] [PubMed]
121. Martin-Biggers, J.; Spaccarotella, K.; Berhaupt-Glickstein, A.; Hongu, N.; Worobey, J.; Byrd-Bredbenner, C. Come and get it! A discussion of family mealtime literature and factors affecting obesity risk. *Adv. Nutr.* **2014**, *5*, 235–247. [CrossRef] [PubMed]
122. Halliday, J.; Palma, C.; Mellor, D.; Green, J.; Renzaho, A. The relationship between family functioning and child and adolescent overweight and obesity: A systematic review. *Int. J. Obes.* **2014**, *38*, 480–493. [CrossRef] [PubMed]
123. Cyril, S.; Halliday, J.; Green, J.; Renzaho, A.M. Relationship between body mass index and family functioning, family communication, family type and parenting style among African migrant parents and children in Victoria, Australia: A parent-child dyad study. *BMC Public Health* **2015**, *15*, 707. [CrossRef] [PubMed]
124. Zeller, M.; Reiter-Purtill, J.; Modi, A.; Gutzwiller, J.; Vannatta, K.; Davies, W. Controlled study of critical parent and family factors in the obesigenic environment. *Obesity* **2007**, *15*, 126–136. [CrossRef] [PubMed]
125. Sigman-Grant, M.; Hayes, J.; VanBrackle, A.; Fiese, B. Childhood obesity: Family Resiliency: A Neglected Perspective in Addressing Obesity in Young Children. *Child. Obes.* **2015**, *11*, 664–673. [CrossRef] [PubMed]
126. Pursey, K.; Burrows, T.; Stanwell, P.; Collins, C. How accurate is web-based self-reported height, weight and body mass index in young adults? *J. Med. Internet Res.* **2014**, *16*, e4. [CrossRef] [PubMed]
127. Chang, L.; Krosnick, J. National surveys via RDD elephone interviewing versus the internet comparing sample representativeness and response quality. *Public Opin. Q.* **2009**, *73*, 641–678. [CrossRef]
128. Sheehan, K.B. Crowdsourcing research: Data collection with Amazon's Mechanical Turk. *Commun. Monogr.* **2018**, *85*, 140–156. [CrossRef]
129. Lefever, S.; Dal, M. Online data collection in academic research: Advantages and limitations. *Br. J. Educ. Technol.* **2007**, *38*, 574–582. [CrossRef]

12

Exploring Relationships between Recurrent Binge Eating and Illicit Substance Use in a Non-Clinical Sample of Women over Two Years

Henry Kewen Lu [1], Haider Mannan [1,2] and Phillipa Hay [2,*]

[1] School of Medicine, Western Sydney University, Penrith NSW 2751, Australia; 17812812@student.westernsydney.edu.au (H.K.L.); H.Mannan@westernsydney.edu.au (H.M.)

[2] Translational Health Research Institute (THRI), School of Medicine, Western Sydney University, Penrith NSW 2751, Australia

* Correspondence: p.hay@westernsydney.edu.au

Abstract: (1) Background: With the new edition of the Diagnostic and Statistical Manual of Mental disorders, 5th Edition (DSM-5), numerous parallels have been drawn between recurrent binge eating (RBE) and substance use disorders, with many authors examining RBE or binge eating disorder (BED) as a "food addiction". The present study aims to clarify the relationship between recurrent binge eating (RBE) and illicit substance use (ISU) through investigating the temporal association between the two problems. (2) Methods: This study was embedded within a larger longitudinal study of non-clinical adult women recruited from Australian tertiary institutions. Participants responded at year 2 and year 4 of follow-up to the Eating Disorder Examination—Questionnaire. ISU was measured using a modified questionnaire taken from the Australian Longitudinal Study on Women's Health. (3) Results: RBE and ISU co-morbidity was 5.88% in this non-clinical sample, and having one condition increased the likelihood of the other. The two conditions had a different trajectory over two years whereby ISU participants had significant risk of developing RBE in addition to or in place of their ISU but the reverse was not found for RBE participants. (4) Conclusion: This unidirectional relationship suggests that in spite of the similarities of RBE and ISU they may be distinct with respect to their co-morbidity over time.

Keywords: recurrent binge eating; illicit substance use; binge eating disorder; longitudinal; co-morbidity; symptom trajectory

---

1. Introduction

1.1. Background

Binge eating disorder (BED) is characterised by recurrent episodes of binge eating (RBE)—defined by an objective overconsumption of food and a sense of loss of control—without the compensatory behaviours which define bulimia nervosa. BED has an estimated lifetime prevalence between 1.9% and 2.8% depending on the population surveyed, making it the most common eating disorder [1–3]. It is categorised within the Feeding and Eating Disorder (ED) chapter of the Diagnostic and Statistical Manual of Mental disorders, Fifth Edition (DSM-5), and is thus distinct from substance use disorders (SUDs). However, parallels have been drawn between BED and SUDs by a number of authors, many of them examining BED as a "food addiction" [1–4]. Criterion A for SUD within the DSM-5 may be divided into groupings of "impaired control, social impairment, risky use and pharmacological criteria" [5]. These are comparable to the BED criteria of "a sense of a lack of control", eating alone due to embarrassment, ongoing overeating despite negative consequences, and eating large amounts of food when not physically hungry.

BED and SUD also share a number of psychological, neurobiological and genetic correlates. Factors such as neuroticism, impulsivity, sensation seeking and mood dysregulation are associated with both BED and SUD [6–8]. Animal models also support the theory that both BED and SUD follow from dysregulation of the same dopaminergic pathways [9,10] and have likewise been able to produce somatic withdrawal symptoms with sucrose cessation [11].

1.2. Co-Morbidity

Literature regarding the co-morbidity shared between RBE/BED and SUD supports the idea that there is an underlying shared pathology between the two conditions. In examining the literature, there are a number of classification issues leading to variability in reported rates of co-morbidity and prior to its recognition in the DSM-5 [5], BED was included as a type of Eating Disorders Not Otherwise Specified (EDNOS) [12]. Complicating matters further, numerous studies either have failed to specify the type of ED they had studied or have classified participants with inconsistent criteria [13]. For many studies RBE has been used to represent BED. For example, in a US national face-to-face survey of 9282 adults, 23% of those who had BED—which was defined as having 3 months or more of RBE—suffered also from a type of SUD [14]. The WHO World Mental Health Surveys support these findings, in which 23.7% of those with BED would have some form of SUD [15]. In exploring the prevalence of SUD, it is noted that the classification of substance abuse is similarly difficult; research in this field varies not only in the scope of substance abuse, ranging from a focus on a single substance to looking at SUDs collectively, but also the severity of substance abuse, studying one-time use as well as physiological dependence [13,16]. Harrop & Marlatt's review [13] reflects these classification inconsistencies with co-morbidity prevalence ranging from 17–46% depending on ED and SUD types.

Illicit Substance Use (ISU) appears to be more common in ED populations than healthy controls; however, more information is needed to clarify the relationship between different types of illicit drugs and ED subgroups [16]. Cannabis [17,18] and opiate [17] use have found to be increased in those with an ED (subgroups combined) compared to controls. Evidence regarding amphetamine usage is inconsistent; one author reports associations of amphetamine usage with dieting and purging behaviour (without binging) [19,20] whilst another did not find increased use of amphetamines when comparing an ED group with the general population [17]. These findings may suggest that amphetamine usage may be associated with dieting and purging rather than with binging behaviour [16].

1.3. Longitudinal Predictors

On the other hand, longitudinal studies seem to suggest that however many similarities there may be between RBE/BED and ISU, they seem to differ in illness trajectories. A five-year longitudinal study of adolescent girls found that depressive symptoms were predictive of higher future levels of eating pathology and substance abuse (broadly defined and including alcohol use); eating pathology itself also predicted increased future substance abuse, with the inverse not being true [21]. Similarly, an Australian cohort study of adolescents and young adults found that even partial anorexia nervosa (AN)/bulimia nervosa (BN) diagnosis (where a participant satisfied two of four or three criteria for AN/BN) was predictive of amphetamine use [22]. The Growing Up Today Study has found that overeating (without a loss of control (LOC)) and RBE (overeating with a sense of a LOC) were both predictors for ISU; however, overeating alone was a stronger predictor for this outcome [23].

Fewer longitudinal papers have focused on predictors of RBE. Vogeltanze-Holm et al., found that the main factors predicting BED (strictly defined) was ISU in the past 12 months (odds ratio (OR) = 5.77, 95% CI = 1.64, 20.34) and more occasions of alcohol use until intoxication in the past 12 months (OR = 1.38, 95% CI = 1.03, 1.85) [24].

Finally, a five-year longitudinal study documenting the natural history of a variety of behavioural addictions over this period found a central effect of time on the problem behaviours, where the prevalence of the behaviours decreased and often resolved without intervention [25]. Excessive eating (examined over four years only) was found to decrease in prevalence at the same rate as comorbid substance use (broadly defined), with a mean 11.7% (SD = 2.3) suffering from comorbid SUD during the four-year time period.

These findings—in particular, that RBE/BED and ISU/SUD may not mutually predict risk for each other—suggest that perhaps distinct higher-order factors are mediating the relationship between RBE/BED and ISU/SUD rather than being controlled by the same underlying factor [13]. In a review of the phenomenology and treatment of behavioural addictions, Grant et al. hypothesises the opposite [26], claiming that one neurobiological dysfunction could give rise to multiple behavioural symptoms. The support for this theory comes from "consummatory cross-sensitisation" where prolonged intake and sensitisation with one substance can lead to increased consumption of another [4]. As a result of this cross-sensitisation, opiate- and stimulant-dependent individuals may have a cross-substitutability of preference for highly palatable foods, leading to reported cravings and binges [9,27].

Although there have been these studies of outcomes and putative symptoms substitution, it is notable that there have been few studies of the impact of comorbidity on other clinical features such as overall psychological distress, health-related quality of life and/or body weight, and findings have been mixed or inconsistent [28]. This may be of clinical importance if co-morbidity was found to be associated with poorer mental health and/or increased likelihood of obesity.

1.4. Aim and Hypotheses

In this study, we aimed to elucidate the nature of co-morbidity by (1) characterising the extent of the overlap of these two features within a non-clinical population, and (2) examining the trajectories of participants with regard to RBE and ISU over a period of two years' time. We hypothesised that there would be significant co-morbidity between the two problems and, furthermore, that participants with RBE and those with ISU will have differing illness trajectories without mutual substitution between the two behaviours. We did not have specific hypotheses in regard to examining general psychological distress or health-related quality of life as these have been little studied in regard to the comorbidity of ISU and RBE.

2. Materials and Methods

2.1. Participants

Participants were 794 women initially recruited in 2004/2005 who were assessed repeatedly over a nine-year period (T0–T9). Any one follow-up assessment was not contingent on having competed any other follow-up. They were recruited through advertisements in four regional universities and vocational colleges (including adult students) in the Australian states of Queensland and Victoria for the purpose of a longitudinal study of community (non-clinical) women with and without eating disorder symptoms. Some participants were recruited via email and responded to the questionnaire online, whilst others were directly approached on campus locations and given hard-copy questionnaires and reply-paid envelopes. Due to these recruitment methods, characteristics of non-responders and overall response rate could not be measured.

ISU was only assessed in T2 and T4 of the longitudinal study. As such, the present study comprises of participants who responded in T2 (n = 357) and those who responded in T4 who also responded in T2 (n = 268). Respondents who had no data for measures of binge eating or substance use in T2 (n = 4) or T4 (n = 9) were excluded. Figure 1 shows the participant flow through T1, T2 and T4 of the longitudinal study.

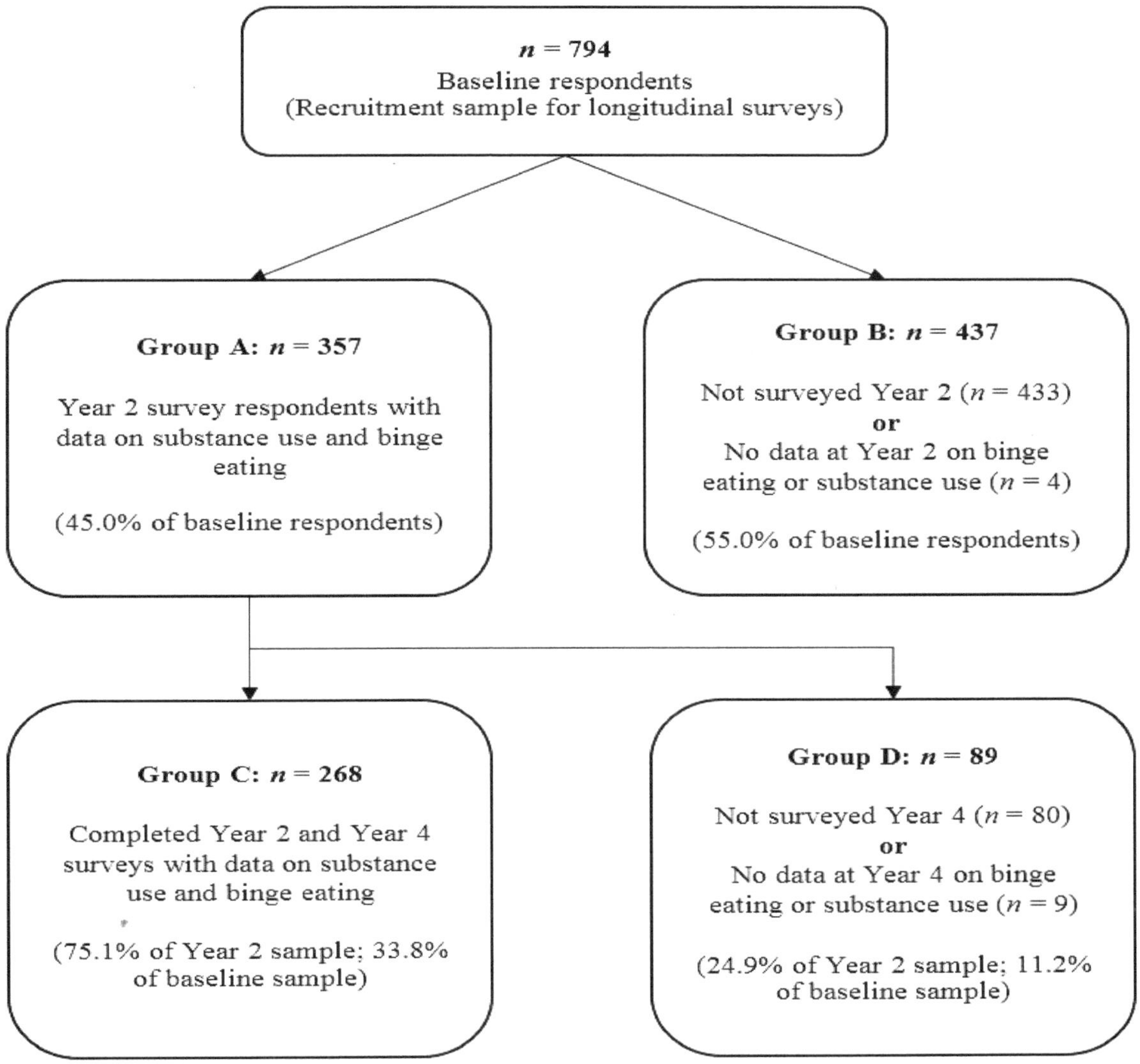

Figure 1. Participant flow from the beginning of the survey.

2.2. Procedures

The study was approved by the human research ethics committees (HREC) of the universities involved, with the Western Sydney University as lead HREC (Approval number 07/240). All participants completed written informed consent forms and there were no children requiring consent from a parent or guardian.

2.3. Measures

2.3.1. Binge Eating

The Eating Disorder Examination Questionnaire (EDE-Q), a self-report questionnaire based on the Eating Disorder Examination (EDE) interview was used in order to assess eating disorder psychopathology. The EDE-Q has been validated in both community and clinical samples of patients with eating disorders and demonstrates close agreement with the EDE overall [29]. However, with regard to the complex features involved with binge eating behaviours the EDE-Q consistently generated higher levels of disturbance relative to the EDE [30].

Four items in the questionnaire targeted binge eating behaviours. The first two assessed objective binge eating (OBE), asking if the respondent had ever consumed what other people would regard as an unusually large amount of food, with a sensation of loss of control, and if so, how many times that had occurred over the past 28 days. This correlates with the DSM-5 criteria for recurrent binge eating episodes (Criterion A) but does not specify a discrete time period [5]. The second two assessed subjective binge eating (SBE), asking if the respondent had consumed a normal amount of food for the circumstances but had experienced a loss of control, and if yes, the number of times that had occurred. This is consistent with binge eating criteria being considered for the incoming International Classification of Diseases, 11th revision (ICD-11) [31], on the basis that people with subjective episodes have similar levels of impairment and distress related to binge eating as well as other psychopathology as do people with objective episodes [32,33]. As such, binge eating was coded as "present" if they had reported "yes" to either an objective or subjective binge for more than four episodes in the past 28 days and is used as the measure in this study of RBE. At the end of the EDE-Q there was a question asking current weight and height from which body mass index (BMI; kg/m^2) scores were derived.

2.3.2. Illicit Substance Use (ISU)

The questionnaire assessed frequency and amount of use of the following illicit substances: cannabis, amphetamines, hallucinogens, barbiturates, "ecstasy/designer drugs/cocaine", "inhalants" and heroin. Participants were asked if they had used any of the illicit substances listed above in the past year, and if yes, the frequency of their current use over a one-month period. These questions were modified from the Australian Longitudinal Study on Women's Health (ALSWH), where their frequency of use was categorised into scores of: 1 = less than monthly, 2 = monthly, 3 = weekly, 4 = two to three times per week, and 5 = daily [34]. The ordinal data gathered by this questionnaire allowed the creation of a new variable for the present study measuring overall ISU, which was calculated by taking the sum of the scores for each of the seven drug categories. A score of zero indicated no ISU, whilst the maximum score of thirty-five indicated that the participant was taking illicit drugs in all seven categories every single day of the week. The score is therefore influenced both by the range of illicit drugs consumed, as well as their frequency. For the purpose of this study, ISU was coded as present if the score was greater than 0, i.e., 1 or more.

2.3.3. Psychological Distress

This was assessed with the Kessler-10 item distress scale (K-10) which was designed to detect cases of anxiety and affective disorders in the general population [35]. It is a 10-item instrument with an ordinal 5-point response to each question. It measures the level of distress and severity associated with psychological symptoms of depression and anxiety. The K10 is extensively used internationally, including in the WHO World Mental Health Survey and by government organizations in Australia, Spain, Colombia and Peru [36]. The advantages of the K-10 are its brief nature and its strong psychometric properties. It focuses on the previous 28 days thus is comparable in time-frame to the EDE-Q.

2.3.4. Health-Related Quality of Life (HRQoL)

HRQoL was assessed with the well-validated 12-item Short Form-12 Health Status Questionnaire (SF-12) [37]. The SF-12 measures the impact of physical and mental ill-health on role limitations. It has been used extensively in research assessing impairment associated with physical and mental health conditions, and has robust psychometric properties, including in an Australian population sample [37,38]. It is a 12-item questionnaire that generates two weighted scales, a Physical Component Summary Scale (PCS) and a Mental Component Summary Scale (MCS), with each a mean of 50 and standard deviation of 10 in normative samples. Higher scores indicate higher levels of functioning.

2.4. Statistical Methods

Data were inspected for normality. Descriptive statistics were employed to report frequencies of socio-demographic variables, general symptoms, binge eating and substance use. Between-group differences were compared using ANOVA with post-hoc Tukey analyses for continuous normal data and Kruskal–Wallis and Mann–Whitney U tests for continuous non-normal data. The chi-squared test was utilised to test differences in distribution between categorical groups and ordinal data. Fisher's exact test was utilised to calculate the p-value for the contingency tables given the small sample size. To determine whether a trajectory based on a transition from year 2 to year 4 was statistically significant, we tested the significance of estimated marginal probability for each trajectory based on the multinomial logistic regression of a multi-category outcome containing all possible combinations of RBE & ISU measured at year 4 conditional on the same outcome at year 2, while controlling for age and mental health-related quality of life both being measured at year 2. While assessing the relationship between a multi-category outcome containing all possible combinations of RBE & ISU measured at year 2 & the same outcome measured at year 4, both the control variables were found to be confounders. Listwise deletion of missing data was applied to the data at year 4 because the percentage missing at time 4 out of a total of 359 cases at time 2 who had any of the four possible RBE & ISU conditions was very low (3.06%), and hence complete case analysis would introduce very little bias. A significance level of $p < 0.05$ was employed for all tests. Analyses were conducted using IBM SPSS Statistics for Windows, version 22.

3. Results

3.1. Participant Features

Of the 357 participants who completed the follow-up survey at T2 (45.0% of baseline respondents), the median age (at T2) was 25 (Interquartile Range (IQR) = 15), 58.0% were unmarried or separated and 52.9% lived with family, friends or alone. The sample was well educated, with 33.9% achieving at least year 12, and 48.5% attaining a bachelor's degree or higher. A large minority of the sample studied full-time (41.5%). Participants with symptoms were overrepresented in this study sample; compared to a previous general population study of Australian women, their Mental Health-Related Quality of Life scores (Short-Form 12 Mental Health Component Scores or SF-12 MCS) were lower and their EDE-Q subscale and global scores were higher, although lower than in clinical samples [39]. (See Section 2.3 for descriptors of these assessment measures.) ISU occurred in 20% ($n = 72$) of participants. Cannabis ($n = 59$, 82%) was the most frequently used substance followed by ecstasy/designer drugs/cocaine ($n = 40$, 56%). Other demographic and clinical features of the 357 participants at T2 can be found in Table 1.

Table 1. Descriptive data of 357 study participants in the present study.

	n	Mean	Standard Deviation	Median	Interquartile Range
Age/years at year 2	354	30.7	11.4	25	15
Body Mass Index (kg/m^2)	342	24.8	5.5	23.5	5.3
Eating Disorder Examination—Questionnaire					
Weight concern subscale	353	2.04	1.54	1.80	2.60
Eating concern subscale	350	0.953	1.18	0.400	1.20
Shape concern subscale	346	2.37	1.58	2.13	2.63
Restraint subscale	352	1.57	1.43	1.20	2.00
Global Score	336	1.74	1.29	1.44	1.95
Illicit substance use frequency [1]	357	0.65	1.72	0	0
Kessler 10 Psychological Distress Scale	351	17.5	6	16	7
Short Form-12 [2] Physical Component Score	348	52.1	8.2	54.5	8.3
Short Form-12 Mental Component Score	348	44.9	11.3	48.6	16.7

[1] Illicit substance use frequency (range none to daily use) was a summed score of the seven drug categories. [2] The Short Form-12 is a measure of Health-Related Quality of Life.

Table 2 compares key characteristics of the four subgroups within the longitudinal study to assess if respondents were significantly different from non-respondents at T2 and T4. These are divided by response status and availability of RBE and ISU data. These groups are also outlined in Figure 1.

Year 2 respondents (Group A) were significantly older (MD = 2.23, SE = 0.74) than those who responded at baseline but were lost to follow-up (Group B), but were not significantly different in the other measures of body mass index (BMI (kg/m^2)) and RBE characteristics. Participants who followed up at both year 2 and year 4 (Group C) were also significantly older (MD = 3.79, SE = 1.38) than their counterparts who did not respond in year 4 (Group D) and similarly, were not significantly different in BMI, RBE or ISU behaviours.

Table 2. Participant characteristics of subgroups within the study.

Feature	Group A [1]	Group B [2]		Group C [3]	Group D [4]	
	Mean (SD) *n*		*t*, *p*	Mean (SD) *n*		*t*, *p*
Age	28.7 (11.4) *354*	26.5 (10.5) *426*	−2.85, 0.005	31.7 (12.02) *266*	27.9 (8.54) *88*	−2.74, 0.006
Body Mass Index (kg/m^2)	24.3 (5.23) *336*	23.7 (5.52) *409*	−1.59, 0.11	24.91 (5.62) *254*	24.5 (5.17) *88*	−6.1, 0.545
	Median (IQR) *n*		*z*, *p*	Median (IQR) *n*		*z*, *p*
OBE/month	0 (0–1) *340*	0 (0–0) *408*	−3.34, 0.001	0 (0–0) *268*	0 (0–0) *89*	−0.62, 0.534
SBE/month	0 (0–2) *340*	0 (0–0) *408*	−2.75, 0.01	0 (0–2) *267*	0 (0–2) *89*	−0.09, 0.928
ISU	n.a. (ISU not assessed at baseline)			0 (0–0) *267*	0 (0–1) *89*	−1.70, 0.089

[1] Participants who responded at T2 (with BE and ISU data), *n* = 357; [2] Participants who responded at baseline, but not at T2 *or* had no BE or ISU data at T2, *n* = 437; [3] Participants who responded at T2 *and* T4 (with BE and ISU data), *n* = 268; [4] Participants who responded at T2 but *not* at T4 *or* had no BE or ISU data at T4, *n* = 94; OBE = objective binge eating episodes; SBE = subjective binge eating episodes; ISU = illicit substance use; BE = binge eating; IQR = Interquartile Range.

3.2. Co-Morbid ISU and RBE in the T2 Cohort

At T2, 226 of 357 (63.3%) respondents had neither RBE nor ISU behaviours; 55 (15.4%) had episodes of RBE *only*; the same number (*n* = 55, 15.4%) engaged in ISU *only*, whilst 21 participants (5.88%) in T2 admitted to engaging in both behaviours.

The majority of participants who were identified as having a problem (either RBE or ISU) had one problem only and not the other (55/76, 72.4%) and this finding was not significant ($\chi^2 = 2.32$, df = 1; $p = 0.09$). As shown in Table 3 it was determined that those who had RBE had significantly higher frequency of ISU compared to those without RBE, and similarly, those who had ISU had significantly higher frequency of RBE compared to those without ISU.

Table 3. Comparative levels of illicit substance use (ISU) and recurrent binge eating (RBE) in participants with and without either problem.

Level of Behaviour	Median, IQ Range, *n*		Mann–Whitney U *Z*, *p*
n = 357	RBE	No RBE	
ISU	1, 0–6, *73*	0, 0–2, *282*	−2.612, 0.009
	ISU	No. ISU	
RBE	0, 0–6, *76*	0, 0–2, *281*	−2.234, 0.026

Furthermore, participants with both ISU and RBE had the highest levels of eating disorder symptoms (global and subscale EDE-Q scores) and psychological distress (K-10 scores) and lowest levels of mental health HRQoL. These differences reached significance only for the findings of global EDE-Q scores compared to those with ISU alone, and K-10 scores compared to those with neither problem. Those with neither problem also had significantly lower EDE-Q global scores than all other groups and lower K-10 scores than those with RBE alone. These differences are shown in Table 4.

Table 4. Comparative clinical features of participants according to their RBE and ISU status.

	Neither [1]	**RBE** [2]	**ISU** [3]	**Both** [4]		**Post-Hoc Tests with $p < 0.05$**
Outcome	mean, SD, *n*				ANOVA F (df), *p*	Tukey test
EDE-Q Global	1.56, 1.21, 210	2.62, 1.38, 59	2.12, 1.43, 49	3.16, 1.23, 21	18.19 (3), <0.001	Neither ≠ Both, ISU, RBE; ISU ≠ Both
EDE-Q Restraint	1.17, 1.20, 219	2.59, 1.44, 59	1.46, 1.41, 50	2.87, 1.43, 23	27.33 (3), <0.001	Neither ≠ Both, RBE; ISU ≠ Both, RBE
EDE-Q Eating Concern	0.52, 0.74, 216	2.11, 1.29, 59	0.69, 0.73, 51	2.46,1.43, 23	70.62 (3), <0.001	Neither ≠ Both, RBE; ISU ≠ Both, RBE
EDE-Q Shape concern	1.86, 1.32, 210	3.82, 1.36, 59	2.01, 1.36, 53	3.89, 1.44, 23	44.24 (3), <0.001	Neither ≠ Both, RBE; ISU ≠ Both, RBE
EDE-Q Weight Concern	1.56, 1.28, 218	3.41, 1.42, 58	1.71, 1.24, 53	3.66, 1.43, 23	43.65 (3), <0.001	Neither ≠ Both, RBE; ISU ≠ Both, RBE
SF-12 MCS	45.94, 10.77, 219	43.04, 11.71, 59	44.31, 1.60, 52	41.09, 11.79, 23	2.13 (3), 0.096	n.a.
SF-12 PCS	52.61, 7.32, 291	51.24, 9.05, 59	53.15, 6.61, 52	51.20, 7.35, 23	0.89 (3), 0.45	n.a.
K-10 score	17.50, 6.23, 218	21.07, 7.65, 60	19.12, 7.8, 52	22.09, 7.99, 23	6.54 (3), <0.001	Neither ≠ RBE, Both
	median, IQ range, *n*				Kruskal–Wallis X^2 (df), *p*	Mann–Whitney U Z, *p*
Body Mass Index (kg/m^2)	23.6, 21.5–26.4 *211*	23.2, 20.8–29.2 *57*	23.5, 20.9–25.0 *50*	23.1, 20.2–25.0 *23*	1.924 (3), 0.588	n.a.

[1] Participants with neither RBE nor ISU features; [2] Participants with RBE only; [3] Participants with ISU features only; [4] Participants with both RBE and ISU features; RBE = Recurrent Binge Eating; ISU = illicit substance use; EDE-Q = Eating Disorder Examination—Questionnaire, SF-12 = Short-Form 12; MCS/PCS = Mental health/physical health component score; K-10 = Kessler 10-item questionnaire.

3.3. Participant Trajectories from T2 to T4

As shown in Table 5, the majority (n = 139, 82.2%) of participants with neither RBE nor ISU in T2 continued to have neither problem in T4, and 12% (n = 21) developed RBE. Almost half (n = 6, 46.2%) of those with both problems in T2 continued to have both problems in T4. Almost half (n = 18, 46.2%) of those with ISU in Year 2 continued to have ISU in year 4 and n = 7 (17.9%) developed an additional problem with RBE and n = 5 (12.8%) transitioned to RBE alone. The majority (n = 26, 57.8%) of those with RBE in T2 had neither problem in T4 and n = 17 (37.8%) continued to have RBE alone.

Table 5. Longitudinal movement of participants between groups (n = 266).

	Year 4 Participants n (%)			
Year 2 Participants	**Neither**	**Both**	**ISU**	**RBE**
Neither [1]	139 (82.2)	2 (1.2)	7 (4.1)	21 (12.4)
Both [2]	2 (15.4)	6 (46.2)	3 (23.1)	2 (15.4)
ISU [3]	9 (23.1)	7 (17.9)	18 (46.2)	5 (12.8)
RBE [4]	26 (57.8)	1 (2.2)	1 (2.2)	17 (37.8)

[1] Participants with neither RBE *nor* ISU features; [2] Participants with both RBE and ISU features; [3] Participants with ISU features only; [4] Participants with RBE only; RBE = Recurrent Binge Eating ISU = illicit substance use.

As shown in Table 6, participants with neither RBE nor ISU at year 2: were significantly more likely ($p < 0.001$) to remain that way or have RBE only by year 4, were significantly more likely ($p < 0.01$) to have ISU only by year 4, but were not significantly more likely to have both RBE and ISU by year 4. The most likely trajectory for those who were neither RBE nor ISU at year 2 was to remain that way by year 4. Participants being both RBE and ISU at year 2: were significantly more likely ($p < 0.05$) to have ISU only or both RBE & ISU by year 4, but were not significantly more likely to have RBE only or neither RBE nor ISU by year 4. The most likely trajectory for those who were both RBE and ISU at year 2 was to remain that way by year 4. Participants being RBE only at year 2 on the contrary: were significantly more likely ($p < 0.05$) to have RBE only or neither RBE nor ISU by year 4, but were not significantly more likely to have ISU only or both RBE & ISU by year 4. The most likely trajectory for those who were RBE only at year 2 was to have neither RBE nor ISU by year 4. For participants being ISU only at year 2 all transitions to year 4 were statistically significant with the most likely trajectory being both ISU only at year 2 and year 4.

Table 6. Estimated marginal probability with 95% confidence interval for each trajectory from year 2 to year 4 based on multinomial logistic regression controlling for age and mental health-related quality of life.

	Year 4 Outcome Estimated Marginal Probability with 95% Confidence Interval			
	Neither RBE nor ISU	**Both RBE & ISU**	**RBE Only**	**ISU Only**
Year 2 Status				
Neither RBE nor ISU	0.825 [a] (0.764, 0.886)	0.009 (−0.005, 0.024)	0.120 [a] (0.068, 0.172)	0.045 [b] (0.012, 0.078)
Both RBE & ISU	0.213 (−0.556, 0.481)	0.334 [c] (0.009, 0.659)	0.139 (−0.052, 0.331)	0.314 [c] (0.007, 0.621)
RBE Only	0.587 [a] (0.432, 0.741)	0.012 (−0.013, 0.036)	0.363 [a] (0.211, 0.515)	0.038 (−0.016, 0.095)
ISU Only	0.270 [b] (0.116, 0.425)	0.137 [c] (0.012, 0.263)	0.116 [c] (0.014, 0.217)	0.477 [a] (0.299, 0.654)

Note: a is $p < 0.001$, b is $p < 0.01$, c is $p < 0.05$ RBE = recurrent binge eating; ISU = illicit substance use.

4. Discussion

The current study investigated the relationship between RBE and ISU in a sample of Australian non-clinical adult women. The co-occurrence of ISU and RBE was examined cross-sectionally and then longitudinally over two years.

4.1. Comorbid Psychopathology

The hypothesis that RBE and ISU co-occur in the setting of a broader community sample was confirmed. Our study found that those with RBE had a higher frequency of ISU as well as the inverse, i.e., those with ISU had higher frequency of RBE. This co-morbidity might be explained by common neurobiological pathways involved in the two conditions [3,4] or may be a reflection of a self-mediated attempt at regulating negative affect [40], as demonstrated by Killeen et al., who found that past 30 day opiate use was correlated with increased EDE-Q scores [41]. Furthermore, our findings support those of Grilo et al. [42], which found that patients with BED with another concurrent psychiatric disorder had elevated levels of eating disorder psychopathology, although in this study this did not reach significance possibly because of small numbers of those with both problems.

4.2. Participant Trajectories and Between-Group Associations

Results from comparing participant numbers as they moved through from year 2 to year 4 demonstrated that participants with ISU were more likely to develop RBE either in addition to, or in place of their ISU, whereas those with RBE were likely to remain unchanged or spontaneously resolve over time, supporting our hypothesis that the two conditions take unique temporal courses and are differentially predictive for each other. Whist our findings are theoretically supportive of the existing literature in distinguishing RBE/BED and ISU/SUD, there are some differences in results. Measelle et al.'s [21] longitudinal study was similar in part to the present study and focussed on a variety of psychiatric disorders in adolescent girls and the temporal associations between symptom domains; in their study they established that there was a unidirectional relationship between BED and SUD—however, in their case pre-existing eating pathology predicted future growth in substance abuse but not the reverse—the opposite conclusion to this present study. This difference might be because of the shorter duration of this study, that Measelle et al. studied substance use more broadly and included alcohol abuse, and that we were studying subthreshold syndromes. Our findings however support the longitudinal findings of Vogeltanz-Holm et al. [24] that the main predictors for BED are ISU and alcohol intoxication. Furthermore, cessation of drug abuse followed by hyperphagia and weight gain is an established phenomenon in human studies [43] and animal models [44], although whether or not this disordered eating persists and develops into RBE/BED is a matter requiring further investigation.

4.3. Strengths and Limitations

The main strengths of this study include the reasonable sample size (n = 268) for the trajectory analysis and a 75.1% rate of retention of participants over the two-year follow-up period. However, the low numbers of those with both ISU and RBE may have limited finding statistical significance. The longitudinal design of the paper adds robustness to the findings presented in the study. However, the voluntary nature of recruitment and follow-up resulted in only 33.8% of baseline respondents being included for analysis, possibly contributing to elevated findings of eating disorder and ISU. Notably, we did not have a full assessment of the criteria for either BED or SUD, or more detailed assessment of RBE over a longer time frame, and did not assess for legal SUDs. Thus, we turned our focus to ISU and did not include legal substances such as alcohol and tobacco on the presumption that the act of breaching the law and risking the consequences of such more strongly implicates disordered substance use. Another important limitation is the non-inclusion of men as they have significantly higher rates of alcohol and drug use disorders; inclusion might produce altered co-morbidity rates and differing trajectories [45]. Further limitations include the single follow-up, self-report assessments of symptoms and BMI.

4.4. Clinical Implications

The key take-away from this study is that many participants with ISU went on to develop RBE, whilst those with RBE had a tendency for their behaviour to resolve over time. This is a relevant piece of information for clinicians in practice as it suggests that early assessment, monitoring and appropriate early intervention is important for individuals with ISU, and that this occurred despite the low threshold for defining ISU in this research. Finally, despite the stated differences between RBE and ISU, taking an addiction framework towards BED may improve current interventions or instigate the development of new treatments [8].

4.5. Future Directions

Studies investigating predictors for binge eating and its temporal associations are limited and, as such, further mixed-gender longitudinal studies conducted over longer periods of time would be warranted to clarify the associations between RBE and ISU. Other relevant aspects inviting possible future study include the investigation of alcohol or tobacco usage and binge eating behaviour as these commonplace drugs are also frequently consumed in excess. As a final point of interest, within the DSM-5, gambling and other behavioural addictions have been included within the same section as SUDs [46]. Given the co-morbidity between BED and SUD, it would be relevant to also consider the possible neurobiological and symptomatic correlates between full-threshold BED and other addictive disorders. It should be kept in mind as well that BED may be a construct distinct from the entity of "food addiction" which may present more similarities with SUD, and as such, further research is required in this area.

5. Conclusions

In this study, RBE and ISU have been found to be comorbid conditions in a non-clinical sample of young adult women, and furthermore, each condition increased the frequency of episodes of the other. Despite their similarities, the two conditions had a diverse trajectory over time, whereby ISU participants had higher likelihood of later developing RBE co-morbidly or in substitution but the reverse was not found for RBE participants. Further studies are indicated of full-spectrum BED and SUDs.

Acknowledgments: The longitudinal research was funded by a grant from the Australian Rotary Health Research Fund to P.H. and colleagues. H.K.L. was supported by a summer research scholarship from the School of Medicine, Western Sydney University.

Author Contributions: H.K.L. and P.H. contributed to the conception, design and aims of the study. H.K.L., H.M. and P.H. conducted the data analysis. H.K.L. drafted the manuscript. All authors read and approved the final manuscript.

References

1. Cassin, S.E.; von Ranson, K.M. Is binge eating experienced as an addiction? *Appetite* **2007**, *49*, 687–690. [CrossRef] [PubMed]
2. Gearhardt, A.N.; White, M.A.; Potenza, M.N. Binge eating disorder and food addiction. *Curr. Drug Abuse Rev.* **2011**, *4*, 201–207. [CrossRef] [PubMed]
3. Schreiber, L.R.; Odlaug, B.L.; Grant, J.E. The overlap between binge eating disorder and substance use disorders: Diagnosis and neurobiology. *J. Behav. Addict.* **2013**, *2*, 191–198. [CrossRef] [PubMed]

4. Smith, D.G.; Robbins, T.W. The neurobiological underpinnings of obesity and binge eating: A rationale for adopting the food addiction model. *Biol. Psychiatry* **2013**, *73*, 804–810. [CrossRef] [PubMed]
5. American Psychiatric Association. Feeding and Eating Disorders. In *Diagnostic and Statistical Manual of Mental Disorders*, 5th ed.; American Psychiatric Association: Washington, DC, USA, 2013.
6. Grant, J.E.; Potenza, M.N.; Weinstein, A.; Gorelick, D.A. Introduction to behavioral addictions. *Am. J. Drug Alcohol. Abuse* **2010**, *36*, 233–241. [CrossRef] [PubMed]
7. Ferriter, C.; Ray, L.A. Binge eating and binge drinking: An integrative review. *Eat Behav.* **2011**, *12*, 99–107. [CrossRef] [PubMed]
8. Schulte, E.M.; Grilo, C.M.; Gearhardt, A.N. Shared and unique mechanisms underlying binge eating disorder and addictive disorders. *Clin. Psychol. Rev.* **2016**, *44*, 125–139. [CrossRef] [PubMed]
9. Avena, N.M.; Rada, P.; Hoebel, B.G. Evidence for sugar addiction: Behavioral and neurochemical effects of intermittent, excessive sugar intake. *Neurosci. Biobehav. Rev.* **2008**, *32*, 20–39. [CrossRef] [PubMed]
10. Johnson, P.M.; Kenny, P.J. Dopamine D2 receptors in addiction-like reward dysfunction and compulsive eating in obese rats. *Nat. Neurosci.* **2010**, *13*, 635–641. [CrossRef] [PubMed]
11. Avena, N.M.; Rada, P.; Hoebel, B.G. Sugar and fat bingeing have notable differences in addictive-like behavior. *J. Nutr.* **2009**, *139*, 623–628. [CrossRef] [PubMed]
12. American Psychiatric Association. Feeding and Eating Disorders. In *Diagnostic and Statistical Manual of Mental Disorders*, 4th ed.; American Psychiatric Association: Washington, DC, USA, 1994.
13. Harrop, E.N.; Marlatt, G.A. The comorbidity of substance use disorders and eating disorders in women: Prevalence, etiology, and treatment. *Addict. Behav.* **2010**, *35*, 392–398. [CrossRef] [PubMed]
14. Hudson, J.I.; Hiripi, E.; Pope, H.G., Jr.; Kessler, R.C. The prevalence and correlates of eating disorders in the National Comorbidity Survey Replication. *Biol. Psychiatry* **2007**, *61*, 348–358. [CrossRef] [PubMed]
15. Kessler, R.C.; Berglund, P.A.; Chiu, W.T.; Deitz, A.C.; Hudson, J.I.; Shahly, V.; Aguilar-Gaxiola, S.; Alonso, J.; Angermeyer, M.C.; Benjet, C.; et al. The prevalence and correlates of binge eating disorder in the World Health Organization World Mental Health Surveys. *Biol. Psychiatry* **2013**, *73*, 904–914. [CrossRef] [PubMed]
16. Gregorowski, C.; Seedat, S.; Jordaan, G.P. A clinical approach to the assessment and management of co-morbid eating disorders and substance use disorders. *BMC Psychiatry* **2013**, *13*, 289. [CrossRef] [PubMed]
17. Calero-Elvira, A.; Krug, I.; Davis, K.; Lopez, C.; Fernandez-Aranda, F.; Treasure, J. Meta-analysis on drugs in people with eating disorders. *Eur. Eat. Disord. Rev. J. Eat. Disord. Assoc.* **2009**, *17*, 243–259. [CrossRef] [PubMed]
18. Root, T.L.; Pisetsky, E.M.; Thornton, L.; Lichtenstein, P.; Pedersen, N.L.; Bulik, C.M. Patterns of co-morbidity of eating disorders and substance use in Swedish females. *Psychol. Med.* **2010**, *40*, 105–115. [CrossRef] [PubMed]
19. Piran, N.; Robinson, S.R. Associations between disordered eating behaviors and licit and illicit substance use and abuse in a university sample. *Addict. Behav.* **2006**, *31*, 1761–1775. [CrossRef] [PubMed]
20. Piran, N.; Robinson, S.R. Patterns of associations between eating disordered behaviors and substance use in two non-clinical samples: A university and a community based sample. *J. Health Psychol.* **2011**, *16*, 1027–1037. [CrossRef] [PubMed]
21. Measelle, J.R.; Stice, E.; Hogansen, J.M. Developmental trajectories of co-occurring depressive, eating, antisocial, and substance abuse problems in female adolescents. *J. Abnorm. Psychol.* **2006**, *115*, 524–538. [CrossRef] [PubMed]
22. Patton, G.C.; Coffey, C.; Carlin, J.B.; Sanci, L.; Sawyer, S. Prognosis of adolescent partial syndromes of eating disorder. *Br. J. Psychiatry* **2008**, *192*, 294–299. [CrossRef] [PubMed]
23. Sonneville, K.R.; Horton, N.J.; Micali, N.; Crosby, R.D.; Swanson, S.A.; Solmi, F.; Field, A.E. Longitudinal associations between binge eating and overeating and adverse outcomes among adolescents and young adults: Does loss of control matter? *JAMA Pediatr.* **2013**, *167*, 149–155. [CrossRef] [PubMed]
24. Vogeltanz-Holm, N.D.; Wonderlich, S.A.; Lewis, B.A.; Wilsnack, S.C.; Harris, T.R.; Wilsnack, R.W.; Kristjanson, A.F. Longitudinal predictors of binge eating, intense dieting, and weight concerns in a national sample of women. *Behav. Ther.* **2000**, *31*, 221–235. [CrossRef]
25. Konkoly Thege, B.; Woodin, E.M.; Hodgins, D.C.; Williams, R.J. Natural course of behavioral addictions: A 5-year longitudinal study. *BMC Psychiatry* **2015**, *15*, 4. [CrossRef] [PubMed]
26. Grant, J.E.; Schreiber, L.R.; Odlaug, B.L. Phenomenology and treatment of behavioural addictions. *Can J. Psychiatry* **2013**, *58*, 252–259. [CrossRef] [PubMed]

27. Cowan, J.; Devine, C. Food, eating, and weight concerns of men in recovery from substance addiction. *Appetite* **2008**, *50*, 33–42. [CrossRef] [PubMed]
28. Long, C.G.; Blundell, J.E.; Finlayson, G. A Systematic Review of the Application And Correlates of YFAS-Diagnosed 'Food Addiction' in Humans: Are Eating-Related 'Addictions' a Cause for Concern or Empty Concepts? *Obes. Facts* **2015**, *8*, 386–401. [CrossRef] [PubMed]
29. Fairburn, C.G.; Beglin, S.J. Assessment of eating disorders: Interview or self-report questionnaire? *Int. J. Eat. Disord.* **1994**, *16*, 363–370. [PubMed]
30. Wilfley, D.E.; Schwartz, M.B.; Spurrell, E.B.; Fairburn, C.G. Assessing the specific psychopathology of binge eating disorder patients: Interview or self-report? *Behav. Res. Ther.* **1997**, *35*, 1151–1159. [CrossRef]
31. Al-Adawi, S.; Bax, B.; Bryant-Waugh, R.; Claudino, A.M.; Hay, P.; Monteleone, P.; Norring, C.; Pike, K.M.; Pilon, D.J.; Herscovici, C.R.; et al. Revision of ICD—Status update on feeding and eating disorders. *Adv. Eat. Disord.* **2013**, *1*, 10–20. [CrossRef]
32. Grilo, C.M.; White, M.A. A controlled evaluation of the distress criterion for binge eating disorder. *J. Consult. Clin. Psychol.* **2011**, *79*, 509–514. [CrossRef] [PubMed]
33. Wolfe, B.E.; Baker, C.W.; Smith, A.T.; Kelly-Weeder, S. Validity and utility of the current definition of binge eating. *Int. J. Eat. Disord.* **2009**, *42*, 674–686. [CrossRef] [PubMed]
34. Womens Health Australia. *The Australian Longitudinal Study on Women's Health: Data Book*, 2nd ed.; Womens Health Australia: Newcastle, UK, 1997.
35. Andrews, G.; Slade, T. Interpreting scores on the Kessler Psychological Distress Scale (K10). *Aust. N. Z. J. Public Health* **2001**, *25*, 494–497. [CrossRef] [PubMed]
36. Vargas Terrez, B.E.; Villamil Salcedo, V.; Rodríguez Estrada, C.; Pérez Romero, J.; Cortés Sotres, J. Validación de la escala Kessler 10 (K-10) en la detección de depresión y ansiedad en el primer nivel de atención. Propiedades psicométricas. *Salud Ment.* **2011**, *34*, 323–331.
37. Ware, J., Jr.; Kosinski, M.; Keller, S.D. A 12-Item Short-Form Health Survey: Construction of scales and preliminary tests of reliability and validity. *Med. Care* **1996**, *34*, 220–233. [CrossRef] [PubMed]
38. Sanderson, K.; Andrews, G. The SF-12 in the Australian population: Cross-validation of item selection. *Aust. N. Z. J. Public Health* **2002**, *26*, 343–345. [CrossRef] [PubMed]
39. Mond, J.M.; Hay, P.J.; Rodgers, B.; Owen, C.; Beumont, P.J. Validity of the Eating Disorder Examination Questionnaire (EDE-Q) in screening for eating disorders in community samples. *Behav. Res. Ther.* **2004**, *42*, 551–567. [CrossRef]
40. Davis, C.; Carter, J.C. Compulsive overeating as an addiction disorder. A review of theory and evidence. *Appetite* **2009**, *53*, 1–8. [CrossRef] [PubMed]
41. Killeen, T.; Brewerton, T.D.; Campbell, A.; Cohen, L.R.; Hien, D.A. Exploring the relationship between eating disorder symptoms and substance use severity in women with comorbid PTSD and substance use disorders. *Am. J. Drug Alcohol. Abuse* **2015**, *41*, 547–552. [PubMed]
42. Grilo, C.M.; White, M.A.; Masheb, R.M. DSM-IV psychiatric disorder comorbidity and its correlates in binge eating disorder. *Int. J. Eat. Disord.* **2009**, *42*, 228–234. [CrossRef] [PubMed]
43. Edge, P.J.; Gold, M.S. Drug withdrawal and hyperphagia: Lessons from tobacco and other drugs. *Curr. Pharm. Des.* **2011**, *17*, 1173–1179. [CrossRef] [PubMed]
44. Orsini, C.A.; Ginton, G.; Shimp, K.G.; Avena, N.M.; Gold, M.S.; Setlow, B. Food consumption and weight gain after cessation of chronic amphetamine administration. *Appetite* **2014**, *78*, 76–80. [CrossRef] [PubMed]
45. Merikangas, K.R.; McClair, V.L. Epidemiology of substance use disorders. *Hum. Genet.* **2012**, *131*, 779–789. [CrossRef] [PubMed]
46. American Psychiatric Association. Substance-Related and Addictive Disorders. In *Diagnostic and Statistical Manual of Mental Disorders*, 5th ed.; American Psychiatric Association: Washington, DC, USA, 2013.

13

Binge-Type Eating in Rats is Facilitated by Neuromedin U Receptor 2 in the Nucleus Accumbens and Ventral Tegmental Area

Ashley E. Smith [1,2], James M. Kasper [1,3], Ara 13 [1], Noelle C. Anastasio [1,3] and Jonathan D. Hommel [1,2,3,*]

1 Center for Addiction Research, University of Texas Medical Branch, Galveston, TX 77555, USA; aesmith@utmb.edu (A.E.S.); jakasper@utmb.edu (J.M.K.); ara13c@gmail.com (Ara 13); ncanasta@utmb.edu (N.C.A.)

2 Department of Neuroscience, Cell Biology and Anatomy, University of Texas Medical Branch, Galveston, TX 77555, USA

3 Department of Pharmacology and Toxicology, University of Texas Medical Branch, Galveston, TX 77555, USA

* Correspondence: jdhommel@utmb.edu

Abstract: Binge-eating disorder (BED) is the most common eating disorder, characterized by rapid, recurrent overconsumption of highly palatable food in a short time frame. BED shares an overlapping behavioral phenotype with obesity, which is also linked to the overconsumption of highly palatable foods. The reinforcing properties of highly palatable foods are mediated by the nucleus accumbens (NAc) and the ventral tegmental area (VTA), which have been implicated in the overconsumption behavior observed in BED and obesity. A potential regulator of binge-type eating behavior is the G protein-coupled receptor neuromedin U receptor 2 (NMUR2). Previous research demonstrated that NMUR2 knockdown potentiates binge-type consumption of high-fat food. We correlated binge-type consumption across a spectrum of fat and carbohydrate mixtures with synaptosomal NMUR2 protein expression in the NAc and VTA of rats. Synaptosomal NMUR2 protein in the NAc demonstrated a strong positive correlation with binge intake of a "lower"-fat (higher carbohydrate) mixture, whereas synaptosomal NMUR2 protein in the VTA demonstrated a strong negative correlation with binge intake of an "extreme" high-fat (0% carbohydrate) mixture. Taken together, these data suggest that NMUR2 may differentially regulate binge-type eating within the NAc and the VTA.

Keywords: binge-eating disorder; BED; obesity; binge-type eating; neuromedin U receptor 2; NMUR2; nucleus accumbens; ventral tegmental area

---

1. Introduction

Binge-eating disorder (BED) is an under-recognized public health problem that is prevalent worldwide [1,2]. In the US, BED affects 3.5% of adult women and 2% of adult men, with a combined lifetime prevalence of 1.4% [1,2]. Although BED is the most common eating disorder, it remains both under-diagnosed and understudied [2]. Therefore, a more mechanistic appreciation of feeding behaviors that contribute to BED is critical to understanding disease etiology, and for identifying potential pharmacotherapeutic targets.

BED is characterized by binge episodes when an individual overconsumes highly-palatable food in a discrete period of time ($\leq$2 h) [3–5]. The frequency of these binge episodes is a hallmark of BED and is used to determine the disease's severity [3–5]. BED is partially attributed to the increased availability of highly palatable food, and also shares physiological, psychological, and epidemiological overlaps with obesity [1,4,6–10].

Obesity is an alarming health crisis that affects 39.8% of adults within the US alone [11]. Obese individuals present a challenging public health problem due to the increased risk of life-threatening co-morbidities [12]. Thus, the health burden of obesity is immense and demands an improved understanding of the feeding behaviors that contribute to obesity. Similar to BED, one of the feeding behaviors that contributes to obesity is the overconsumption of highly palatable food.

Highly palatable food, including high-fat food, is both energy dense and highly reinforcing in humans and rodents [13]. These reinforcing properties promote overconsumption behavior that is potentiated by dysregulation in portion control [14–17]. In fact, individuals with BED ascribe higher reinforcement value to high-fat food than individuals without BED [18]. The reinforcing properties of food are largely encoded by brain regions within the mesolimbic "reward" pathway, which includes the nucleus accumbens (NAc) and the ventral tegmental area (VTA) [19,20]. Both the NAc and the VTA have been implicated in BED and obesity [2,9,19–25]. Reinforcement value is mediated by the NAc—a key neuroanatomical region that regulates hedonic feeding, or food intake in the absence of a caloric deficit [9,19,20]. The VTA is also linked to reinforcement value, and affects obesogenic diet consumption [26].

Overall, BED and obesity share multifaceted feeding behaviors involving multiple brain circuits that regulate a complex interplay of emotions, food intake, and food reinforcement. These feeding behaviors can be probed using animal models designed for quantifying specific aspects of these diseases. Models of binge-type eating have been validated in rodents, demonstrating success in studying the overconsumption behavior characteristic of both BED and obesity [27–35]. The intermittent access model provides ad libitum access to regular chow and water, with limited presentation of a highly palatable food, which simulates a binge episode, similar to that observed in BED and obesity [27,29,30,32,33,35]. While this model can recreate and quantify food intake during a binge episode, it does not replicate the psychological aspects of BED, such as feelings of loss of control and feelings of shame and guilt [2–5]. Nonetheless, this model is helpful in understanding neural mechanisms underlying binge-type consumption and identifying potential regulators of this specific maladaptive feeding behavior.

Here, we investigate a novel mediator of binge-type eating, the neuropeptide receptor neuromedin U receptor 2 (NMUR2). NMUR2 is a G protein-coupled receptor predominantly expressed throughout the mammalian central nervous system. This receptor is known to regulate food intake and body weight [36–40]. For example, NMUR2-knockout mice are hyperphagic and demonstrate increased food intake patterns [41]. Additionally, deletion of hypothalamic NMUR2 via viral-mediated RNAi resulted in increased motivation for high-fat food and potentiated binge-type eating [32,42]. These studies indicate that NMUR2 regulates food intake—a process that is dysregulated in BED and obesity. Interestingly, the role of NMUR2 in reinforcement brain centers such as the NAc and VTA in binge-type eating has not been explored.

Importantly, the endogenous expression of NMUR2 is highly variable among individuals and among various brain regions [41,43,44]. Neuroanatomical variability and individual differences in NMUR2 expression may underlie aspects of individual differences observed in BED and obesity [45]. The purpose of the current study was to explore relationships between synaptosomal NMUR2 expression in the NAc and the VTA—key brain regions associated with reinforcement—in a rodent model of binge-type eating across a spectrum of dietary fat and carbohydrate contents. Our findings revealed a strong positive correlation between the intake of "lower"-fat (i.e., higher carbohydrate) food and synaptosomal NMUR2 protein expression in the NAc, and a strong negative correlation between the intake of "extreme" high-fat (0% carbohydrate) food and synaptosomal NMUR2 protein expression in the VTA.

2. Materials and Methods

2.1. Animals

Male Sprague-Dawley rats (Harlan, Houston, TX, USA) weighing 225–250 g were used in all experiments. Animals were housed individually in a temperature (i.e., 21–23 °C) and humidity (40%–50%) controlled environment with a standard 12 h light–dark cycle (lights on between 06:00 and 18:00 h). All animals were given ad libitum access to normal chow (17% fat by kcal; Teklad LM-485 Mouse/Rat Sterilizable Diet; Teklad Diets, Madison, WI, USA) and water in their home cages, including during binge sessions. Upon arrival, animals were allowed to acclimate to the room for seven days prior to handling and experimental procedures. All experiments were conducted in accordance with the NIH Guide for Use and Care of Laboratory Animals (2011), and with approval from the Institutional Animal Use and Care Committee at the University of Texas Medical Branch.

2.2. NMUR2 Immunohistochemistry

Rats ($n = 4$) were anesthetized with 1%–5% isoflurane, perfused with phosphate buffered saline for 5 min, followed by 4% paraformaldehyde (PFA) for 15 min. Brains were removed and sliced into 40 micronsections using a cryostat. NAc and VTA sections were stained as described in previous studies [33,43,46]. Briefly, sections were washed twice in 1× PBS, and then antigen-unmasked with 1% SDS for 5 min. Next, sections were blocked in donkey serum and incubated in 1:150 primary antibody rabbit αNMUR2 (NBP1-02351, Novus Biologicals, Littleton, CO, USA) overnight. The following day, sections were washed three times in 1X PBS, then incubated with 1:200 donkey αrabbit IgG Alexa Fluor 568 (A10042, Invitrogen, Carlsbad, CA, USA). Images were acquired using Leica True Confocal Scanner SPE in confocal mode and Leica Application Suite × software (Leica Microsystems, Wetzlar, Germany).

2.3. Binge Study Design

Our binge-type eating protocol was based on previously published models [27,29,32,33,35]. Briefly, male Sprague-Dawley rats ($n = 10$) were maintained on a diet of normal chow (17% fat by kcal) and water. Rats were not restricted from feeding prior to the binge period, and had ad libitum access to normal chow and water throughout the study, including during the binge period. Two days prior to experiments, animals were exposed to a mixture of 60% fat by kcal and 40% carbohydrate by kcal to minimize food neophobia. Fat–carbohydrate mixtures were prepared and weighed immediately before the binge period. Vegetable shortening (Crisco, Orrville, OH, USA) comprised of 100% fat by energy (110 kcal/12 g serving with 110 kcal from fat; 9.16 kcal/g) was mixed with marshmallow creme (Kraft, Chicago, IL, USA), containing 100% carbohydrate by energy (45 kcal/13 g serving with 0 kcal from fat; 3.46 kcal/g) to create a total of five fat mixtures of varying fat–carbohydrate content. The fat–carbohydrate mixtures were prepared as follows: 2.18 g fat and 23.12 g carbohydrate were mixed for 20% fat/80% carbohydrate/0% protein by energy, 4.36 g fat and 17.34 g carbohydrate were mixed for 40% fat/60% carbohydrate/0% protein by energy, 6.55 g fat and 11.56 g carbohydrate were mixed for 60% fat/40% carbohydrate/0% protein by energy, 8.73 g fat and 5.78 g carbohydrate were mixed for 80% fat/20% carbohydrate/0% protein by energy, and 10 g fat and 0 g carbohydrate was used for 100% fat/0% carbohydrate/0% protein by energy. One limitation is that the marshmallow creme does contain any flavoring. However, the consistency and texture of the marshmallow creme were required to promote homogeneity among the mixtures.

Rats were randomized into five groups using a Latin square design, with each animal receiving all fat–carbohydrate mixtures in a randomized order. Each group was presented with mixtures of 20% fat (80% carbohydrate), 40% fat (60% carbohydrate), 60% fat (40% carbohydrate), 80% fat (20% carbohydrate), and 100% fat (0% carbohydrate) for a period of 5 days. Exposure to fat–carbohydrate mixtures occurred during binge 1 at the first 2-h of the dark cycle (18:00–20:00) and binge 2 at 2-h near the end of the light cycle (14:00–16:00). For all exposures, fat–carbohydrate mixtures were weighed prior to presentation and then immediately after the 2-h binge period. Differences in food weight were interpreted as total grams consumed or total calories consumed during the binge period.

2.4. NAc and VTA Protein Extraction

After the completion of binge studies, rats (n = 10) were anesthetized with 1%–5% isoflurane, and brains were removed. Both NAc and VTA were microdissected from each rat, using guidance from a rat brain atlas [26,44,47], then stored at −80 °C until protein extraction. The crude synaptosomal protein fraction was isolated as previously published to identify long-term changes in protein expression [48]. NAc and VTA tissue were homogenized in ice-cold Krebs-sucrose buffer containing protease inhibitors (P8340, Millipore Sigma, St. Louis, MO, USA) and phosphatase inhibitors (P5726, P0044 Millipore Sigma, St. Louis, MO, USA). The crude synaptosomal protein fractionation protocol enriches samples for pre- and postsynaptic proteins (i.e., presynaptic terminals, postsynaptic membranes, etc.) [49]. Samples were centrifuged for 10 min at 100 g at 4 °C to pellet the nuclear protein fraction. The supernatant was centrifuged for 20 min at 16,000 g at 4 °C to separate the crude synaptosomal protein fraction (pellet). The NAc and VTA synaptosomal protein fractions were used for all further analyses. After extraction, total protein concentration was determined using a Pierce BCA Protein Assay Kit (23225, Thermo Fisher, Waltham, MA, USA).

2.5. NAc and VTA NMUR2 Protein Expression

NAc (n = 10) and VTA (n = 10) samples were assayed for NMUR2 protein expression using the Wes^{TM} (ProteinSimple, San Jose, CA, USA) automated Western blotting system. Wes^{TM} is a capillary electrophoresis-based immunoblotting instrument, and was optimized for receptor quantification in brain tissues [48,50]. Wes^{TM} reagents (biotinylated molecular weight marker, streptavidin-HRP fluorescent standards, luminol-S, hydrogen peroxide, sample buffer, DTT, stacking matrix, separation matrix, running buffer, wash buffer, matrix removal buffer, secondary antibodies, antibody diluent, and capillaries) were obtained from the manufacturer (ProteinSimple) and used according to the manufacturer's specifications with minor modifications. NMUR2 polyclonal antibody (NBP1-02351, Novus Biologicals, Littleton, CO, USA) was diluted 1:50 in antibody diluent.

Samples were prepared and subjected to capillary electrophoresis-based immunoblotting as described previously [49]. Briefly, 2 μg of protein was denatured in 0.1× sample buffer and 5× master mix at 95 °C for 5 min. Then, samples and primary antibody were dispensed into a prefilled microplate (ProteinSimple). Capillary electrophoresis (375 V, 25 min, 25 °C) and immunodetection were completed using the following settings: separation matrix load, 200 s; stacking matrix load, 15 s; sample load, 9 s; antibody diluent, 30 min; primary antibody incubation, 60 min; secondary antibody incubation, 30 min; and chemiluminescent signal exposure for 15, 30, 120, 240, and 480 s. Data were analyzed using Compass Software (ProteinSimple). The Western blot analysis signal was defined as the area under the curve (AUC) for the NMUR2 peak at 48 kDa and representative "virtual blot" electrophoretic images for NMUR2 were automatically generated by the Compass Software (ProteinSimple).

2.6. Statistical Analysis

Binge-type eating across a spectrum of fat–carbohydrate contents in binge 1 and binge 2 was analyzed by repeated measures one-way ANOVA and Bonferroni's multiple comparisons. All comparisons were made to the intake of a 20% fat mixture. Correlations between binge-type eating across a spectrum of fat–carbohydrate contents and NMUR2 protein expression in the NAc and the VTA were analyzed by linear regression. All statistical analyses were performed in GraphPad Prism 7.0a (GraphPad Software Inc., La Jolla, CA, USA) with an experiment-wise error rate of $\alpha = 0.05$.

3. Results

3.1. NMUR2 is Expressed Presynaptically in the NAc and the VTA

Previous work demonstrated that NMUR2 is expressed postsynaptically in the hypothalamus and presynaptically in the NAc [32,46]. We confirmed NAc and VTA localization of NMUR2 with immunohistochemistry. We observed a "beads on a string" staining pattern indicative of presynaptic NMUR2 expression in the NAc and in the VTA (Figure 1).

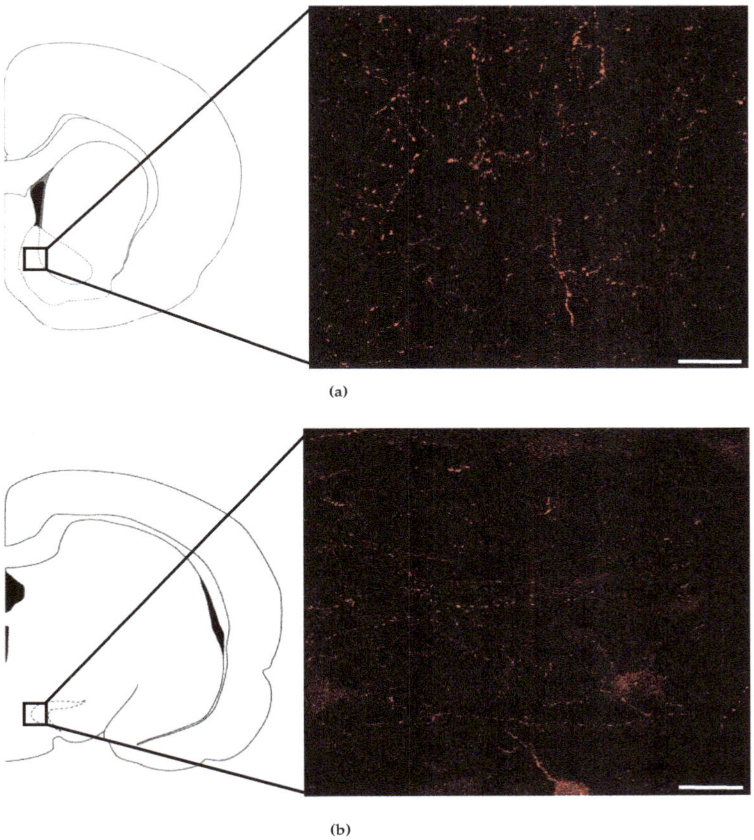

Figure 1. Neuropeptide receptor neuromedin U receptor 2 (NMUR2)immunostaining in the nucleus accumbens (NAc) and the ventral tegmental area (VTA). (**a**) Representative image of NMUR2 immunostaining in the NAc (bregma +1.92); (**b**) Representative image of NMUR2 immunostaining in the VTA (bregma −4.80). Images were acquired from the regions indicated at in confocal mode, scale bar = 25 μm.

3.2. Fat Content and Binge-Type Eating

Using our binge-type eating paradigm, we quantified how much rats would consume during a 2-h binge period (Figure 2). Figure 2 illustrates binge intake across a spectrum of fat–carbohydrate contents during binge 1 and binge 2. Comparisons were made within each binge to the intake of a 20% fat (80% carbohydrate) mixture. In binge 1, rats consumed significantly fewer grams of the 100% fat (0% carbohydrate) mixture ($p = 0.0003$) compared to the 20% fat (80% carbohydrate) mixture (Figure 2). In binge 2, rats consumed significantly more grams of the 60% fat (40% carbohydrate) mixture ($p = 0.010$) compared to the 20% fat (80% carbohydrate) mixture (Figure 2). Notably, common Western diet foods contain percentages of fat that fall at the peak of the curve, including French fries (42% fat), potato chips (56% fat), cheesecake (63% fat), and peanut butter (78% fat), which gives context for the percentages of fat used in our rodent studies.

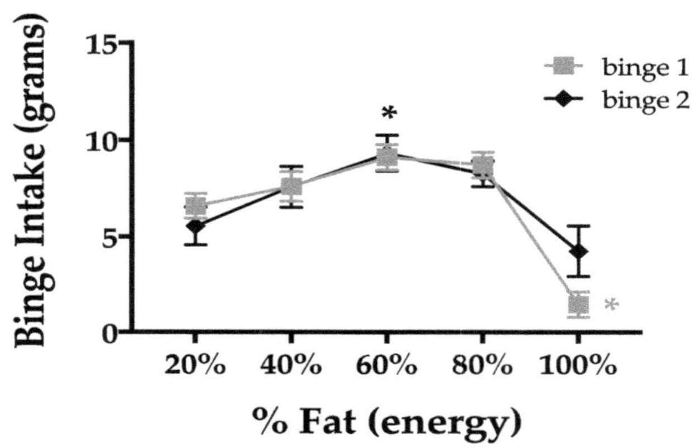

Figure 2. Rat binge-type eating across a spectrum of fat–carbohydrate contents. Binge-type eating in rats was highest at 60% fat (40% carbohydrate) and lowest at 80% fat (20% carbohydrate) compared to 20% fat (80% carbohydrate). * $p < 0.05$.

3.3. Binge-Type Intake and NAc NMUR2 Protein Expression

To determine the relationship between binge-type intake and NMUR2 expression in the NAc, we quantified NAc NMUR2 synaptosomal protein (Figure 3a), and correlated it to fat intake during the binge period (Figure 3b–f). Interestingly, NAc NMUR2 expression demonstrated a strong positive correlation with binge intake of a "lower"-fat (higher carbohydrate) mixture, specifically 20% fat (80% carbohydrate) (p = 0.047) and 40% fat (60% carbohydrate) ($p < 0.001$) (Figure 3b–c). As fat content increased and carbohydrate content decreased, the relationship diminished. However, no significant correlation was observed when NAc NMUR2 was correlated to total calories consumed to account for energy density. In addition, we found no significant correlation between NAc NMUR2 and binge intake of a 60% (40%) (p = 0.86), 80% (20%) (p = 0.084), or 100% (0%) (p = 0.86) fat (carbohydrate) mixture (Figure 3d–f).

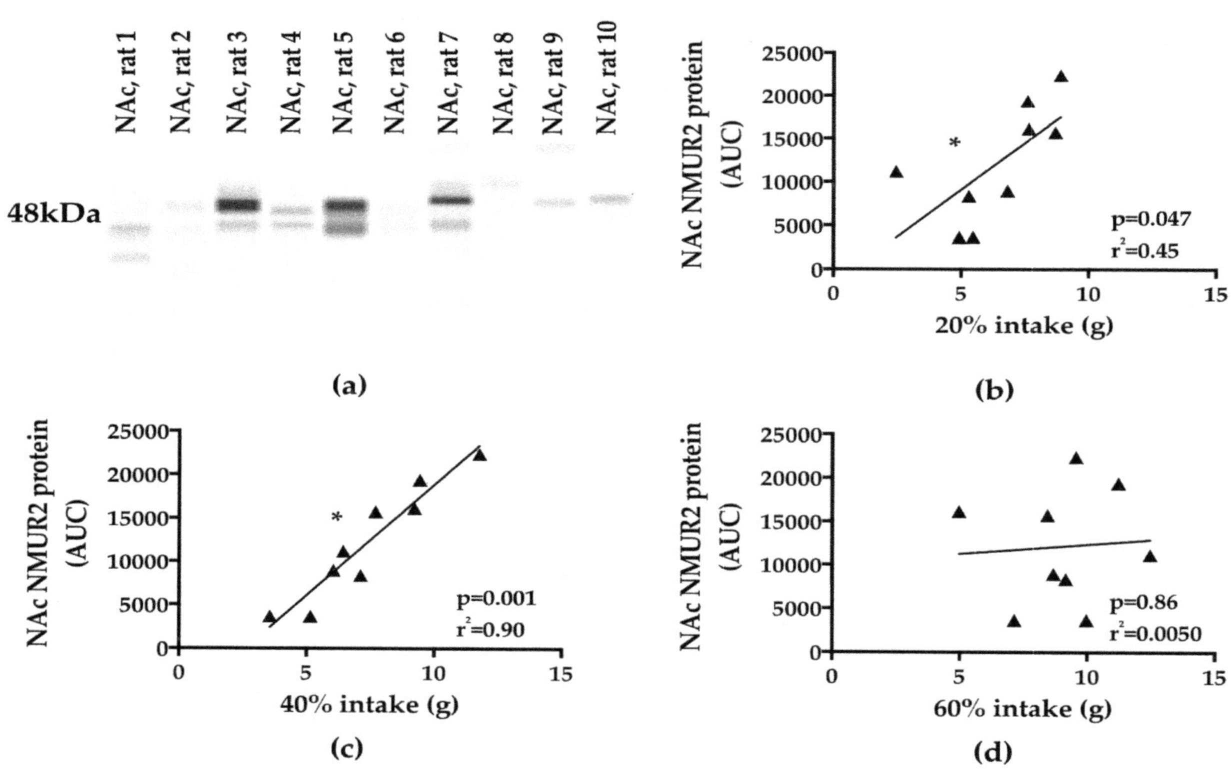

Figure 3. *Cont.*

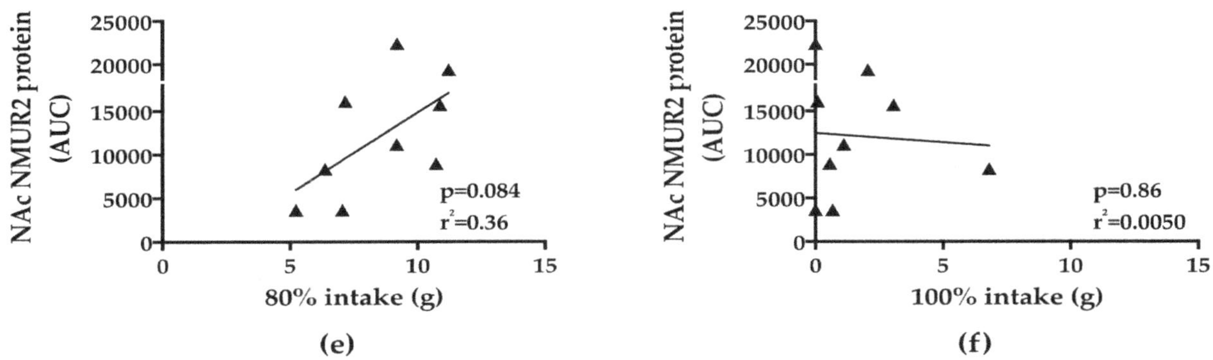

Figure 3. NAc NMUR2 protein expression was positively correlated with binge-type eating. (**a**) representative Western blot image for NMUR2 synaptosomal protein from NAc samples; (**b**) NAc NMUR2 expression was positively correlated with intake of a 20% fat (80% carbohydrate) mixture; (**c**) NAc NMUR2 expression was positively correlated with intake of a 40% fat (60% carbohydrate) mixture; (**e**) NAc NMUR2 expression was not correlated with intake of a 60% fat (40% carbohydrate) mixture; (**f**) NAc NMUR2 expression was not correlated with intake of an 80% fat (20% carbohydrate) mixture; (**g**) NAc NMUR2 protein expression was not correlated with intake of a 100% fat (0% carbohydrate) mixture. AUC: area under the curve. * $p < 0.05$.

3.4. Binge-Type Intake and VTA NMUR2 Protein Expression

Next, we quantified VTA NMUR2 synaptosomal protein (Figure 4a). We correlated VTA NMUR2 synaptosomal protein to fat intake during the binge period (Figure 4b–f). No significant correlation was observed between VTA NMUR2 and binge intake of a 20% (80%) ($p = 0.11$), 40% (60%) ($p = 0.37$), 60% (40%) ($p = 0.95$), or 80% (20%) ($p = 0.26$) fat (carbohydrate) mixture (Figure 4b–e). VTA NMUR2 demonstrated a strong negative correlation with binge intake of an "extreme" high-fat mixture of 100% fat (0% carbohydrate) ($p = 0.034$) (Figure 4f). Interestingly, the slope of the trend line transitioned from a positive slope value for the lower-fat mixtures (higher carbohydrate) to a negative slope for the higher-fat mixtures (lower carbohydrate).

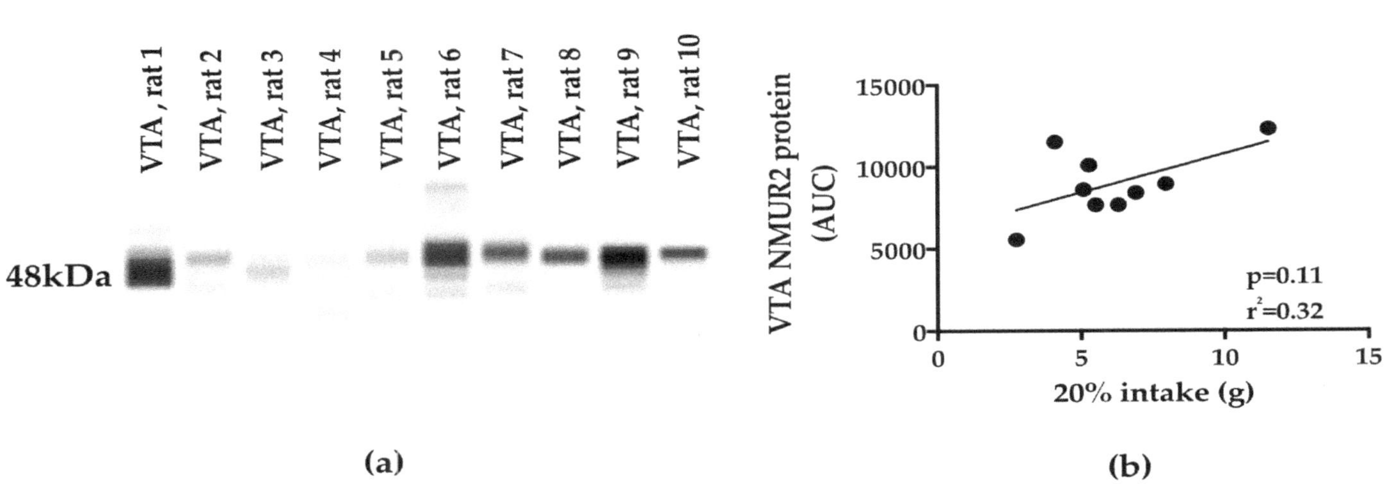

Figure 4. *Cont.*

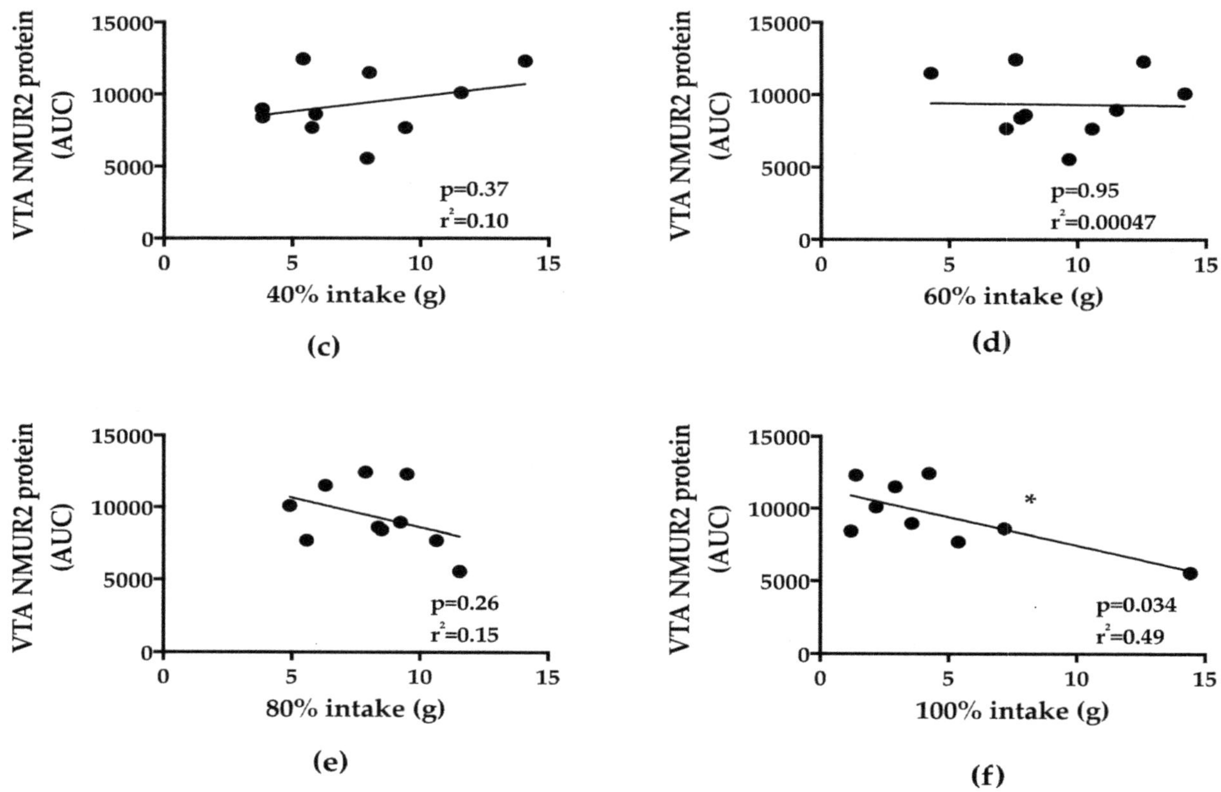

Figure 4. VTA NMUR2 protein expression was negatively correlated with binge-type eating. (**a**) representative Western blot image for NMUR2 synaptosomal protein from VTA samples; (**b**) VTA NMUR2 expression was not correlated with intake of a 20% fat (80% carbohydrate) mixture; (**c**) VTA NMUR2 expression was not correlated with intake of a 40% fat (60% carbohydrate) mixture; (**d**) VTA NMUR2 expression was not correlated with intake of a 60% fat (40% carbohydrate) mixture; (**e**) VTA NMUR2 expression was not correlated with intake of an 80% fat (20% carbohydrate) mixture; (**f**) VTA NMUR2 expression was negatively correlated with intake of a 100% fat (0% carbohydrate) mixture. * $p < 0.05$.

4. Discussion

In the present study, we assessed the synaptic localization of NMUR2 in the NAc and the VTA. Our results support previous studies indicating synaptic NMUR2 expression in the NAc. Additionally, these results extend our knowledge by demonstrating Western blot staining of NMUR2 in synaptosomal VTA fractions, and by visualizing punctate staining patterns for NMUR2 in the VTA, consistent with synaptic localization [46]. Our NMUR2 antibody has previously been shown to stain NMUR2-expressing cell bodies in the PVN, suggesting that the staining pattern is not an antibody limitation [32]. In the NAc, NMUR2 is localized to synapses that express a neuronal marker of GABAergic signaling, which supports a role for NMUR2 in inhibitory signaling [46]. Additional studies are needed to determine the functional role of NMUR2 in the mesoaccumbens circuit, including its effects on BED and obesity.

We used an animal model of binge-type eating to quantify binge intake in rats. This model only simulated a binge episode, similar to that observed in BED and obesity [27,29,30,32,33,35]. One of the major limitations of our study is the inability of our model to replicate all clinical aspects of BED. While our model can quantify food intake during a binge episode, it does not replicate the psychological aspects of BED, such as feelings of loss of control and feelings of shame and guilt [2–5]. Nonetheless, this model is helpful in understanding neural mechanisms underlying binge-type consumption and identifying potential regulators of this specific overconsumption behavior. During our studies, animals were maintained on their normal chow consisting of 17% fat by kcal which does not promote overconsumption and maintains a healthy energy balance. However, energy-dense diets are reinforcing and are significantly preferred by rodents. The fat–carbohydrate mixtures were designed to contain the preferred higher energy density, which promotes overeating and improves the translational relevance in which humans binge on energy-dense foods [13,35,51–53].

Using this model, we quantified binge-type consumption across a spectrum of fat–carbohydrate mixtures and correlated it to synaptosomal NMUR2 protein expression in the NAc and the VTA in rats. To our knowledge, we are the first to quantify synaptosomal NMUR2 protein in the NAc and VTA and the first to explore relationships between NMUR2 expression and binge intake. Our results demonstrated a strong positive correlation between synaptosomal NMUR2 protein expression in the NAc and binge intake of a "lower"-fat (higher carbohydrate) mixture of 20% fat (80% carbohydrate) and 40% fat (60% carbohydrate). This region-specific effect of NAc NMUR2 facilitated the binge-type intake of a "lower"-fat (higher carbohydrate) mixture, especially food around 40% fat (60% carbohydrate), which is commonly overconsumed in humans [13,51–54]. Synaptosomal VTA NMUR2 protein expression demonstrated a strong negative correlation with the binge intake of an "extreme" high fat mixture, particularly 100% fat (0% carbohydrate). Contrary to NAc NMUR2, this finding implicates VTA NMUR2 as an inhibitor of binge intake of "extreme" high-fat, low-carbohydrate food. Thus, VTA NMUR2 may act as a "behavioral brake" on the binge intake of high-fat, low-carbohydrate food.

Overall, our findings demonstrate key relationships and brain-region-specific differences in synaptosomal NMUR2 protein expression, and establish NMUR2 as a regulator of binge-type intake in rats in the NAc and the VTA. Binge-type eating changes based on fat–carbohydrate content and NMUR2 expression varies not only across animals, but across brain regions. Interestingly, binge-type intake could be based on fat content, carbohydrate content, or fat-to-carbohydrate ratio, and future studies should delineate the role of NMUR2 in fat and carbohydrate preference. Thus, endogenous NMUR2 may be a driver of individual differences in binge-type eating. Although the observed high degree of inter-animal variability and inter-brain region variability of NMUR2 can limit data interpretation based on averaged differences in NMUR2, it also raises the possibility that NMUR2 protein contributes to individual differences for binge-type food intake in humans.

The clinical implications of our findings establish NMUR2 as a novel regulator of binge-type eating and therefore as a potential druggable candidate for the overconsumption behavior observed in BED and obesity. Recently, we showed that small-molecule NMUR2 agonists successfully suppressed high-fat food intake in rats, which supports NMUR2 as a viable therapeutic target [55]. Future studies will continue to investigate the contribution of NMUR2 in the NAc and the VTA at molecular, neural, and pharmacological levels, including investigating the effects of these small-molecule NMUR2 agonists on binge-type eating.

5. Conclusions

The overconsumption behavior observed in BED and obesity is poorly understood, and demands more mechanistic and molecular studies. NMUR2 facilitates binge-type eating in rats by promoting the binge intake of "lower"-fat diets via the NAc while suppressing the intake of "extreme" higher fat diets via the VTA. Therefore, NMUR2 represents a promising druggable target, and has already been shown to successfully alter feeding behavior [55–57]. The current study demonstrates key relationships between NMUR2 expression in "reward" centers of the brain and binge-type behavior that will contextualize the interpretation of future research determining the therapeutic potential of NMUR2 to regulate overconsumption behavior.

Author Contributions: Conceptualization, A.E.S., J.M.K., and J.D.H.; Methodology, A.E.S. and N.C.A.; Formal analysis, A.E.S. and J.D.H.; Investigation, A.E.S. and J.M.K; Visualization, A.E.S.; Writing—original draft preparation, A.E.S.; Writing—review and editing, A.E.S., J.M.K., Ara 13, N.C.A., and J.D.H.; Supervision, J.D.H.; Funding acquisition, J.D.H.

Acknowledgments: We acknowledge Erica D. Holliday, for assistance with statistical analysis, Reyna Collura for assistance with graphical design.

References

1. Kessler, R.C.; Berglund, P.A.; Chiu, W.T.; Deitz, A.C.; Hudson, J.I.; Shahly, V.; Aguilar-Gaxiola, S.; Alonso, J.; Angermeyer, M.C.; Benjet, C.; et al. The prevalence and correlates of binge eating disorder in the world health organization world mental health surveys. *Biol. Psychiatry* **2013**, *73*, 904–914. [CrossRef] [PubMed]
2. Guerdjikova, A.I.; Mori, N.; Casuto, L.S.; McElroy, S.L. Binge eating disorder. *Psychiatr. Clin. N. Am.* **2017**, *40*, 255–266. [CrossRef] [PubMed]
3. American Psychiatric Association. *Feeding and Eating Disorders*; American Psychiatric Publishing: Washington, DC, USA, 2013.
4. *Eating Disorders and Obesity a Comprehensive Handbook*, 3rd ed.; The Guilford Press: New York, NY, USA, 2017.
5. American Psychiatric Association. *Diagnostic and Statistical Manual of Mental Disorders*; American Psychiatric Publishing: Washington, DC, USA, 2013.
6. De Zwaan, M. Binge eating disorder and obesity. *Int. J. Obes. Relat. Metab. Disord.* **2001**, *25*, S51–S55. [CrossRef] [PubMed]
7. Berridge, K.C. 'Liking' and 'wanting' food rewards: Brain substrates and roles in eating disorders. *Physiol. Behav.* **2009**, *97*, 537–550. [CrossRef] [PubMed]
8. Berridge, K.C.; Ho, C.Y.; Richard, J.M.; DiFeliceantonio, A.G. The tempted brain eats: Pleasure and desire circuits in obesity and eating disorders. *Brain Res.* **2010**, *1350*, 43–64. [CrossRef] [PubMed]
9. Volkow, N.D.; Wang, G.J.; Tomasi, D.; Baler, R.D. The addictive dimensionality of obesity. *Biol. Psychiatry* **2013**, *73*, 811–818. [CrossRef] [PubMed]
10. Rancourt, D.; McCullough, M.B. Overlap in eating disorders and obesity in adolescence. *Curr. Diab. Rep.* **2015**, *15*, 78. [CrossRef]
11. Hales, C.M.; Carroll, M.D.; Fryar, C.D.; Ogden, C.L. Prevalence of obesity among adults and youth: United States, 2015–2016. *NCHS Data Brief.* **2017**, *219*, 1–8.
12. National Institutes of Health, National Heart, Lung, and Blood Institute. Managing Overweight and Obesity in Adults, Systematic Evidence Review from the Obesity Expert Panel. Available online: https://www.nhlbi.nih.gov/sites/default/files/media/docs/obesity-evidence-review.pdf (accessed on 1 December 2018).
13. Drewnowski, A.; Almiron-Roig, E. Human perceptions and preferences for fat-rich foods. In *Fat Detection: Taste, Texture, and Post Ingestive Effects*; Montmayeur, J., le Coutre, J., Eds.; CRC Press/Taylor & Francis: Boca Raton, FL, USA, 2010.
14. Rippin, H.L.; Hutchinson, J.; Jewell, J.; Breda, J.J.; Cade, J.E. Portion size of energy-dense foods among french and uk adults by bmi status. *Nutrients* **2018**. [CrossRef]
15. Lyons, J.; Walton, J.; Flynn, A. Larger food portion sizes are associated with both positive and negative markers of dietary quality in irish adults. *Nutrients* **2018**, *10*, 1929. [CrossRef]
16. Carstairs, S.A.; Caton, S.J.; Blundell-Birtill, P.; Rolls, B.J.; Hetherington, M.M.; Cecil, J.E. Can reduced intake associated with downsizing a high energy dense meal item be offset by increased vegetable variety in 3–5-year-old children? *Nutrients* **2018**. [CrossRef] [PubMed]
17. Reale, S.; Kearney, C.M.; Hetherington, M.M.; Croden, F.; Cecil, J.E.; Carstairs, S.A.; Rolls, B.J.; Caton, S.J. The feasibility and acceptability of two methods of snack portion control in United Kingdom (UK) preschool children: Reduction and replacement. *Nutrients* **2018**. [CrossRef] [PubMed]
18. Schebendach, J.; Broft, A.; Foltin, R.W.; Walsh, B.T. Can the reinforcing value of food be measured in bulimia nervosa? *Appetite* **2013**, *62*, 70–75. [CrossRef] [PubMed]
19. Volkow, N.D.; Wang, G.J.; Tomasi, D.; Baler, R.D. Obesity and addiction: Neurobiological overlaps. *Obes. Rev.* **2013**, *14*, 2–18. [CrossRef] [PubMed]

20. Volkow, N.D.; Wise, R.A. How can drug addiction help us understand obesity? *Nat. Neurosci.* **2005**, *8*, 555–560. [CrossRef] [PubMed]
21. Davis, C.; Carter, J.C. Compulsive overeating as an addiction disorder. A review of theory and evidence. *Appetite* **2009**, *53*, 1–8. [CrossRef]
22. Dichter, G.S.; Damiano, C.A.; Allen, J.A. Reward circuitry dysfunction in psychiatric and neurodevelopmental disorders and genetic syndromes: Animal models and clinical findings. *J. Neurodev. Disord.* **2012**, *4*, 19.
23. Witt, A.A.; Lowe, M.R. Hedonic hunger and binge eating among women with eating disorders. *Int. J. Eat. Disord.* **2014**, *47*, 273–280. [CrossRef]
24. Satta, V.; Scherma, M.; Piscitelli, F.; Usai, P.; Castelli, M.P.; Bisogno, T.; Fratta, W.; Fadda, P. Limited access to a high fat diet alters endocannabinoid tone in female rats. *Front. Neurosci.* **2018**, *12*, 40. [CrossRef]
25. Corwin, R.L.; Wojnicki, F.H.; Zimmer, D.J.; Babbs, R.K.; McGrath, L.E.; Olivos, D.R.; Mietlicki-Baase, E.G.; Hayes, M.R. Binge-type eating disrupts dopaminergic and gabaergic signaling in the prefrontal cortex and ventral tegmental area. *Obesity* **2016**, *24*, 2118–2125. [CrossRef]
26. Hommel, J.D.; Trinko, R.; Sears, R.M.; Georgescu, D.; Liu, Z.W.; Gao, X.B.; Thurmon, J.J.; Marinelli, M.; DiLeone, R.J. Leptin receptor signaling in midbrain dopamine neurons regulates feeding. *Neuron* **2006**, *51*, 801–810. [CrossRef] [PubMed]
27. Corwin, R.L.; Wojnicki, F.H. Binge eating in rats with limited access to vegetable shortening. *Curr. Protoc. Neurosci.* **2006**. [CrossRef]
28. Wojnicki, F.H.; Babbs, R.K.; Corwin, R.L. Reinforcing efficacy of fat, as assessed by progressive ratio responding, depends upon availability not amount consumed. *Physiol. Behav.* **2010**, *100*, 316–321. [CrossRef] [PubMed]
29. Corwin, R.L.; Avena, N.M.; Boggiano, M.M. Feeding and reward: Perspectives from three rat models of binge eating. *Physiol. Behav.* **2011**, *104*, 87–97. [CrossRef] [PubMed]
30. Corwin, R.L.; Babbs, R.K. Rodent models of binge eating: Are they models of addiction? *ILAR J.* **2012**, *53*, 23–34. [CrossRef] [PubMed]
31. Babbs, R.K.; Wojnicki, F.H.; Corwin, R.L. Assessing binge eating. An analysis of data previously collected in bingeing rats. *Appetite* **2012**, *59*, 478–482. [CrossRef] [PubMed]
32. Benzon, C.R.; Johnson, S.B.; McCue, D.L.; Li, D.; Green, T.A.; Hommel, J.D. Neuromedin u receptor 2 knockdown in the paraventricular nucleus modifies behavioral responses to obesogenic high-fat food and leads to increased body weight. *Neuroscience* **2014**, *258*, 270–279. [CrossRef]
33. Price, A.E.; Stutz, S.J.; Hommel, J.D.; Anastasio, N.C.; Cunningham, K.A. Anterior insula activity regulates the associated behaviors of high fat food binge intake and cue reactivity in male rats. *Appetite* **2018**, *133*, 231–239. [CrossRef]
34. Price, A.E.; Anastasio, N.C.; Stutz, S.J.; Hommel, J.D.; Cunningham, K.A. Serotonin 5-ht2c receptor activation suppresses binge intake and the reinforcing and motivational properties of high-fat food. *Front. Pharmacol.* **2018**, *9*, 821. [CrossRef]
35. Kasper, J.M.; Johnson, S.B.; Hommel, J.D. Fat preference: A novel model of eating behavior in rats. *J. Vis. Exp.* **2014**, e51575. [CrossRef]
36. Howard, A.D.; Wang, R.; Pong, S.S.; Mellin, T.N.; Strack, A.; Guan, X.M.; Zeng, Z.; Williams, D.L.; Feighner, S.D.; Nunes, C.N.; et al. Identification of receptors for neuromedin u and its role in feeding. *Nature* **2000**, *406*, 70–74. [CrossRef] [PubMed]
37. Shan, L.; Qiao, X.; Crona, J.H.; Behan, J.; Wang, S.; Laz, T.; Bayne, M.; Gustafson, E.L.; Monsma, F.J.; Hedrick, J.A. Identification of a novel neuromedin u receptor subtype expressed in the central nervous system. *J. Biol. Chem.* **2000**, *275*, 39482–39486. [CrossRef] [PubMed]
38. Hosoya, M.; Moriya, T.; Kawamata, Y.; Ohkubo, S.; Fujii, R.; Matsui, H.; Shintani, Y.; Fukusumi, S.; Habata, Y.; Hinuma, S.; et al. Identification and functional characterization of a novel subtype of neuromedin u receptor. *J. Biol. Chem.* **2000**, *275*, 29528–29532. [CrossRef] [PubMed]
39. Raddatz, R.; Wilson, A.E.; Artymyshyn, R.; Bonini, J.A.; Borowsky, B.; Boteju, L.W.; Zhou, S.; Kouranova, E.V.; Nagorny, R.; Guevarra, M.S.; et al. Identification and characterization of two neuromedin u receptors differentially expressed in peripheral tissues and the central nervous system. *J. Biol. Chem.* **2000**, *275*, 32452–32459. [CrossRef] [PubMed]
40. Brighton, P.J.; Szekeres, P.G.; Willars, G.B. Neuromedin u and its receptors: Structure, function, and physiological roles. *Pharmacol. Rev.* **2004**, *56*, 231–248. [CrossRef] [PubMed]

41. Egecioglu, E.; Ploj, K.; Xu, X.; Bjursell, M.; Salomé, N.; Andersson, N.; Ohlsson, C.; Taube, M.; Hansson, C.; Bohlooly-Y, M.; et al. Central nmu signaling in body weight and energy balance regulation: Evidence from nmur2 deletion and chronic central nmu treatment in mice. *Am. J. Physiol. Endocrinol. Metab.* **2009**, *297*, E708–E716. [CrossRef] [PubMed]
42. McCue, D.L.; Kasper, J.M.; Hommel, J.D. Regulation of motivation for food by neuromedin u in the paraventricular nucleus and the dorsal raphe nucleus. *Int. J. Obes.* **2017**, *41*, 120–128. [CrossRef] [PubMed]
43. Gartlon, J.; Szekeres, P.; Pullen, M.; Sarau, H.M.; Aiyar, N.; Shabon, U.; Michalovich, D.; Steplewski, K.; Ellis, C.; Elshourbagy, N.; et al. Localisation of nmu1r and nmu2r in human and rat central nervous system and effects of neuromedin-u following central administration in rats. *Psychopharmacology* **2004**, *177*, 1–14. [CrossRef] [PubMed]
44. Kasper, J.; Smith, A.; Hommel, J. Cocaine-evoked locomotor activity correlates with the expression of neuromedin-u receptor 2 in the nucleus accumbens. *Front. Behav. Neurosci.* **2018**. In press. [CrossRef]
45. Zander, M.E.; De Young, K.P. Individual differences in negative affect and weekly variability in binge eating frequency. *Int. J. Eat. Disord.* **2014**, *47*, 296–301. [CrossRef]
46. Kasper, J.M.; McCue, D.L.; Milton, A.J.; Szwed, A.; Sampson, C.M.; Huang, M.; Carlton, S.; Meltzer, H.Y.; Cunningham, K.A.; Hommel, J.D. Gamma-aminobutyric acidergic projections from the dorsal raphe to the nucleus accumbens are regulated by neuromedin u. *Biol. Psychiatry* **2016**, *80*, 878–887. [CrossRef] [PubMed]
47. Paxinos, G.; Watson, C. *The Rat Brain in Stereotaxic Coordinates*, 6th ed.; Elsevier: Amsterdam, The Netherlands, 2007.
48. Anastasio, N.C.; Stutz, S.J.; Fink, L.H.; Swinford-Jackson, S.E.; Sears, R.M.; DiLeone, R.J.; Rice, K.C.; Moeller, F.G.; Cunningham, K.A. Serotonin (5-ht) 5-ht2a receptor (5-ht2ar):5-ht2cr imbalance in medial prefrontal cortex associates with motor impulsivity. *ACS Chem. Neurosci.* **2015**, *6*, 1248–1258. [CrossRef] [PubMed]
49. Breukel, A.I.; Besselsen, E.; Ghijsen, W.E. Synaptosomes. A model system to study release of multiple classes of neurotransmitters. *Methods Mol. Biol.* **1997**, *72*, 33–47. [PubMed]
50. Fink, L.H.; Anastasio, N.C.; Fox, R.G.; Rice, K.C.; Moeller, F.G.; Cunningham, K.A. Individual differences in impulsive action reflect variation in the cortical serotonin 5-ht2a receptor system. *Neuropsychopharmacology* **2015**, *40*, 1957–1968. [CrossRef] [PubMed]
51. Drewnowski, A.; Grinker, J.A.; Hirsch, J. Obesity and flavor perception: Multidimensional scaling of soft drinks. *Appetite* **1982**, *3*, 361–368. [CrossRef]
52. Drewnowski, A.; Greenwood, M.R. Cream and sugar: Human preferences for high-fat foods. *Physiol. Behav.* **1983**, *30*, 629–633. [CrossRef]
53. Drewnowski, A. Taste preferences and food intake. *Annu. Rev. Nutr.* **1997**, *17*, 237–253. [CrossRef]
54. Yanovski, S.Z.; Leet, M.; Yanovski, J.A.; Flood, M.; Gold, P.W.; Kissileff, H.R.; Walsh, B.T. Food selection and intake of obese women with binge-eating disorder. *Am. J. Clin. Nutr.* **1992**, *56*, 975–980. [CrossRef]
55. Sampson, C.M.; Kasper, J.M.; Felsing, D.E.; Raval, S.R.; Ye, N.; Wang, P.; Patrikeev, I.; Rytting, E.; Zhou, J.; Allen, J.A.; et al. Small-molecule neuromedin u receptor 2 agonists suppress food intake and decrease visceral fat in animal models. *Pharmacol. Res. Perspect.* **2018**, *6*, e00425. [CrossRef]
56. Kaisho, T.; Nagai, H.; Asakawa, T.; Suzuki, N.; Fujita, H.; Matsumiya, K.; Nishizawa, N.; Kanematsu-Yamaki, Y.; Dote, K.; Sakamoto, J.I.; et al. Effects of peripheral administration of a neuromedin u receptor 2-selective agonist on food intake and body weight in obese mice. *Int. J. Obes.* **2017**, *41*, 1790–1797. [CrossRef]
57. Kanematsu-Yamaki, Y.; Nishizawa, N.; Kaisho, T.; Nagai, H.; Mochida, T.; Asakawa, T.; Inooka, H.; Dote, K.; Fujita, H.; Matsumiya, K.; et al. Potent body weight-lowering effect of a neuromedin u receptor 2-selective pegylated peptide. *J. Med. Chem.* **2017**, *60*, 6089–6097. [CrossRef] [PubMed]

Early Maladaptive Schemas and Cognitive Distortions in Adults with Morbid Obesity: Relationships with Mental Health Status

Felipe Q. da Luz [1,2,3,*], Amanda Sainsbury [1,2], Phillipa Hay [4], Jessica A. Roekenes [1], Jessica Swinbourne [1], Dhiordan C. da Silva [3] and Margareth da S. Oliveira [3]

1 The Boden Institute of Obesity, Nutrition, Exercise & Eating Disorders, Sydney Medical School, Charles Perkins Centre, The University of Sydney, NSW 2006, Australia; amanda.salis@sydney.edu.au (A.S.); jess.roekenes@gmail.com (J.A.R.); jessica.swinbourne@sydney.edu.au (J.S.)

2 School of Psychology, Faculty of Science, The University of Sydney, NSW 2006, Australia

3 Faculty of Psychology, Pontifical Catholic University of Rio Grande do Sul, Av. Ipiranga 6681, Porto Alegre/RS, CEP 90619-900, Brazil; dhiordanc@gmail.com (D.C.d.S.); marga@pucrs.br (M.d.S.O.)

4 Centre for Health Research and School of Medicine, The University of Western Sydney, Locked Bag 1797, Penrith NSW 2751, Australia; p.hay@westernsydney.edu.au

* Correspondence: felipe.quintodaluz@sydney.edu.au

Academic Editor: Scott J. Hunter

Abstract: Dysfunctional cognitions may be associated with unhealthy eating behaviors seen in individuals with obesity. However, dysfunctional cognitions commonly occur in individuals with poor mental health independently of weight. We examined whether individuals with morbid obesity differed with regard to dysfunctional cognitions when compared to individuals of normal weight, when mental health status was controlled for. 111 participants—53 with morbid obesity and 58 of normal weight—were assessed with the Mini-Mental State Examination, Young Schema Questionnaire, Cognitive Distortions Questionnaire, Depression, Anxiety and Stress Scale, and a Demographic and Clinical Questionnaire. Participants with morbid obesity showed higher scores in one (insufficient self-control/self-discipline) of 15 early maladaptive schemas and in one (labeling) of 15 cognitive distortions compared to participants of normal weight. The difference between groups for insufficient self-control/self-discipline was not significant when mental health status was controlled for. Participants with morbid obesity showed more severe anxiety than participants of normal weight. Our findings did not show clinically meaningful differences in dysfunctional cognitions between participants with morbid obesity or of normal weight. Dysfunctional cognitions presented by individuals with morbid obesity are likely related to their individual mental health and not to their weight.

Keywords: obesity; morbid obesity; psychology; dysfunctional cognition; mental health

1. Introduction

Schema Theory proposes that some individuals can develop dysfunctional patterns of beliefs and unhelpful perceptions of the world and themselves [1]. These beliefs and perceptions usually develop during childhood or adolescence as a result of psychologically harmful experiences involving family members or other significant individuals, and for this reason are referred to as early maladaptive schemas. According to this theory, early maladaptive schemas develop in response to unmet core emotional needs, namely: secure attachment to others, autonomy/competence, freedom to express emotions, spontaneity, and realistic limits/self-control. It was previously suggested that as a result of this process, people can develop different types of psychological disorders and engage in a continuum of dysfunctional behaviors [1].

There is some evidence that early maladaptive schemas can relate to dysfunctional eating behaviors. For example, the unhealthy eating behaviors seen in patients with eating disorders were found to be associated with the presence of early maladaptive schemas [2]. One study [3] evaluated the presence of early maladaptive schemas in participants with obesity and found that they showed more severe early maladaptive schemas than participants of normal weight, notably the early maladaptive schemas of social isolation/alienation and defectiveness/shame. Another study [4] found that the early maladaptive schemas of isolation/alienation, emotional inhibition, abandonment/instability and unrelenting standards/hypercriticalness negatively influenced aspects of identity amongst individuals with obesity. Additionally, a higher presence of the following early maladaptive schemas were found amongst adolescents with overweight or obesity in comparison to adolescents of normal weight: social isolation/alienation, defectiveness/shame, emotional deprivation, failure to achieve, dependence/incompetence, and subjugation [5], as well as emotional deprivation, abandonment/instability, subjugation and insufficient self-control/self-discipline [6]. Additionally, another study [7] involving adolescents with overweight found that those who experienced a loss of control over eating had a greater severity of the early maladaptive schemas of social isolation/alienation, abandonment/instability, unrelenting standards/hypercriticalness, mistrust/abuse, failure to achieve and subjugation, in contrast with those that did not experience loss of control over eating.

Another set of dysfunctional cognitive processes, named cognitive distortions, plays an important role in maintaining the negative core beliefs that form early maladaptive schemas, through the perceptual distortion of facts [1]. Cognitive distortions are common thoughts that happen quickly, involuntarily, and in a distorted manner [8]. Some specific types of cognitive distortions have been suggested to be experienced by individuals with obesity [9]. These distorted thoughts occur, for example, when someone thinks that the desire to eat is irresistible ("magnification"), that they are "losers" because they are obese ("labeling") or that people reject them because they are overweight ("mind reading"). One study found that dichotomous thinking (a type of cognitive distortion) about food, weight and eating was predictive of weight regain, and that a general dichotomous thinking pattern (not necessarily related to food, weight or eating) was an even better predictor of weight regain [10]. Two other studies [11,12] assessed vulnerability to a specific cognitive distortion, namely thought-shape fusion, in participants with obesity and participants of normal weight. This type of cognitive distortion occurs when the imagination of the consumption of high-energy food generates the feeling of being fat and negative moral judgment. In these studies, individuals with obesity were less vulnerable to thought-shape fusion than individuals of normal weight, thus revealing differences in cognitive processes between groups. Studies have further examined the correlation of cognitive distortions with binge eating disorder. A small ($n = 42$) exploratory study [13] reported that participants with obesity, whether or not they had binge eating disorder, showed more cognitive distortions than participants of normal weight. In contrast, another study [14] found that individuals with obesity and comorbid binge eating disorder were more affected by dichotomous thinking than individuals with obesity but without binge eating disorder. The studies above suggest that individuals with obesity, especially those with comorbid binge eating disorder, experience more of some types of cognitive distortions than individuals of normal weight.

Other studies, however, emphasize the relationship between dysfunctional cognitions and mental health status independently of the occurrence of eating or weight disorders. For example, there is evidence that early maladaptive schemas predict depression [15], are associated with complex cases of mood and anxiety disorders [16], and are vulnerability factors for the development of symptoms of depression and anxiety amongst individuals experiencing stressful situations [17]. There are also indications that early maladaptive schemas predict occupational stress [18]. Both early maladaptive schemas and cognitive distortions were found to be significantly associated with emotional problems, namely depression and anxiety [19]. In regards to cognitive distortions specifically, a study found that participants with depression showed strong negative interpretations of metaphors [20]. Cognitive distortions also predict depression and anxiety amongst children and adolescents [21]. Additionally, the cognitive model proposes that cognitive distortions, together with neurobiological correlates, influence how people cope with stressful situations and develop depression [22]. All of the studies discussed in this paragraph show a clear association of the occurrence of dysfunctional cognitions and mental health problems, irrespective of the weight of the participants. Therefore, it is possible that the observation that individuals with obesity experience more early maladaptive schemas or cognitive distortions than individuals of normal weight could be mediated by the fact that participants with obesity frequently experience symptoms of mental illness [23], and not because of their elevated weight.

In summary, dysfunctional thinking styles, known as early maladaptive schemas and cognitive distortions, have been found in individuals with eating disorders, overweight or obesity. However, it is possible that these findings are associated with the mental health status of the participants and not necessarily with their obesity. Our study thus aimed to further examine this issue. Therefore, we sought to clarify whether individuals with morbid obesity show higher levels of dysfunctional cognitions than individuals of normal weight, and if so, if this is related to their individual mental health condition. Ultimately, this understanding could aid in the development of effective psychological and behavioral assessments and subsequent interventions, tailored specifically for individuals with morbid obesity.

2. Methods

2.1. Ethical Considerations

The study was conducted in accordance with the Declaration of Helsinki. This project was approved by the Research Ethics Committees of the Pontifical Catholic University of Rio Grande do Sul (Brazil) (CAAE: 07888612.4.0000.5336) and the Conceição Hospital Group where the participants were assessed. Informed consent was obtained from participants.

2.2. Participants

Participants were included if they had morbid obesity (BMI $\geq$ 40 kg/m^2) or normal weight (BMI: 18.5–24.9 kg/m^2) [24], were aged between 18 and 65 years, and had at least five years of education. The exclusion criterion was low cognitive performance (score $\leq$ 23) as assessed by the Mini Mental State Examination (MMSE) [25], as this could compromise comprehension and hence the accuracy in answering questionnaires. Two potential participants were excluded from the study because of this criterion.

There were 111 participants in this study, 53 (47.7%) with morbid obesity and 58 (52.3%) of normal weight. Participants with morbid obesity were recruited from the hospital bariatric surgery clinic and were classified as such by the medical team. Participants of normal weight were recruited through advertisements within the hospital. Participants' weight and height were recorded based on self-report. The groups were comparable with regards to sex, age, education, marital status and economic criteria of participants (see Table 1). Participants were not compensated for their participation in this research.

Table 1. Demographic details and body mass index of the participants with morbid obesity versus participants of normal weight.

Variables	Group				p
	Morbid Obesity (n = 53)		Normal Weight (n = 58)		
	n	%	n	%	
Sex					
Female	41	77.4	45	77.6	>0.999 $^{\Phi}$
Male	12	22.6	13	22.4	
Age (years)					
Mean $\pm$ standard deviation (range)	42.3 $\pm$ 9.6 (25–59)		38.7 $\pm$ 13.9 (18–65)		0.072 $^{£}$
Median (interquartile range)	42.0 (35.0–42.5)		38.5 (26.0–52.0)		
Highest education completed					

Table 1. *Cont.*

Variables	Group				p
	Morbid Obesity (n = 53)		Normal Weight (n = 58)		
	n	%	n	%	
Primary	24	45.3	24	41.4	0.678 ¶
Secondary/Tertiary	29	54.7	34	58.6	
Marital status					
Single	12	22.6	18	31.0	
Married	36	67.9	36	62.1	0.580 ¶
Separated/Divorced/Widowed	5	9.4	4	6.9	
Brazilian economic criteria					
Highest affluence	24	45.3	36	62.1	0.089 ¶
Lowest affluence)	29	54.7	22	37.9	
Body mass index (kg/m^2)					
Mean ± standard deviation	48.9 ± 6.3		22.1 ± 1.8		

Φ: Pearson's chi-square test with continuity correction; £: Students t-test for independent groups; ¶: Fisher's Exact Test for Monte Carlo simulation.

2.3. Questionnaires and Interviews

All questionnaires and interviews were conducted or overseen by the first author, in the bariatric surgery clinic of the hospital. The assessments of participants with morbid obesity occurred before bariatric surgery.

2.3.1. Mini Mental State Examination (MMSE)

The MMSE was used to assess mental state and cognitive deficits in potential participants [25]. The questions in this examination are divided into seven categories to assess specific cognitive functions: time orientation, place orientation, attention, basic calculation, word recognition and memorization, language and visual ability. The scores for examination can range from 0 to 30 points, with scores equal to or higher than 24 indicating normal cognition [25].

2.3.2. Young Schema Questionnaire (YSQ)

The YSQ is a self-report questionnaire that aims to identify the occurrence of early maladaptive schemas. This questionnaire has been used for research into core beliefs associated with psychological disturbances [26]. It is available in both a long and short version (205 and 75 items, respectively). Both versions of the YSQ have good psychometric properties, as indicated by statistically significant internal consistency [1]. Indeed, Cronbach's alpha is greater than 0.80 for each of the subscales on both versions [27]. The questionnaire's short form (YSQ-S2) was validated for use in Brazil (Cronbach's alpha = 0.95) [28] and was used in this study. The YSQ-S2 consists of a 75-item questionnaire assessing 15 types of early maladaptive schemas (groups of 5 items assess each of the 15 schemas). Participants are asked to answer the degree that they emotionally feel that the statements describe them according to the following options: 1—Completely untrue of me; 2—Mostly untrue of me; 3—Slightly more true than untrue; 4—Moderately true of me; 5—Mostly true of me and 6—Describes me perfectly. High scores in the items that relate to a specific early maladaptive schema indicate greater severity.

2.3.3. Cognitive Distortions Questionnaire (CD-Quest)

The CD-Quest is a self-report questionnaire that assesses a combination of the last week's frequency (no, occasional, much of the time or almost all of the time) and intensity (no, a little, much or very much) with which participants engaged in 15 common types of cognitive distortions [29]. Participants can score from 0 to 5 in each cognitive distortion, with higher scores indicating greater occurrence of the cognitive distortion. This instrument has been validated in Brazil and was found to have robust psychometric properties (Cronbach's alpha = 0.85) [30].

2.3.4. Depression, Anxiety and Stress Scale (DASS-21)

The DASS-21 measures symptoms of depression, anxiety and psychological stress in clinical and nonclinical groups. It has good internal consistency and concurrent validity [31]. In the current study, the short version with 21 items was used. This instrument has adequate internal consistency, with a Cronbach's alpha of 0.94 for the depression scale, 0.87 for the anxiety scale and 0.91 for the stress scale [31]. The DASS-21 has been validated for use in Brazil and the following Cronbach's alpha values were found for the depression, anxiety and stress scales, respectively: 0.92, 0.86 and 0.90 [32]. The DASS-21 provides specific scores for depression, anxiety and stress. Higher scores indicate greater severity of the symptoms.

2.3.5. Demographic and Clinical Questionnaire

Demographic and clinical features were assessed by a structured interview developed for this study. Questions included date of birth, marital status, education level, economic status, and use of psychiatric medications. The Brazilian Economic Criteria were used to classify economic status according to the following categories (highest to lowest affluence): A, B, C, D and E [33], computed from quantification of household assets and income.

2.4. Statistical Analysis

Descriptive statistics were used to describe the results in terms of absolute and relative distribution, as well as central tendency and variability measures. Age distribution was compared using the Kolmogorov-Smirnov test [34].

For bivariate analysis of categorical variables, the Pearson's chi-square test ($\chi 2$) was used. Fisher's exact test was performed in contingency tables where at least 25% of cell values presented an expected frequency of less than 5. Monte Carlo simulation was used when at least one variable had polytomous characteristics. For correlational analysis of continuous variables, the Spearman ranked correlations test (Spearman rho, r_S) was employed because of non-normality of data. For between-group comparisons of non-parametric ordinal or continuous variables, the Mann-Whitney U test was used.

On data inspection, all early maladaptive schemas and cognitive distortions correlated significantly with levels of depression, anxiety and stress as measured with the DASS-21 (all $r_S > 0.40$, all $p > 0.001$). Thus, Multivariable logistic regression analysis was applied to test the strength of association between the dependent variable (obesity, using binary yes/no, with the reference category being 'participants with obesity') and independent variables (early maladaptive schemas and cognitive distortions) that were found to be significant or approaching significance at a level of 5% when univariate tests were performed and adjusted for levels of depression, anxiety and stress. A significance level of $p < 0.05$ was employed for all tests. Analyses were conducted using the SPSS for Windows version 20 (Armonk, NY, USA).

3. Results

3.1. Early Maladaptive Schemas in Participants with Morbid Obesity Versus Participants of Normal Weight

As shown in Table 2, scores for the early maladaptive schema of insufficient self-control/self-discipline were significantly higher in participants with morbid obesity compared to participants of normal weight, as assessed using the YSQ-S2. High scores on this early maladaptive schema indicate beliefs of insufficient control over emotions or impulses and beliefs of not having enough capacity to deal with boredom or frustration in order to complete tasks [1]. There were no other statistically significant differences between participants with morbid obesity and participants of normal weight with respect to scores on early maladaptive schemas (see Table 2).

Table 2. Early maladaptive schemas as assessed by the YSQ-S2 in participants with morbid obesity versus participants of normal weight.

YSQ-S	Groups						p §
	Morbid Obesity (n = 53)			Normal Weight (n = 58)			
	Mean	Standard Deviation	Median	Mean	Standard Deviation	Median	
Emotional deprivation	2.5	1.5	2.0	2.0	1.3	1.5	0.08
Abandonment/instability	2.6	1.6	2.0	2.5	1.6	1.6	0.44
Mistrust/abuse	2.4	1.5	2.0	2.2	1.3	1.8	0.58
Social isolation/alienation	2.0	1.4	1.4	1.9	1.3	1.3	0.57
Defectiveness/shame	1.5	1.2	1.0	1.3	0.8	1.0	0.77
Failure	1.7	1.2	1.2	1.6	1.0	1.2	0.72
Dependence/incompetence	1.7	1.1	1.2	1.5	0.7	1.4	0.91
Vulnerability to harm	2.0	1.2	1.6	2.1	1.3	1.6	0.86
Enmeshment	1.7	1.0	1.2	2.0	1.2	1.7	0.16
Subjugation	1.8	1.1	1.4	1.8	1.2	1.2	0.53
Self-sacrifice	4.1	1.5	4.2	3.7	1.6	3.9	0.29
Emotional inhibition	2.5	1.6	1.8	1.9	1.2	1.6	0.11
Unrelenting standards	3.1	1.5	3.0	2.7	1.1	2.5	0.15
Entitlement/grandiosity	2.6	1.4	2.4	2.3	1.2	1.8	0.22
Insufficient self-control/self-discipline	2.5	1.4	2.4	2.0	1.2	1.6	0.01

YSQ-S: Young Schema Questionnaire—short form. §: Values compared using the Mann-Whitney U test.

3.2. Cognitive Distortions in Participants with Morbid Obesity Versus Participants of Normal Weight

Participants with morbid obesity showed a statistical trend ($p = 0.05$) for higher scores on the cognitive distortion of labeling in comparison with participants of normal weight (see Table 3). Labeling is a type of cognitive distortion that occurs when someone gives derogatory or demeaning names to themselves or others (e.g., "I am a failure") [29]. There were no other statistically significant differences between participants with morbid obesity and participants of normal weight, with respect to scores on cognitive distortions.

Table 3. Cognitive distortions as assessed by the CD-Quest in participants with morbid obesity versus participants of normal weight.

CD-Quest (¥)	Group						p §
	Morbid Obesity (n = 53)			Normal Weight (n = 58)			
	Mean	Standard Deviation	Median	Mean	Standard Deviation	Median	
All-or-nothing thinking	1.5	1.9	0.0	1.3	1.7	0.0	0.60
Fortune-telling	1.2	1.7	0.0	1.1	1.5	0.0	0.91
Disqualifying	0.5	1.0	0.0	0.5	1.2	0.0	0.45
Emotional reasoning	1.9	2.0	1.0	1.8	1.8	1.0	0.93
Labeling	1.4	1.7	1.0	0.8	1.3	0.0	0.05
Magnification/minimization	0.8	1.3	0.0	0.7	1.3	0.0	0.67
Mental filter	0.9	1.5	0.0	1.1	1.5	0.0	0.22
Mind reading	1.3	1.5	1.0	1.1	1.6	0.0	0.39
Overgeneralization	1.0	1.5	0.0	1.2	1.6	0.0	0.37
Personalization	0.8	1.4	0.0	0.8	1.2	0.0	0.58
Should statements	2.4	1.9	2.0	1.9	1.7	2.0	0.21
Jumping to conclusions	1.4	1.8	1.0	1.4	1.6	1.0	0.69
Blaming	1.6	1.9	1.0	1.3	1.7	0.0	0.45
What if...?	1.4	1.9	0.0	1.8	1.9	1.0	0.30
Unfair comparisons	1.2	1.8	0.0	1.0	1.5	0.0	0.98
CD-Quest Total	19.1	15.7	16.0	17.7	14.4	15.0	0.74

CD-Quest: Cognitive Distortions Questionnaire. §: Values compared using the Mann-Whitney U test; ¥: Asymmetrically distributed variable.

3.3. Depression, Anxiety and Stress Symptoms in Participants with Morbid Obesity Versus Participants of Normal Weight

No significant differences between groups were found on scores of symptoms of depression or stress. However, participants with morbid obesity showed significantly higher scores on anxiety symptoms in comparison to participants of normal weight (see Table 4). Median and interquartile range were used (instead of mean and standard deviation) to analyze differences between participants with morbid obesity and participants of normal weight, because data on levels of depression, anxiety and stress were highly skewed.

Table 4. Levels of depression, anxiety and stress scores on the DASS-21 in participants with morbid obesity compared to participants of normal weight.

DASS-21	Group		Z, *p*
	Morbid Obesity (n = 53)	Normal Weight (n = 58)	
Depression			
Mean ± standard deviation	9.7 ± 10.2 (0–40.0)	7.3 ± 9.9 (0–42.0)	
Median (interquartile range)	6.0 (2.0–14.0)	4.0 (0–10.5)	−1.58, 0.14
Anxiety			
Mean ± standard deviation (range)	12.6 ± 11.9 (0–42.0)	8.1 ± 10.1 (0–42.0)	
Median (interquartile range)	8.0 (2.0–23.0)	4.0 (0–12.5)	−2.37, 0.018
Stress			
Mean ± standard deviation (range)	16.1 ± 13.4 (0–42.0)	13.1 ± 11.1 (0–42.0)	
Median (interquartile range)	14.0 (4.0–30.0)	9.0 (3.5–20.0)	−0.953, 0.34

Z = Z score from the Mann-Whitney U test, conducted on the non-parametric median and interquartile range statistics.

3.4. Comparative Analysis by Binary Logistic Regression to Predict Morbid Obesity

Logistic regression analysis revealed that the difference in scores of the early maladaptive schema of insufficient self-control/self-discipline between participants with morbid obesity and participants of normal weight was no longer significant when adjustment was made for levels of depression, anxiety and stress. The difference in scores of the cognitive distortion of labeling between participants with morbid obesity and participants of normal weight however was significant when adjustment was made for levels of depression, anxiety and stress (see Table 5).

Table 5. Results of multivariable (logistic regression) analysis with presence or absence of morbid obesity as dependent variable * (Model Nagelkerke R^2 = 0.15).

Predictor (Independent) Variable	Exp (B)	95% Confidence Interval	*p*
Early maladaptive schema: insufficient self-control/self-discipline	0.70	0.47; 1.05	0.09
Cogntive distortion: Labelling	0.69	0.49; 0.96	0.03
Anxiety	0.92	0.85; 0.99	0.03
Depression	1.05	0.97; 1.13	0.25
Stress	1.06	0.99; 1.13	0.10

* The reference category (specified as 'participants with obesity') is such that a value of Exp (B) (also referred to as the odds ratio) of less than 1 implies that the predictor variable is higher in participants with obesity.

3.5. Psychiatric Medication Use in Participants with Morbid Obesity Versus Participants of Normal Weight

Data from the demographic and clinical questionnaire showed that the group of participants with morbid obesity had a significantly higher number of users of psychiatric medication at the time of the assessment in comparison to participants of normal weight (28 out of 53 or 54% of participants with morbid obesity versus 8 out of 58 or 14% of the participants of normal weight, χ^2 = 19.98, $p < 0.001$).

4. Discussion

The main aim of this study was to compare the occurrence of early maladaptive schemas and cognitive distortions in participants with morbid obesity versus those of normal weight, and to examine if mental health status could influence potential differences between groups in the occurrence of these dysfunctional cognitions. Higher occurrences of the early maladaptive schema of insufficient self-control/self-discipline and a statistical trend towards higher occurrence of the cognitive distortion of labeling were found in participants with morbid obesity compared to participants of normal weight. However, after controlling for symptoms of depression, of anxiety, and stress, participants with morbid obesity and participants of normal weight did not differ statistically in regards to scores on early maladaptive schemas. These findings support a previous study that found that an individual's responses in the YSQ-S are influenced by their emotional state while completing the questionnaire [35].

Furthermore, even before controlling for mental health status, the statistical differences of early maladaptive schemas and cognitive distortions found amongst participants with morbid obesity compared to participants of normal weight were small (1 out of 15 types of early maladaptive schemas and 1 out of 15 types of cognitive distortions). These are slight differences that may have been found due to chance. These findings do not indicate significant clinical differences in the occurrence of dysfunctional cognitions between those with morbid obesity and those of a normal weight.

We did not find statistically significant differences between participants with morbid obesity and participants of normal weight in regards to symptoms of depression and stress. However, significant differences were found in the presence of anxiety symptoms between groups. These findings contradict a systematic review and meta-analysis that found an association between obesity and depression, particularly amongst women [36]. The levels of depression symptoms in the participants with morbid obesity in our sample were possibly low since more than half (54%) of our participants with morbid obesity were being treated with psychiatric medication at the time of the assessment. Although stress-induced eating habits seem to have an important role in the development of obesity [37], in our study, no differences in the level of stress symptoms were found between groups. Our findings regarding the higher anxiety symptoms amongst participants with morbid obesity are consistent with the outcomes from a systematic review and meta-analysis that found a positive association between anxiety disorders and obesity [38]. A previous study found that individuals with obesity, especially those with comorbid binge eating disorders, tend to eat in response to unpleasant emotional states [39].

An additional finding of our study is that the participants with morbid obesity used significantly more psychiatric medication than the participants of normal weight. This may have been influenced by the fact that the participants with morbid obesity were patients of the bariatric surgery clinic and therefore were regularly seen by the medical team, and such medical attention did not necessarily occur for participants of normal weight. This finding is compatible with a previous study [40] that found high psychiatric medication use amongst individuals with morbid obesity (40.7% of their sample). A controversial issue regarding the prescription of psychiatric medication for individuals with morbid obesity is the effect of these medicines on weight. A recent systematic review reported that body fat accumulation is a common side effect of psychotropic medication [41]. Therefore, it is possible that the higher use of psychiatric medication contributed to the excess weight of the participants with morbid obesity, albeit this was not the focus of the current study.

The current findings have relevance to clinical practice. Lifestyle interventions aimed at promoting healthy eating habits and appropriate levels of physical activity are routinely recommended for people with morbid obesity, due to their role in reducing the medical complications related to morbid obesity and in improving psychological health [42]. However, further psychological therapy may be required for some individuals with morbid obesity. Their mental health status should be assessed, and those with depression, anxiety and/or psychological distress may be considered for further assessment of early maladaptive schemas and cognitive distortions and these (if present) may need to be addressed with specific psychotherapy, such as cognitive and/or schema therapy [1,8].

Limitations of this study include the use of self-report assessment of early maladaptive schemas and cognitive distortions, as some people may have difficulty identifying their own dysfunctional thoughts [43]. A second limitation is that participants with morbid obesity may have tried to express socially desirable responses in an attempt to allay social stigma [44], or for fear of a psychological evaluation that could deny or delay their referral for bariatric surgery [45] (although they were told that their responses would be confidential). A third limitation of this study is that types of psychiatric medication used by the participants, psychotherapeutic treatment and psychiatric diagnosis were not assessed. Future research in this field should include participants with obesity that are not seeking treatment, and examine causal effects of anxiety symptoms and use of psychiatric drugs amongst individuals with morbid obesity.

5. Conclusions

In conclusion, higher occurrence of dysfunctional cognitions (the early maladaptive schema of insufficient self-control/self-discipline and the cognitive distortion of labeling) amongst participants with morbid obesity in comparison to participants of normal weight was small and the early maladaptive schema of insufficient self-control/self-discipline was no longer statistically significant once symptoms of depression, anxiety and stress were controlled for. Dysfunctional cognitions presented by individuals with morbid obesity are probably related to their individual mental health status and not to their weight disorder.

Acknowledgments: This work was supported by the CAPES Foundation, Ministry of Education of Brazil, via scholarships to Felipe Quinto da Luz and via the National Health and Medical Research Council (NHMRC) of Australia via a Project Grant and Senior Research Fellowship to Amanda Sainsbury. Our thanks also go to Sanja Lujic for statistical advice.

Author Contributions: Felipe Quinto da Luz and Margareth da Silva Oliveira conceived and designed the study. Felipe Quinto da Luz collected the data. Felipe Quinto da Luz, Amanda Sainsbury, Phillipa Hay, Jessica Ann Roekenes, Jessica Swinbourne, Dhiordan Cardoso da Silva and Margareth da Silva Oliveira analyzed the data and wrote the paper.

References

1. Young, J.E.; Klosko, J.S.; Weishaar, M.E. *Schema Therapy: A Practitioner's Guide*; Guilford Publications: New York, NY, USA, 2003.
2. Unoka, Z.; Tölgyes, T.; Czobor, P. Early Maladaptive Schemas and Body Mass Index in Subgroups of Eating Disorders: A Differential Association. *Compr. Psychiatry* **2007**, *48*, 199–204. [CrossRef] [PubMed]
3. Anderson, K.; Rieger, E.; Caterson, I. A Comparison of Maladaptive Schemata in Treatment-Seeking Obese Adults and Normal-Weight Control Subjects. *J. Psychosom. Res.* **2006**, *60*, 245–252. [CrossRef] [PubMed]
4. Poursharifi, H.; Bidadian, M.; Bahramizadeh, H.; Salehinezhad, M.A. The Relationship between Early Maladaptive Schemas and Aspects of Identity in Obesity. *Procedia Soc. Behav. Sci.* **2011**, *30*, 517–523. [CrossRef]
5. Vlierberghe, L.V.; Braet, C. Dysfunctional Schemas and Psychopathology in Referred Obese Adolescents. *Clin. Psychol. Psychother.* **2007**, *14*, 342–351. [CrossRef]
6. Turner, H.M.; Rose, K.S.; Cooper, M.J. Schema and Parental Bonding in Overweight and Nonoverweight Female Adolescents. *Int. J. Obes. Relat. Metab. Disord.* **2005**, *29*, 381–387. [CrossRef] [PubMed]
7. Vlierberghe, L.V.; Braet, C.; Goossens, L. Dysfunctional Schemas and Eating Pathology in Overweight Youth: A Case–Control Study. *Int. J. Eat. Disord.* **2009**, *42*, 437–442. [CrossRef] [PubMed]
8. Beck, J.S. *Cognitive Therapy: Basics and Beyond*; Guilford Press: New York, NY, USA, 1995.
9. Beck, J.S. *The Beck Diet Solution: Train Your Brain to Think Like a Thin Person*; Oxmoor House, Inc.: New York, NY, USA, 2012.
10. Byrne, S.M.; Cooper, Z.; Fairburn, C.G. Psychological Predictors of Weight Regain in Obesity. *Behav. Res. Ther.* **2004**, *42*, 1341–1356. [CrossRef] [PubMed]
11. Coelho, J.S.; Jansen, A.; Bouvard, M. Cognitive Distortions in Normal-Weight and Overweight Women: Susceptibility to Thought-Shape Fusion. *Cognit. Ther. Res.* **2012**, *36*, 417–425. [CrossRef]
12. Coelho, J.S.; Siggen, M.J.; Dietre, P.; Bouvard, M. Reactivity to Thought–Shape Fusion in Adolescents: The Effects of Obesity Status. *Pediatr. Obes.* **2013**, *8*, 439–444. [CrossRef] [PubMed]
13. Volery, M.; Carrard, I.; Rouget, P.; Archinard, M.; Golay, A. Cognitive Distortions in Obese Patients with or without Eating Disorders. *Eat. Weight Disord.* **2006**, *11*, 123–126. [CrossRef]
14. Ramacciotti, C.E.; Elisabetta, C.; Bondi, E.; Burgalassi, A.; Massimetti, G.; Dell'Osso, L. Shared Psychopathology in Obese Subjects with and without Binge-Eating Disorder. *Int. J. Eat. Disord.* **2008**, *41*, 643–649. [CrossRef] [PubMed]

15. Halvorsen, M.; Wang, C.E.; Eisemann, M.; Waterloo, K. Dysfunctional Attitudes and Early Maladaptive Schemas as Predictors of Depression: A 9-Year Follow-up Study. *Cognit. Ther. Res.* **2010**, *34*, 368–379. [CrossRef]
16. Hawke, L.D.; Provencher, M.D. Early Maladaptive Schemas: Relationship with Case Complexity in Mood and Anxiety Disorders. *J. Cogn. Psychother.* **2013**, *27*, 359–369. [CrossRef]
17. Cámara, M.; Calvete, E. Early Maladaptive Schemas as Moderators of the Impact of Stressful Events on Anxiety and Depression in University Students. *J. Psychopathol. Behav. Assess.* **2012**, *34*, 58–68. [CrossRef]
18. Bamber, M.; McMahon, R. Danger-Early Maladaptive Schemas at Work!: The Role of Early Maladaptive Schemas in Career Choice and the Development of Occupational Stress in Health Workers. *Clin. Psychol. Psychother.* **2008**, *15*, 96–112. [CrossRef] [PubMed]
19. Leung, P.W.L.; Poon, M.W.L. Dysfunctional Schemas and Cognitive Distortions in Psychopathology: A Test of the Specificity Hypothesis. *J. Child Psychol. Psychiatry* **2011**, *42*, 755–765. [CrossRef]
20. Bartczak, M.; Bokus, B. Cognitive Representations (Metaphorical Conceptualizations) of Past, Future, Joy, Sadness and Happiness in Depressive and Non-Depressive Subjects: Cognitive Distortions in Depression at the Level of Notion. *J. Psycholinguist. Res.* **2015**, *44*, 159–185. [CrossRef] [PubMed]
21. Weems, C.F.; Berman, S.L.; Silverman, W.K.; Saavedra, L.M. Cognitive Errors in Youth with Anxiety Disorders: The Linkages between Negative Cognitive Errors and Anxious Symptoms. *Cognit. Ther. Res.* **2001**, *25*, 559–575. [CrossRef]
22. Beck, A.T. The Evolution of the Cognitive Model of Depression and Its Neurobiological Correlates. *Am. J. Psychiatry* **2008**, *165*, 969–977. [CrossRef] [PubMed]
23. Müller, A.; Mitchell, J.E.; Sondag, C.; de Zwaan, M. Psychiatric Aspects of Bariatric Surgery. *Curr. Psychiatry Rep.* **2013**, *15*, 1–8. [CrossRef] [PubMed]
24. World Health Organization. *Obesity: Preventing and Managing the Global Epidemic: Report of a WHO Consultation*; World Health Organization Technichal Report Series: Geneva, Switzerland, 2000.
25. Folstein, M.F.; Folstein, S.E.; McHugh, P.R. "Mini-Mental State". A Practical Method for Grading the Cognitive State of Patients for the Clinician. *J. Psychiat. Res.* **1975**, *12*, 189–198. [CrossRef]
26. Renner, F.; Lobbestael, J.; Peeters, F.; Arntz, A.; Huibers, M. Early Maladaptive Schemas in Depressed Patients: Stability and Relation with Depressive Symptoms over the Course of Treatment. *J. Affect. Disord.* **2012**, *136*, 581–590. [CrossRef] [PubMed]
27. Waller, G.; Meyer, C.; Ohanian, V. Psychometric Properties of the Long and Short Versions of the Young Schema Questionnaire: Core Beliefs among Bulimic and Comparison Women. *Cognit. Ther. Res.* **2001**, *25*, 137–147. [CrossRef]
28. Cazassa, M.; Oliveira, M. Validação Brasileira Do Questionário De Esquemas De Young: Forma Breve. *Estud. Psicol.* **2012**, *29*, 23–31. [CrossRef]
29. De Oliveira, I.R. *Trial-Based Cognitive Therapy: A Manual for Clinicians*; Routledge: London, UK, 2014; pp. 28–35.
30. De Oliveira, I.R.; Seixas, C.; Osório, F.L.; Crippa, J.A.S.; Abreu, J.N.; Menezes, I.G.; Pidgeon, A.; Sudak, D.; Wenzel, A. Evaluation of the Psychometric Properties of the Cognitive Distortions Questionnaire (Cd-Quest) in a Sample of Undergraduate Students. *Innov. Clin. Neurosci.* **2015**, *12*, 20–27. [PubMed]
31. Antony, M.M.; Bieling, P.J.; Cox, B.J.; Enns, M.W.; Swinson, R.P. Psychometric Properties of the 42-Item and 21-Item Versions of the Depression Anxiety Stress Scales in Clinical Groups and a Community Sample. *Psychol. Assess.* **1998**, *10*, 176–181. [CrossRef]
32. Vignola, R.C.B.; Tucci, A.M. Adaptation and Validation of the Depression, Anxiety and Stress Scale (Dass) to Brazilian Portuguese. *J. Affect. Disord.* **2014**, *155*, 104–109. [CrossRef] [PubMed]
33. Associação Brasileira de Empresas de Pesquisa. Critério De Classificação Econômica Brasil. Available online: www.abep.org/Servicos/Download.aspx?id=07 (accessed on 3 November 2016).
34. Everitt, B.; Dunn, G. *Applied Multivariate Data Analysis*; Wiley: London, UK, 1991.
35. Stopa, L.; Waters, A. The Effect of Mood on Responses to the Young Schema Questionnaire: Short Form. *Psychol. Psychother.* **2005**, *78*, 45–57. [CrossRef] [PubMed]
36. De Wit, L.; Luppino, F.; van Straten, A.; Penninx, B.; Zitman, F.; Cuijpers, P. Depression and Obesity: A Meta-Analysis of Community-Based Studies. *Psychiatry Res.* **2010**, *178*, 230–235. [CrossRef] [PubMed]
37. Dallman, M.F. Stress-Induced Obesity and the Emotional Nervous System. *Trends Endocrinol. Metab.* **2010**, *21*, 159–165. [CrossRef] [PubMed]

38. Gariepy, G.; Nitka, D.; Schmitz, N. The Association between Obesity and Anxiety Disorders in the Population: A Systematic Review and Meta-Analysis. *Int. J. Obes.* **2010**, *34*, 407–419. [CrossRef] [PubMed]
39. Zeeck, A.; Stelzer, N.; Linster, H.W.; Joos, A.; Hartmann, A. Emotion and Eating in Binge Eating Disorder and Obesity. *Eur. Eat. Disord. Rev.* **2011**, *19*, 426–437. [CrossRef] [PubMed]
40. Mitchell, J.E.; Selzer, F.; Kalarchian, M.A.; Devlin, M.J.; Strain, G.W.; Elder, K.A.; Marcus, M.D.; Wonderlich, S.; Christian, N.J.; Yanovski, S.Z. Psychopathology before Surgery in the Longitudinal Assessment of Bariatric Surgery-3 (Labs-3) Psychosocial Study. *Surg. Obes. Relat. Dis.* **2012**, *8*, 533–541. [CrossRef] [PubMed]
41. Dent, R.; Blackmore, A.; Peterson, J.; Habib, R.; Kay, G.P.; Gervais, A.; Taylor, V.; Wells, G. Changes in Body Weight and Psychotropic Drugs: A Systematic Synthesis of the Literature. *PLoS ONE* **2012**, *7*, e36889. [CrossRef] [PubMed]
42. Stanton, R.; Reaburn, P. Exercise and the Treatment of Depression: A Review of the Exercise Program Variables. *J. Sci. Med. Sport* **2014**, *17*, 177–182. [CrossRef] [PubMed]
43. Beck, A.T. *Cognitive Therapy of Depression*; Guilford Press: New York, NY, USA, 1979.
44. Lee, L.; Shapiro, C.M. Psychological Manifestations of Obesity. *J. Psychosom. Res.* **2003**, *55*, 477–479. [CrossRef]
45. Ambwani, S.; Boeka, A.G.; Brown, J.D.; Byrne, T.K.; Budak, A.R.; Sarwer, D.B.; Fabricatore, A.N.; Morey, L.C.; O'Neil, P.M. Socially Desirable Responding by Bariatric Surgery Candidates During Psychological Assessment. *Surg. Obes. Relat. Diseas.* **2013**, *9*, 300–305. [CrossRef] [PubMed]

15

Obesity with Comorbid Eating Disorders: Associated Health Risks and Treatment Approaches

Felipe Q. da Luz [1,2,3,*], Phillipa Hay [4], Stephen Touyz [2] and Amanda Sainsbury [1,2]

1 The Boden Institute of Obesity, Nutrition, Exercise & Eating Disorders, Faculty of Medicine and Health, Charles Perkins Centre, The University of Sydney, Camperdown, NSW 2006, Australia; Amanda.salis@sydney.edu.au
2 Faculty of Science, School of Psychology, the University of Sydney, Camperdown, NSW 2006, Australia; Stephen.touyz@sydney.edu.au
3 CAPES Foundation, Ministry of Education of Brazil, Brasília, DF 70040-020, Brazil
4 Translational Health Research Institute (THRI), School of Medicine, Western Sydney University, Locked Bag 1797, Penrith, NSW 2751, Australia; P.hay@westernsydney.edu.au
* Correspondence: Felipe.quintodaluz@sydney.edu.au

Abstract: Obesity and eating disorders are each associated with severe physical and mental health consequences, and individuals with obesity as well as comorbid eating disorders are at higher risk of these than individuals with either condition alone. Moreover, obesity can contribute to eating disorder behaviors and vice-versa. Here, we comment on the health complications and treatment options for individuals with obesity and comorbid eating disorder behaviors. It appears that in order to improve the healthcare provided to these individuals, there is a need for greater exchange of experiences and specialized knowledge between healthcare professionals working in the obesity field with those working in the field of eating disorders, and vice-versa. Additionally, nutritional and/or behavioral interventions simultaneously addressing weight management and reduction of eating disorder behaviors in individuals with obesity and comorbid eating disorders may be required. Future research investigating the effects of integrated medical, psychological and nutritional treatment programs addressing weight management and eating disorder psychopathology in individuals with obesity and comorbid eating disorder behaviors—such as binge eating—is necessary.

Keywords: obesity; eating disorders; binge eating; dieting; treatment

---

1. Introduction

Obesity is commonly associated with health complications. Individuals with obesity are at high risk of several physical diseases, such as certain cancers, diabetes, hypertension, heart disease, stroke, as well as being at increased risk of mortality [1–7]. Obesity is also often associated with mental health problems and psychosocial difficulties. Indeed, women with obesity tend to report worse mental health than women without obesity [8]. Moreover, women tend to experience more mental health complications associated with obesity than men [9], albeit mental health problems associated with obesity (e.g., anxiety) occur in both women and men [9]. One factor that can be detrimental to the mental health of individuals with obesity is exposure to well-documented discriminatory attitudes and behaviors in different areas, such as employment, education and healthcare [10]. Additionally, discrimination against individuals with higher body mass index (BMI) can be particularly problematic because it can induce strong dissatisfaction with one's body weight and/or shape, which is a risk factor for the development of comorbid eating disorder behaviors [11].

The eating disorders that have been most frequently studied in individuals with obesity are binge eating disorder and bulimia nervosa. Binge eating disorder is defined in the current Diagnostic and Statistical Manual of Mental Disorders (DSM-5) by recurrent binge eating episodes occurring at least once a week for the past 3 months, and associated with marked distress [12]. The DSM-5 criteria for binge eating disorder also require that individuals experience at least three of the following five features: eating much more quickly than normal; eating until feeling excessively full; overeating when not feeling physically hungry; eating alone because of embarrassment related to the amount of food consumed; and feeling disgusted, depressed, or very guilty after the binge eating episodes [12]. Bulimia nervosa is characterized by self-evaluation that is excessively influenced by body weight and shape, recurrent binge eating, and recurrent unhealthy compensatory behaviors to prevent weight gain (i.e., self-induced vomiting; misuse of laxatives, diuretics or other medications; fasting; excessive exercise) [12]. The DSM-5 criteria for bulimia nervosa require that the binge eating episodes and compensatory unhealthy behaviors have occurred at least once per week for the past 3 months [12]. In addition to binge eating disorder and bulimia nervosa, individuals with obesity can also experience "other specified feeding or eating disorder" when presentations cause significant distress or impairment but do not completely meet the DSM-5 criteria for a specific eating disorder [12]. For example, according to the DSM-5, a person may have binge eating disorder of low frequency and/or limited duration. In this case, the person meets the DSM-5 criteria for binge eating disorder, except that binge eating has occurred less than once a week and/or for less than 3 months [12].

There is a significant co-occurrence of eating disorders, particularly binge eating disorder, in individuals with higher BMI. In Latin America, for example, the prevalence of binge eating disorder was 16–52% in individuals with obesity (BMI $\geq$ 30 kg/m^2) attending weight loss programs [13]. In the United States, a study with a nationally-representative sample of 9282 people assessed in 2001–2003 found that 42% of individuals that had had a binge eating disorder at any stage in their life had obesity at the time of the survey [14]. A more recent study in the United States, with a sample of 36,306 participants assessed in 2012–2013, found that relative to those with no history of eating disorders, participants who met criteria for binge eating disorder in the last 12 months, or at any time in their lives, had significantly increased odds of having obesity or extreme obesity [15]. On the flip side, a study with a clinical sample of 1383 individuals with current eating disorders, including 123 with binge eating disorder and 551 with bulimia nervosa, found that 87% of individuals with binge eating disorder, and 33% of individuals with bulimia nervosa, had also had obesity at some point in their lives [16]. These studies show a significant co-occurrence of obesity and eating disorders, and are consistent with the hypothesis that these conditions can potentially contribute to and/or exacerbate each other. Additionally, obesity with comorbid eating disorder behaviors, such as binge eating, may be a growing problem. In a population-representative sample of 9053 people in Australia between the years of 1995 to 2015, there were significant increases in the prevalence of obesity and eating disorder behaviors independently; however, the greatest increases were in the prevalence of individuals with obesity and comorbid binge eating or very strict dieting (7.3 fold and 11.5 fold, respectively) [17]. The increases in the prevalence of obesity and comorbid eating disorder behaviors mentioned above may be related to a potential contribution of binge eating to obesity [14,18,19], as well as to the social expectancy for people with obesity to lose excess weight [17]. The potentially growing prevalence of individuals with obesity and comorbid eating disorder behaviors is concerning due to the medical and psychosocial risks that these individuals are exposed to.

2. Health Risks of Obesity with Comorbid Eating Disorders

Individuals with obesity and comorbid eating disorders are at high risk of several medical and psychosocial complications. A study with 152 treatment-seeking individuals with obesity found that those with binge eating disorder had higher BMIs, more severe levels of depression and obsessive-compulsive symptoms, and stronger feelings of inadequacy and inferiority than those without binge eating disorder [20]. Similarly, bariatric surgery candidates with comorbid binge eating disorder had significantly more mood and anxiety disorders than bariatric surgery candidates without binge eating disorder (27% versus 5% for mood disorders, and 27% versus 8% for anxiety disorders, respectively) [21]. Indeed, 40% of bariatric surgery candidates with comorbid binge eating disorder had a mood or anxiety disorder, with some participants having both a mood and an anxiety disorder [21]. Similarly, gastric bypass surgery candidates with binge eating disorder had more disordered eating attitudes and behaviors, as well as worse physical, emotional and social quality of life, than gastric bypass surgery candidates without binge eating disorder [22]. Not only is binge eating in individuals with obesity associated with poor mental health and poor quality of life, but binge eating can also hinder weight loss in individuals with morbid obesity. For instance, a systematic review found that individuals submitted to bariatric surgery that had clinically significant binge eating before and after the surgery had worse weight loss outcomes than those without pre-surgical binge eating, or than those who stopped binge eating after the surgery [23]. The occurrence of obesity in individuals with eating disorders is also associated with greater mental health complications. For instance, individuals with eating disorders that had had obesity at any stage in their lives had higher eating disorder severity and greater general psychopathology than those with eating disorders that had never had obesity [16]. Finally, obesity with comorbid binge eating can be functionally detrimental. For example, individuals with obesity and comorbid binge eating had greater work-related impairment in productivity than those with obesity only, or binge eating only, or than those of normal weight without binge eating [24]. Thus, individuals with obesity and comorbid eating disorders are at higher risk of medical and psychosocial complications than individuals with only one or the other condition. However, the most appropriate treatment approaches for individuals experiencing these combined conditions is a controversial topic amongst healthcare professionals.

3. The Potential Benefits and Harms of Dieting to Lose Weight

There are often theoretical and clinical debates amongst healthcare professionals regarding the most appropriate treatment approaches for individuals with obesity and comorbid eating disorders. The most controversial aspect of this debate relates to potential benefits and harms of dieting to lose weight. Healthcare professionals specializing in obesity often recommend dieting to their patients or clients with overweight or obesity, encouraging them to reduce and then maintain a healthy weight. Conversely, healthcare professionals specializing in eating disorders, especially those working mainly with individuals with anorexia nervosa and bulimia nervosa, are often concerned about the use of diets driven by idealization of thinness [25].

The negative perception that some healthcare professionals may sustain regarding dieting is understandable when one considers that strict dieting is often a core symptom of eating disorders such as anorexia nervosa and bulimia nervosa [11]. For example, the trans-diagnostic cognitive-behavioral model of eating disorders, which is used to guide the "gold standard" treatment for binge eating disorder and bulimia nervosa, namely cognitive behavior therapy—enhanced (CBT-E), shows strict dieting as a central behavioral component in the maintenance of eating disorders [11]. Furthermore, concerns regarding dieting are derived from studies that found relationships between dieting and eating disorder symptoms [26–28]. A classic study in this field, namely the Keys' study, found that young healthy men submitted to prolonged periods of semi-starvation experienced symptoms that were similar to those experienced by people with eating disorders, such as preoccupation with food, binge eating, distress and depression [26]. Additionally, literature reviews of studies including clinical and non-clinical samples suggest that cognitive restraint can make dieters vulnerable to disinhibition and consequent binge eating [27], and that dietary restriction can lead to binge eating, emotional alterations, distractibility and preoccupation with food and eating [28]. Notwithstanding that dieting can be associated with these negative consequences, one literature review concluded that some dietary restriction (i.e., the consumption of certain foods in moderation) may be necessary for individuals with obesity or for those at risk of developing weight-related health problems in order to reduce the health consequences of overweight [28].

Although there are some important concerns regarding the safety of dieting, the relationship between dieting and binge eating is not clear-cut and needs to be further examined. For instance, a study with 166 patients with bulimia nervosa at admission for residential treatment found that a significant proportion of them (43%) were *not* currently dieting to lose weight or to avoid weight gain [29]. Additionally, this study also found that those who were dieting to lose weight reported lower binge eating frequency in comparison to non-dieters [29]. In line with this, a literature review of studies on different levels of dietary restraint, and retrospective and prospective studies examining the effects of dieting on eating behavior, did not find consistent evidence supporting the view that medically supervised dietary restriction exacerbates binge eating disorder [30]. It is possible that other factors besides dieting need to be present in order to increase the risk for eating disorder behaviors. For example, a prospective study with a population-based sample of 1827 adolescents and young adults and a 10-year follow-up period, found that symptoms of depression and low self-esteem in dieters were important elements increasing the risk of binge eating [31]. Moreover, a narrative review concluded that while dieting may contribute to eating disorders, other factors mediate this relationship, namely a family history of eating disorders, mood disorders, problems with substance/alcohol use, personality characteristics, problematic family interactions, and biological vulnerability [32]. Finally, a systematic review showed that clinically supervised severe energy restriction to treat obesity—as in that used with total meal replacement diets such as very low energy diets—mostly did not cause binge eating, and even reduced binge eating in those with pre-treatment binge eating behaviors [33]. These findings are in line with a previous literature review which showed that moderate dietary energy restriction in combination with behavioral weight loss therapy does not seem to induce binge eating in overweight adults without pre-treatment binge eating, and can reduce binge eating in those with pre-treatment binge eating behaviors [34]. Taken together, these findings suggest that the relationship between dieting and binge eating may be significantly influenced by several other variables, e.g., degree of psychological support and medical need for weight loss. Notably, the young men in the Key's experiment (see above) were not in medical need of weight loss. Whilst they considered themselves extremely well supervised from a medical perspective [26], psychological effects were less well understood and they would go to great lengths to avoid the shame of dismissal from the trial and the stigma of being a "cheater" when they had broken the diet [29]. The complexity of the relationship between dieting to lose weight and eating disorder behaviors and weight stigma potentially contributes to disagreements amongst healthcare professionals regarding the most appropriate treatment approaches for individuals with obesity and comorbid eating disorders.

4. Treatments for Obesity with Comorbid Eating Disorders

Previous studies have examined the effects of treating individuals with obesity and comorbid eating disorders with weight loss or eating disorder treatments, alone or in combination [35–38]. One study investigated the effects of cognitive behavior therapy (CBT), behavioral weight loss therapy, or a sequential approach of CBT followed by behavioral weight loss therapy on body weight and binge eating [38]. This study showed that at 12-month follow-up, 51% of participants submitted to CBT, 36% of those submitted to behavioral weight loss therapy, and 40% of those submitted to CBT followed by behavioral weight loss therapy, had achieved binge eating remission [39]. It also showed that at 12 months, CBT induced significantly greater reduction in binge eating than behavioral weight loss therapy, and that behavioral weight loss therapy induced significantly greater weight loss than CBT [38]. Moreover, participants who exhibited remission from binge eating had significantly greater reductions in BMI compared to participants who did not [38]. Nonetheless, the reduction in BMI induced by behavioral weight loss therapy was relatively small (i.e., -2.1 kg/m^2) [38], and the combination of CBT with other obesity treatments could potentially induce greater weight loss. In line with this, another study found significant reductions in body weight (average loss of 12 kg) and binge eating at 6 months from treatment commencement in individuals submitted to a diet allowing 7100 kJ (1700 kcal) per day, combined with CBT, sertraline (a serotonin reuptake inhibitor) and topiramate (an anti-convulsant sometimes used in the treatment of obesity) [35].This same study did not show any significant change in body weight or binge eating in the comparison groups of individuals submitted to a 7100 kJ (1700 kcal) per day diet, CBT and sertraline (without topiramate), or in those submitted to nutritional counselling and CBT [35]. We could thus conclude from this study that complex treatments including dietary intervention, CBT and a combination of pharmaceuticals can induce substantial reductions in body weight and binge eating. Another study assessed the addition of CBT to 16 sessions of group behavioral weight loss therapy in 116 women with overweight/obesity and comorbid binge eating disorder [36]. In this study, the serotonin reuptake inhibitor fluoxetine (or placebo) was also investigated. Thus, participants were randomized to one of the following four groups, with all groups receiving the same behavioral weight loss therapy: (1) CBT + fluoxetine; (2) CBT + placebo; (3) fluoxetine; or (4) placebo [36]. This study showed that participants in the groups that included CBT had significantly greater reductions in binge eating frequency, and greater abstinence from binge eating, than participants in groups that did not include CBT [36]. Additionally, this study found that participants reporting abstinence from binge eating at the end of treatment ($n = 54$) exhibited greater weight loss in comparison to those who did not report abstinence from binge eating ($n = 62$) (i.e., a weight loss of 6.2 kg versus weight gain of 0.7 kg, respectively) [36]. From these findings it thus seems that CBT is particularly important for binge eating reduction and abstinence, and that binge eating abstinence may be necessary for successful weight loss. While CBT appears to be an essential element of treatment, another study suggests that there is some flexibility in the types of dietary interventions that can be combined with CBT in order to reduce body weight and binge eating. Indeed, in another study involving 50 individuals with obesity and comorbid binge eating disorder, participants were randomized to CBT + a diet of low energy density, or CBT + general nutrition counselling [37]. This study found that 13 out of the 43 participants that completed their assigned intervention lost at least 5% of their initial body weight, and reduced binge eating episodes by 55–75%, with no significant differences in outcomes between participants in the two groups [37]. Overall, the above-mentioned studies showed that certain combinations of obesity treatments with CBT for eating disorders can induce significant reduction of binge eating and weight loss in individuals with obesity and comorbid eating disorders.

While some scientific studies have examined the effects of combining obesity treatments with eating disorder treatments [35–37], most of the current treatment programs for obesity or eating disorders still target only one or the other condition. For example, CBT-E is suitable for use in binge eating disorder, however, it does not encourage weight loss for those with overweight or obesity and comorbid binge eating disorder [11], nor does it result in substantial weight loss [38,39]. In the same way, a recent systematic review and meta-analysis on the effectiveness of treatments for binge eating disorder found that therapist-led CBT induced greater reduction of binge eating frequency in comparison to behavioral weight loss therapy; however, greater body weight reduction was achieved with behavioral weight loss therapy in comparison to CBT [39]. According to this systematic review, at the end of treatment, participants submitted to CBT reduced BMI by an average of 0.41 kg/m^2 (which is not clinically significant), whereas participants submitted to behavioral weight loss therapy reduced BMI by an average of 2.2 kg/m^2 (which is clinically significant) [39]. Furthermore, another review of treatments for binge eating disorder concluded that weight loss treatments should be offered only to individuals with obesity that do not engage in binge eating [40]. This contrasts with a study which found that behavioral weight loss therapy, although not designed to thoroughly address eating disorder psychopathology, concomitantly reduced binge eating and body weight in individuals with obesity and comorbid binge eating disorder [38]. Additionally, a systematic review and meta-analyses found a lack of treatments aiming to simultaneously assist weight management and reduce eating disorder behaviors in individuals with obesity and comorbid bulimia nervosa [41]. According to that systematic review and meta-analysis, it is necessary to develop and test integrated treatments for obesity with bulimia nervosa due to the rise in prevalence of individuals with obesity and comorbid bulimia nervosa [41]. In line with this, we have been involved with the development of a new integrated treatment, named HAPIFED (a **H**ealthy **AP**proach to we**I**ght management and **F**ood in **E**ating **D**isorders), which aims to simultaneously aid weight management (i.e., via a moderate to slow rate of weight loss) and to reduce eating disorder behaviors in individuals with obesity and comorbid eating disorders [42]. The feasibility and acceptability of this intervention was shown in a pilot study that used 20 sessions of group multidisciplinary therapy [42], and this treatment is currently under examination in a randomized controlled trial comparing 30 sessions of group therapy of either HAPIFED or CBT-E [43]. Moreover, the effectiveness of HAPIFED in "real world" clinics is also currently been investigated [44].

Integrated treatments, such as HAPIFED, may be particularly attractive to individuals with obesity and comorbid eating disorders. For instance, a systematic review found that only an estimated 23% of individuals with eating disorders sought treatment for their eating disorder, whereas 30–73% of individuals with eating disorders sought treatments for their overweight or obesity (13). This tendency for individuals with eating disorders to seek weight loss treatments instead of eating disorder treatments could potentially be used to facilitate treatment of a significant proportion of individuals with eating disorders that are overweight or have obesity. In addition to potentially improving treatment adherence, integrated treatments for obesity with comorbid eating disorders may also promote greater physical and mental health benefits than treatments focused on only one or the other condition. For instance, individuals with clinically significant binge eating are more susceptible to difficulties achieving a healthy body weight after undergoing a weight loss treatment (i.e., bariatric surgery) in comparison to those without clinically significant binge eating [23]. Therefore, it is important to further investigate integrated treatment options aiming to simultaneously reduce body weight and eating disorder behaviors and to discuss these studies with healthcare professionals working with clients with obesity or eating disorders. This is especially important given that healthcare professionals working in the fields of obesity or eating disorders frequently have different professional backgrounds (i.e., psychological versus medical versus nutritional).

5. Conclusions

Individuals with obesity and comorbid eating disorders are at higher risk for several medical and psychosocial complications than individuals with either condition alone. The co-occurrence of obesity with comorbid eating disorders, particularly binge eating disorder, requires attention of healthcare professionals working with clients with either of these conditions. Healthcare professionals specialized in obesity treatment and not addressing eating disorder behaviors of their clients—when these are present—will likely see unsuccessful weight loss interventions in the long-term due to continued binge eating. On the flip side, healthcare professionals specialized in eating disorders and not addressing weight management with their clients with comorbid overweight or obesity may see a reduced interest from their clients, potentially resulting in disengagement from (or lack of engagement at all in) the eating disorder treatment, seeking instead weight loss treatments that do not address their eating disorder behaviors. While these healthcare professionals may sometimes disagree on the potential benefits and harms of recommending weight loss diets to their clients, healthcare professionals working in either of these fields of obesity or eating disorders can acknowledge the common goal of promoting healthy eating behaviors, healthy relationships of their clients with their bodies, and positive personal health goals of weight loss. We contend, it is vital to develop and test innovative medical, psychological, and nutritional treatment options that simultaneously address obesity as well as comorbid eating disorders. Such integrated treatments can potentially induce greater improvements in health—and in more people—than treatments targeting only one or the other condition.

Author Contributions: F.Q.d.L. conceived, reviewed the literature discussed in the paper and wrote his paper P.H. co-conceived and co-wrote the paper and contributed additional literature, S.T. co-conceived and co-wrote the paper and A.S. co-conceived and c0-wrote this paper.

References

1. Wang, Y.C.; McPherson, K.; Marsh, T.; Gortmaker, S.L.; Brown, M. Health and economic burden of the projected obesity trends in the USA and the UK. *Lancet* **2011**, *378*, 815–825. [CrossRef]
2. Zhang, H.; Rodriguez-Monguio, R. Racial disparities in the risk of developing obesity-related diseases: A cross-sectional study. *Ethn. Dis.* **2012**, *22*, 308–316. [PubMed]
3. Dehal, A.; Garrett, T.; Tedders, S.H.; Arroyo, C.; Afriyie-Gyawu, E.; Zhang, J. Body mass index and death rate of colorectal cancer among a national cohort of U.S. Adults. *Nutr. Cancer* **2011**, *63*, 1218–1225. [CrossRef] [PubMed]
4. Vranian, M.; Blaha, M.; Silverman, M.; Michos, E.; Minder, C.; Blumenthal, R.; Nasir, K.; de Carvalho, J.M.; Santos, R. The interaction of fitness, fatness, and cardiometabolic risk. *J. Am. Coll. Cardiol.* **2012**, *59*, E1754. [CrossRef]
5. Ma, Y.; Hébert, J.R.; Manson, J.E.; Balasubramanian, R.; Liu, S.; Lamonte, M.J.; Bird, C.E.; Ockene, J.K.; Qiao, Y.; Olendzki, B.; et al. Determinants of racial/ethnic disparities in incidence of diabetes in postmenopausal women in the U.S.: The Women's Health Initiative 1993–2009. *Diabetes Care* **2012**, *35*, 2226–2234. [CrossRef] [PubMed]
6. Kitahara, C.M.; Flint, A.J.; de Gonzalez, A.B.; Bernstein, L.; Brotzman, M.; MacInnis, R.J.; Moore, S.C.; Robien, K.; Rosenberg, P.S.; Singh, P.N.; et al. Association between class iii obesity (bmi of 40–59 kg/m^2) and mortality: A pooled analysis of 20 prospective studies. *PLoS Med.* **2014**, *11*, e1001673. [CrossRef] [PubMed]
7. Tanamas, S.K.; Ng, W.L.; Backholer, K.; Hodge, A.; Zimmet, P.Z.; Peeters, A. Quantifying the proportion of deaths due to body mass index- and waist circumference-defined obesity: Mortality attributable to obesity. *Obesity* **2016**, *24*, 735–742. [CrossRef] [PubMed]
8. Magallares, A.; Pais-Ribeiro, J.L. Mental health and obesity: A meta-analysis. *Appl. Res. Qual. Life* **2014**, *9*, 295–308. [CrossRef]
9. Tronieri, J.S.; Wurst, C.M.; Pearl, R.L.; Allison, K.C. Sex differences in obesity and mental health. *Curr. Psychiatry Rep.* **2017**, *19*, 29. [CrossRef] [PubMed]
10. Puhl, R.; Brownell, K.D. Bias, discrimination, and obesity. *Obes. Res.* **2001**, *9*, 788–805. [CrossRef] [PubMed]
11. Fairburn, C. *Cognitive Behavior Therapy and Eating Disorders*; Guilford: New York, NY, USA, 2008.
12. American Psychiatric Association. *Diagnostic and Statistical Manual of Mental Disorders*, 5th ed.; American Psychiatric Association: Washington, DC, USA, 2013.
13. Palavras, M.A.; Kaio, G.H.; Mari, J.; Claudino, A.M. A review of latin american studies on binge eating disorder. *Rev. Bras. Psiquiatr.* **2011**, *33*, s81–s94. [CrossRef] [PubMed]
14. Hudson, J.I.; Hiripi, E.; Pope, H.G., Jr.; Kessler, R.C. The prevalence and correlates of eating disorders in the national comorbidity survey replication. *Biol. Psychiatry* **2007**, *61*, 348–358. [CrossRef] [PubMed]
15. Udo, T.; Grilo, C.M. Prevalence and correlates of dsm-5 eating disorders in nationally representative sample of united states adults. *Biol. Psychiatry* **2018**. [CrossRef] [PubMed]
16. Villarejo, C.; Fernandez-Aranda, F.; Jimenez-Murcia, S.; Penas-Lledo, E.; Granero, R.; Penelo, E. Lifetime obesity in patients with eating disorders: Increasing prevalence, clinical and personality correlates. *Eur. Eat. Disord. Rev.* **2012**, *20*, 250–254. [CrossRef] [PubMed]
17. Da Luz, F.Q.; Sainsbury, A.; Mannan, H.; Touyz, S.; Mitchison, D.; Hay, P. Prevalence of obesity and comorbid eating disorder behaviors in south australia from 1995 to 2015. *Int. J. Obes.* **2017**, *41*, 1148–1153. [CrossRef] [PubMed]
18. Fairburn, C.G.; Doll, H.A.; Welch, S.L.; Hay, P.J.; Davies, B.A.; O'Connor, M.E. Risk factors for binge eating disorder: A community-based, case-control study. *Arch. Gen. Psychiatry* **1998**, *55*, 425–432. [CrossRef] [PubMed]
19. Raman, J.; Smith, E.; Hay, P. The clinical obesity maintenance model: An integration of psychological constructs including mood, emotional regulation, disordered overeating, habitual cluster behaviours, health literacy and cognitive function. *J. Obes.* **2013**, *2013*, 240128. [CrossRef] [PubMed]
20. Poli, R.; Maninetti, L.; Bodini, P.; Agrimi, E. Obesity, binge eating, obstruction sleep apnea and psychopathological features. *Clin. Neuropsychiatry* **2012**, *9*, 166–170.
21. Jones-Corneille, L.; Wadden, T.; Sarwer, D.; Faulconbridge, L.; Fabricatore, A.; Stack, R.; Cottrell, F.; Pulcini, M.; Webb, V.; Williams, N. Axis i psychopathology in bariatric surgery candidates with and without binge eating disorder: Results of structured clinical interviews. *Obes. Surg.* **2012**, *22*, 389–397. [CrossRef] [PubMed]

22. Hsu, L.K.G.; Mulliken, B.; McDonagh, B.; Krupa Das, S.; Rand, W.; Fairburn, C.G.; Rolls, B.; McCrory, M.A.; Saltzman, E.; Shikora, S.; et al. Binge eating disorder in extreme obesity. *Int. J. Obes. Relat. Metab. Disord.* **2002**, *26*, 1398–1403. [CrossRef] [PubMed]
23. Niego, S.H.; Kofman, M.D.; Weiss, J.J.; Geliebter, A. Binge eating in the bariatric surgery population: A review of the literature. *Int. J. Eat. Disord.* **2007**, *40*, 349–359. [CrossRef] [PubMed]
24. Striegel, R.H.; Bedrosian, R.; Wang, C. Comparing work productivity in obesity and binge eating. *Int. J. Eat. Disord.* **2012**, *45*, 995–998. [CrossRef] [PubMed]
25. Sainsbury, A.; Hay, P. Call for an urgent rethink of the 'health at every size' concept. *J. Eat. Disord.* **2014**, *2*, 8. [CrossRef] [PubMed]
26. Keys, A.; Brozek, J.; Henschel, A. *The Biology of Human Starvation*; University of Minnesota Press: Minneapolis, MN, USA, 1950; Volume 2.
27. Polivy, J.; Herman, C.P. Dieting and binging. A causal analysis. *Am. Psychol.* **1985**, *40*, 193–201. [CrossRef] [PubMed]
28. Polivy, J. Psychological consequences of food restriction. *J. Am. Diet. Assoc.* **1996**, *96*, 589–592. [CrossRef]
29. Lowe, M.R.; Witt, A.A.; Grossman, S.L. Dieting in bulimia nervosa is associated with increased food restriction and psychopathology but decreased binge eating. *Eat. Behav.* **2013**, *14*, 342–347. [CrossRef] [PubMed]
30. Howard, C.E.; Porzelius, L.K. The role of dieting in binge eating disorder: Etiology and treatment implications. *Clin. Psychol. Rev.* **1999**, *19*, 25–44. [CrossRef]
31. Goldschmidt, A.B.; Wall, M.; Loth, K.A.; Le Grange, D.; Neumark-Sztainer, D. Which dieters are at risk for the onset of binge eating? A prospective study of adolescents and young adults. *J. Adolesc. Health* **2012**, *51*, 86–92. [CrossRef] [PubMed]
32. Hsu, L.K. Can dieting cause an eating disorder? *Psychol. Med.* **1997**, *27*, 509–513. [CrossRef] [PubMed]
33. Da Luz, F.Q.; Hay, P.; Gibson, A.A.; Touyz, S.W.; Swinbourne, J.M.; Roekenes, J.A.; Sainsbury, A. Does severe dietary energy restriction increase binge eating in overweight or obese individuals? A systematic review. *Obes. Rev.* **2015**, *16*, 652–665. [CrossRef] [PubMed]
34. Yanovski, S.Z.; Billington, C.J.; Epstein, L.H.; Goodwin, N.J.; Hill, J.O.; Pi-Sunyer, F.X.; Rolls, B.J.; Stern, J.S.; Wadden, T.A.; Weinsier, R.L.; et al. Dieting and the development of eating disorders in overweight and obese adults. *Arch. Intern. Med.* **2000**, *160*, 2581–2589.
35. Brambilla, F.; Samek, L.; Company, M.; Lovo, F.; Cioni, L.; Mellado, C. Multivariate therapeutic approach to binge-eating disorder: Combined nutritional, psychological and pharmacological treatment. *Int. Clin. Psychopharmacol.* **2009**, *24*, 312–317. [CrossRef] [PubMed]
36. Devlin, M.J.; Goldfein, J.A.; Petkova, E.; Jiang, H.; Raizman, P.S.; Walk, S.; Mayer, L.; Carino, J.; Bellace, D.; Kamenetz, C.; et al. Cognitive behavioral therapy and fluoxetine as adjuncts to group behavioral therapy for binge eating disorder. *Obesity* **2005**, *13*, 1077–1088. [CrossRef] [PubMed]
37. Masheb, R.M.; Grilo, C.M.; Rolls, B.J. A randomized controlled trial for obesity and binge eating disorder: Low-energy-density dietary counseling and cognitive-behavioral therapy. *Behav. Res. Ther.* **2011**, *49*, 821–829. [CrossRef] [PubMed]
38. Grilo, C.M.; Masheb, R.M.; Wilson, G.T.; Gueorguieva, R.; White, M.A. Cognitive-behavioral therapy, behavioral weight loss, and sequential treatment for obese patients with binge-eating disorder: A randomized controlled trial. *J. Consult. Clin. Psychol.* **2011**, *79*, 675–685. [CrossRef] [PubMed]
39. Peat, C.M.; Berkman, N.D.; Lohr, K.N.; Brownley, K.A.; Bann, C.M.; Cullen, K.; Quattlebaum, M.J.; Bulik, C.M. Comparative effectiveness of treatments for binge-eating disorder: Systematic review and network meta-analysis. *Eur. Eat. Disord. Rev.* **2017**, *25*, 317–328. [CrossRef] [PubMed]
40. Dingemans, A.E.; Bruna, M.J.; Van Furth, E.F. Binge eating disorder: A review. *Int. J. Obes.* **2002**, *26*, 299–307. [CrossRef] [PubMed]
41. Palavras, M.A.; Hay, P.; Dos Santos, C.A.; Claudino, A. The efficacy of psychological therapies in reducing weight and binge eating in people with bulimia nervosa and binge eating disorder who are overweight or obese-a critical synthesis and meta-analyses. *Nutrients* **2017**, *9*, 299. [CrossRef] [PubMed]
42. Da Luz, F.Q.; Swinbourne, J.; Sainsbury, A.; Touyz, S.; Palavras, M.; Claudino, A.; Hay, P. Hapifed: A healthy approach to weight management and food in eating disorders: A case series and manual development. *J. Eat. Disord.* **2017**, *5*, 29. [CrossRef] [PubMed]

43. Palavras, M.A.; Hay, P.; Touyz, S.; Sainsbury, A.; da Luz, F.; Swinbourne, J.; Estella, N.M.; Claudino, A. Comparing cognitive behavioural therapy for eating disorders integrated with behavioural weight loss therapy to cognitive behavioural therapy-enhanced alone in overweight or obese people with bulimia nervosa or binge eating disorder: Study protocol for a randomised controlled trial. *Trials* **2015**, *16*, 578. [PubMed]
44. Australian New Zealand Clinical Trials Regisitry. *The Real Happy Trial: A Multi-Centre, Prospective, Open-Label, Non-Comparative Assessment of the Real-World Effectiveness of Hapifed (A Healthy Approach to Weight Management and Food in Eating Disorders) in Reducing Weight and Treating the Symptoms of Binge Eating in Participants with Overweight/Obesity and Binge Eating Disorder, Bulimia Nervosa or Other Specified Feeding and Eating Disorders*; ACTRN12617001020370; ANZCTR: Camperdown, Australia, 2017.

16

Profile of Free Fatty Acids and Fractions of Phospholipids, Cholesterol Esters and Triglycerides in Serum of Obese Youth with and without Metabolic Syndrome

Juliana Bermúdez-Cardona and Claudia Velásquez-Rodríguez *

Research Group in Food and Human Nutrition, Universidad de Antioquia (UdeA), Calle 70 No. 52-21 Medellín 050010238, Colombia; juliana.bermudez@udea.edu.co

* Correspondence: claudia.velasquez@udea.edu.co

Abstract: The study evaluated the profile of circulating fatty acids (FA) in obese youth with and without metabolic syndrome (MetS) to determine its association with nutritional status, lifestyle and metabolic variables. A cross-sectional study was conducted in 96 young people, divided into three groups: obese with MetS (OBMS), obese (OB) and appropriate weight (AW). FA profiles were quantified by gas chromatography; waist circumference (WC), fat folds, lipid profile, high-sensitivity C-reactive protein, glucose, insulin, the homeostasis model assessment (HOMA index), food intake and physical activity (PA) were assessed. The OBMS group had significantly greater total free fatty acids (FFAs), palmitic-16:0 in triglyceride (TG), palmitoleic-16:1*n*-7 in TG and phospholipid (PL); in the OB group, these FAs were higher than in the AW group. Dihomo-gamma-linolenic (DHGL-20:3*n*-6) was higher in the OBMS than the AW in PL and FFAs. Linoleic-18:2*n*-6 in TG and PL had the lowest proportion in the OBMS group. WC, PA, total FFA, linoleic-18:2*n*-6 in TG and DHGL-20:3*n*-6 in FFAs explained 62% of the HOMA value. The OB group presented some higher proportions of FA and biochemical values than the AW group. The OBMS had proportions of some FA in the TG, PL and FFA fractions that correlated with disturbances of MetS.

Keywords: obesity; metabolic syndrome; fatty acids; serum; youth

---

1. Introduction

Obesity is a pandemic that affects 34.3% of the adult population, generating an increase in the prevalence of chronic diseases [1]. Obesity is also present in youth; in 2013, the prevalence of overweight reached 22.6% in girls and 23.9% in boys in industrialized countries [2]. In Latin America, it is estimated that there are between 16.5 and 22.1 million obese adolescents, with a prevalence of overweight of 17% in Colombia, 20% in Brazil, and 35% in Mexico and Chile [3].

Obesity, mainly abdominal, induces metabolic disturbances, such as insulin resistance (IR), glucose intolerance, decreased high-density lipoproteins (HDL-C), elevated triglycerides (TG) and increased blood pressure, which together make up Metabolic Syndrome (MetS) [4].

In states of chronic excess energy, both subcutaneous and visceral adipocytes undergo hypertrophy and saturation of their storage capacity, along with infiltration and activation of macrophages; these events result in an increased release of fatty acids (FAs) and pro-inflammatory substances, such as tumor necrosis factor (TNF)α and interleukin (IL)-6, which generates tissue dysfunction and metabolic damage [5,6].

The release of pro-inflammatory substances and free FAs (FFAs) could be the connection between central obesity and metabolic disturbances. Once released into the portal circulation, FAs invade organs, such as the liver, where the excessive deposit of triglycerides affects lipoprotein synthesis and may induce simple steatosis or fatty liver (FL), which may be complicated by liver inflammation (non-alcoholic steatohepatitis, NASH), alterations that induce the development of non-alcoholic fatty liver disease (NAFLD), which is widely considered to be the liver expression of metabolic syndrome [7,8]. The FFAs also affect the pancreas where they impair insulin production (lipotoxicity); in addition, they simultaneously generate IR in muscle and adipose tissue through the activation of pathways such as protein kinase C (PKCθ) [6,9].

The FA profile can be modulated with food, as some FAs, such as linoleic-18:2*n*-6 and αlinolenic-18:3*n*-3, are not synthesized by humans and reflect dietary intake. Thus, circulating FA levels and cell membrane compositions depend on this intake. In serum, the FA profile specifically reflects the intake of the last two to six weeks, and tissue FAs represent the dietary patterns of months or years [10]. Blood levels of FAs, such as palmitoleic-16:1*n*-7 and DHGL-20:3*n*-6, are less dependent on intake and could reflect endogenous metabolism (lipogenesis) [11,12].

Research in adults has demonstrated the relationship between an altered FA profile, obesity, IR and MetS [13,14]. This profile is characterized by high percentages of saturated fatty acids (SFAs), such as palmitic-16:0 and stearic-18:0, and monounsaturated FAs (MUFAs), such as palmitoleic-16:1*n*-7, and decreased percentages of polyunsaturated fatty acids (PUFAs), including arachidonic acid (ARA-20:4*n*-6) and docosahexaenoic acid (DHA-22:6*n*-3) [14,15].

In obese individuals, a decrease in PUFAs may be due to a deficit in the synthesis and elongation of essential FAs, caused by metabolic disturbances arising from obesity, such as hyperinsulinemia; a high SFA intake and a low PUFA intake, especially omega-3 [16]. However, the FA profile in adults is affected by intervening variables, such as atheromatous disease, advanced metabolic disorders and long-term exposure to unfavorable lifestyle factors (*i.e.*, a sedentary lifestyle, overeating, and alcohol and tobacco consumption) [17].

In youth, describing the circulating FA profile could contribute to a better understanding of the obesity-IR-MetS relationship, given that confounding factors are less involved in metabolic analyses at early ages. However, the results in youth are also conflicting, possibly because fractions from which circulating FAs are recovered are different and not comparable among studies. Some obtain FA from cholesterol esters (CE) and others from phospholipids (PL), fractions in which FAs are mainly recovered from HDL-C and low-density lipoprotein (LDL-C), respectively, which are influenced by consumption [18]. Other studies recover FAs from TG, which is the fraction of highest proportion in circulation and mainly reflects endogenous synthesis of FAs produced from energetic nutrients (carbohydrates and fats) that travel in very-low-density lipoproteins (VLDL) [19]. Finally, others report FFAs released from adipose tissue and carried by albumin, which could be an indirect marker of the FA composition of adipose tissue in states of obesity if recovered after a 10- to 12-h fast [18,20]. Given the differences between fractions and modulations of the FA profile by diet, comparisons of results and the establishment of a consensus on FA profiles are complex. Therefore, the objective of this study is to evaluate the profile of circulating FAs in obese youth with and without MetS between 10 and 18 years old and to determine its association with nutritional status, lifestyle and components of MetS.

2. Materials and Methods

Study design: A cross-sectional study was developed that included 96 youth, boys and girls, 10 to 18 years old, selected from a previous population study [21].

The sample size necessary to form three groups was defined with the software Primer®, considering an alpha error of 0.05, a power of 85% and an expected minimum difference between the case and control groups in the concentrations of different FAs according to reports from other studies: Palmitic-16:0 in CE [22] and FFAs [23]; Palmitoleic-16:1*n*-7 in PL, CE and TG [22,24]; Stearic-18:0 in PL [22] and FFAs [23]; and DHGL-20:3*n*-6 in PL [24,25] and CE [22], which indicated a number of 32 youth per group.

The groups were formed as follows: (1) obese with MetS (OBMS): body mass index (BMI) >98 percentile [26] and diagnosis of MetS; (2) obese (OB): BMI >98 percentile and without MetS; and (3) appropriate weight (AW): BMI between the 15–85 percentile and none of the components of MetS. Groups were matched one to one by age, gender, pubertal maturation and socioeconomic stratum.

MetS was diagnosed when the affected youth had three or more of the following criteria: TG ⩾110 mg/dL, HDL-C ⩽40 mg/dL, fasting blood glucose ⩾100 mg/dL, blood pressure ⩾90 percentile and waist circumference (WC) ⩾90 percentile [27].

Youth who consumed drugs for metabolic disturbances of MetS or nutritional supplements, who had diabetes mellitus (DM) II, who were elite athletes or who were pregnant or lactating were excluded from the study.

Anthropometric evaluation: weight and height were measured; BMI was calculated (kg/m^2) and was classified according to the 2007 World Health Organization (WHO) standard [26]; fat fold measurements were taken at the triceps and subscapular areas, % of body fat was calculated and classified according to Lohman [28]; and WC was taken and classified according to Fernández [29]. Measurements were performed with equipment and techniques for international use [28].

Food consumption: The 24-h recall was distributed on different weekdays. A second recall was consequently distributed among a random subsample constituted by 20% of the study population (19 adolescents) to calculate intra-individual variation [30,31]. The Evaluation Program of Dietary Intake (EVINDI-v4) was used [32]. The nutrient report was processed using the PC version of the Software for Intake Distribution Estimation (SIDE) program, Iowa State University, version 1.0, June 2004.

Physical activity (PA): The 3-day Physical Activity Recall (3DPAR) method was applied [33]. Metabolic equivalent (METs) values of each activity were obtained from the Compendium of Physical Activities of the American College of Sports Medicine [34]. The PA of 3–6 METs was classified as moderate to vigorous intensity (MVPA), and vigorous PA (VPA) was classified as >6 METs [35].

Time dedicated to watching television and playing video games: The reported times were converted into hours/day and were classified into two categories: less than three hours and three or more hours per day [36].

Clinical and biochemical tests: Pubertal maturation was evaluated and classified by self-report according to Tanner's methodology [37,38].

Blood pressure was taken with a mercury sphygmomanometer (Riester®) and was classified according to Fourth Task Force methodology [39].

An antecubital venous blood sample was taken following a 10- to 12-h fast, and serum was obtained and stored at −80 °C. Total cholesterol (TC), HDL-C, LDL-C and TG were determined by spectrophotometry in an RA-50 photocolorimeter (Bayer, series 71663, Dublin, Ireland) using specific enzymatic colorimetric kits (BioSystems Reagents and Instruments, Barcelona, Spain). Blood glucose and insulin were determined by micro-particle enzyme immunoassay (MEIA) [40]. IR was estimated by the mathematical model of the HOMA (Homeostasis Model Assessment) index using the HOMA Calculator Version 2.2.2 software, copyrighted by the Diabetes Trials Unit of the University of Oxford. IR was defined as a HOMA ⩾3.1, based on three criteria: 3.1 was the HOMA in the 95 percentile in the population under study [21], 3.1 was the cutoff point established by others authors [41,42]. hsCRP was determined by immunoturbidimetry and was classified as low cardiovascular risk <1 mg/L, average risk 1-3 mg/L and high risk >3 mg/L [43].

Profile of circulating FFAs: Lipid extraction from serum was performed according to the Folch method [44]. For separation of CE, TG and PL fractions, the methodology by solid-phase extraction (SPE) of Agren J [45] and Kaluzny M [46] was used. To the dry extract of each fraction, hexane and boron trifluoride (BF_3) in 20% methanol were added, and the mixture was heated between 80 °C and 90 °C for one hour. [47]. Chromatographic analysis was performed in an Agilent 6890N gas chromatograph with a flame ionization detector (FID), TR-CN100 column, 60 m × 0.25 mm × 0.2 µm ID, oven temperature program beginning at 90 °C × 7 min, increased at a rate of 5 °C/min to 240 °C for

15 min, detector temperature of 300 °C, and He carrier gas at a flow of 1.1 mL/min. FA identification was performed by comparisons of retention times with the standard FAME Mix of 37 components (Supelco, Bellefonte, PA). The results are presented as relative amounts of each FA.

Total concentrations of SFA, MUFA and PUFA were calculated from the sum of each FA from 14 to 22 carbons of each family, in each fraction. The product/precursor ratios were calculated as an indirect indicator of the activity of the desaturase enzymes. These ratios were as follows: stearoyl CoA desaturase = Palmitoleic-16:1*n*-7/Palmitic-16:0 and Oleic-18:1*n*-9/Stearic-18:0, delta-5 desaturase = ARA-20:4*n*-6/DHGL-20:3*n*-6 and delta-6 desaturase = DHGL-20:3*n*-6/Linoleic-18:2*n*-6, as previously reported [10,13,48].

Ethical management: The investigation was classified as having a minimum risk according to the Colombian Ministry of Health, Resolution 008439, Article 11 of October 1993. The study was approved by the University of Antioquia Bioethics Committee. Informed consent was signed by the youth and their parents and included the Helsinki declaration.

Statistical analysis: Normality was established with the Shapiro-Wilk test. The difference among groups was performed by analysis of variance (ANOVA) or Kruskall-Wallis. For comparisons between two groups, Scheffe or Mann-Whitney U tests were performed. Qualitative variables were expressed with frequencies; quantitative variables, with means and standard deviations or medians and interquartile ranges. For associations of qualitative variables Chi^2 and Odds Ratium were used, while Pearson *R* or Spearman *Rho* were used for quantitative variables. A stepwise multiple linear regression model was applied to explain the HOMA (dependent variable in logarithmic units) with WC, average METs, linoleic-18:2*n*-6 in TG, DHGL-20:3*n*-6 in FFAs and total FFAs as independent variables; the model was adjusted by food intake variables: daily intake of calories, simple carbohydrates, saturated fat, monounsaturated fat and polyunsaturated fat. R^2 and ANOVA determined the fit of the model, and fulfillment of assumptions (Durbin Watson, normality of residuals, inflation factor of the variance and independence) was checked. Finally, the β values of the crude and the adjusted model were transformed with antilogarithm to express in units of the dependent variable: HOMA, in Table 5. A $p < 0.05$ was considered significant. Statistical analysis was performed using the program Statistical Package for the Social Sciences (SPSS®) V 21.0.

3. Results

Matched variables between groups did not show significant differences (Table 1).

Table 1. Matched characteristics of the study groups.

		OBMS $n = 32$	OB $n = 32$	AW $n = 32$	p *,†
Age (Me, IQR)		13.9 (4.8)	14.2 (4.1)	14.0 (4.2)	0.93 *
Gender (%)	Boys	56.3	56.3	56.3	1.00 †
	Girls	43.8	43.8	43.8	
Pubertal Maturation (%)	Prepubescent	12.5	12.5	12.5	0.99 †
	Pubescent	25.0	21.9	25.0	
	Post-pubescent	62.5	65.6	62.5	
Socioeconomic Stratum (%)	Low	53.1	53.1	50.0	0.84 †
	Medium	37.5	31.3	38.5	
	High	9.4	15.6	11.5	

OBMS: obesity with metabolic syndrome; OB: obesity; AW: Appropriate weight; Me: medians; IQR: interquartile ranges; * Kruskal Wallis; † Pearson Chi squared.

Both obese groups showed similar behaviors for fat percentage and inflammation. The risk of mild chronic inflammation (high-sensitivity C-reactive protein (hsCRP > 1 mg/dL)) in obese youth was 2.6 times greater than in the appropriate weight (AW) group (odds ratio 2.6; confidence interval 1.27–5.54; $p = 0.001$), only this risk was significant; hsCRP correlated with fat percentage ($r = 0.51$

$p = 0.001$). The obese with MetS (OBMS) group had higher BMI, WC, blood glucose, insulin, HOMA and TG and lower HDL-C compared to the other two groups ($p = 0.001$). A total of 97.3% of the OBMS group simultaneously had high TG and low HDL-C, according to the criteria used in the diagnosis of MetS in this study. Of the OBMS, 53.1% simultaneously had high WC and HOMA; both variables were correlated ($Rho = 0.71$; $p < 0.001$) (Table 2).

Table 2. Anthropometric, biochemical, food intake and physical activity variables of the study groups [1].

	OBMS $n = 32$	OB $n = 32$	AW $n = 32$	p *,†
		Anthropometric		
BMI kg/m^2	31.1 ± 5.0 [a, 2]	27.1 ± 2.9 [b]	20.2 ± 2.3 [c]	<0.001 *
Waist circumference cm	91.2 ± 10.9 [a]	80.5 ± 5.6 [b]	67.6 ± 5.4 [c]	<0.001 *
Subscapular fold mm	29.9 ± 10.9 [a]	25.5 ± 8.1 [a]	11.5 ± 3.5 [b]	<0.001 *
Triceps fold mm	25.2 ± 6.7 [a]	23.6 ± 6.2 [a]	12.9 ± 4.1 [b]	<0.001 *
% fat	38.1 (18.7) [a]	34.7 (15.8) [a]	22.2 (14.2) [b]	<0.001 †
		Biochemical		
Blood glucose mg/dL	90.3 ± 8.2 [a]	83.7 ± 7.5 [b]	83.3 ± 6.9 [b]	<0.001 *
Insulin mU/L	25.7 (12.4) [a]	11.5 (7.8) [b]	7.1(4.1) [c]	<0.001 †
HOMA	3.2 (1.7) [a]	1.5 (1.0) [b]	0.9(0.5) [c]	<0.001 †
Cholesterol (mg/dL)	192.6 ± 50.3 [a]	172.3 ± 34.5	162.1 ± 27.9 [b]	<0.001 *
Triglycerides (mg/dL)	162 (94) [a]	92 (37) [b]	71 (32) [c]	<0.001 †
HDL-C (mg/dL)	38 (6) [a]	45 (15) [b]	54 (15) [c]	<0.001 †
LDL-C (mg/dL)	99 (61) [a]	88 (37) [a]	79 (31) [b]	<0.001 †
hsCRP (mg/dL)	1.7 (2.9) [a]	0.9 (2.5) [a]	0.4 (0.7) [b]	<0.001 †
		Nutrient consumption/day		
Kilocalories	2238 (436) [a]	2007 (264) [a]	2442 (229) [b]	<0.001 †
Total fat (g)	79.5 (14.6) [a]	70.3 (12.5) [b]	96.9 (44.0) [c]	<0.001 †
Saturated fat (g)	31.3 (9.2)	28.5 (8.3) [a]	36.4 (20.1) [b]	0.015 †
Monounsaturated fat (g)	26.7 (5.1) [a]	25.5 (3.5) [a]	30.0 (1.7) [b]	<0.001 †
Polyunsaturated fat (g)	16.3 (1.6) [a]	15.4 (1.5) [b]	15.7 (1.8) [c]	0.004 †
Total carbohydrates (g)	294 (50) [a]	276 (57) [a]	329 (36) [b]	<0.001 †
Complex carbohydrates (g)	232 (58) [a]	222 (51) [a]	263 (28) [b]	<0.001 †
Fiber (g)	14 ± 2 [a]	14 ± 3 [a]	16 ± 1 [b]	0.001 *
		Physical activity		
METs/day	61.5 (15.4)	61.1 (10.0)	62.8 (14.7)	0.88 †
MVPA Blocks	1.3 (3.60)	1.3 (2.3)	1.0 (2.5)	0.317 †
VPA Blocks	0.1 (1.0)	0.3 (1.0)	0.0 (1.3)	0.991 †
Hours of TV/day	3.6 ± 1.7	3.8 ± 2.7	3.3 ± 3.1	0.57 *

OBMS: obesity with metabolic syndrome; OB: obesity; AW: Appropriate weight; BMI: Body Mass Index; HOMA: Homeostasis Model Assessment; HDL-C: high-density lipoprotein; LDL-C: low-density lipoprotein; hsCRP: high-sensitivity C-reactive protein; MET: Metabolic equivalent; MVPA: moderate to vigorous physical activity; VPA: vigorous physical activity; [1] Averages ± standard deviations and medians (interquartile ranges); [2] Different letters between lines show significant differences between groups; * ANOVA with Scheffé or † Kruskal-Wallis with Mann–Whitney U post-test.

In the TG fraction, the OBMS group has a significantly higher proportion of SFAs compared to the other groups ($p = 0.001$); additionally, the OB group had a higher proportion of SFAs compared to the AW ($p = 0.028$). Total MUFAs was significantly greater in the OBMS group compared to the AW group ($p = 0.003$). The proportion of palmitoleic-16:1n-9 for OBMS and OB was higher than AW ($p = 0.009$). Of the total PUFAs represented in this case by linoleic-18:2n-6, the OBMS group had the lowest proportion among the three groups ($p = 0.001$), followed by the OB group, with the highest being AW ($p = 0.042$) (Table 3). In this fraction, palmitic-16:0 correlated directly with the HOMA ($Rho = 0.55$ $p = 0.001$) and serum TG ($Rho = 0.66$ $p = 0.001$) and inversely with HDL-C ($Rho = -0.52$ $p = 0.001$). Linoleic-18:2n-6 was correlated inversely with the HOMA ($Rho = -0.56$ $p = 0.001$) and serum TG ($Rho = -0.70$ $p = 0.001$) and directly with HDL-C ($Rho = 0.49$ $p = 0.001$) (Table S1).

Table 3. Major fatty acids in lipid fractions of youth according to the study groups [1].

FA (% Total FA)	OBMS $n = 32$	OB $n = 32$	AW $n = 32$	p *,†
Triglycerides				
SFA sum	38.3 (7.1) [a, 2]	34.6 (8.9) [b]	30.8 (7.6) [c]	<0.001 †
Palmitic-16:0	29.7 ± 4.0 [a]	26.4 ± 3.7 [b]	23.6 ± 3.3 [c]	<0.001 *
Stearic-18:0	6.2 (3.8)	7.4 (4.1)	7.2 (3.8)	0.42 †
MUFA sum	36.1 ± 5.2 [a]	33.5 ± 5.0	31.7 ± 5.0 [b]	0.003 *
Palmitoleic-16:1*n*-7 [3]	4.5 (2.0) [a]	4.1 (1.4) [a]	3.0 (1.6) [b]	0.009 †
Oleic-18:1*n*-9	32.1 ± 4.3	30.7 ± 3.9	30.1 ± 4.3	0.14 *
PUFA sum	-	-	-	-
Linoleic-18:2*n*-6	25.6 ± 5.8 [a]	32.2 ± 6.3 [b]	36.4 ± 7.5 [c]	<0.001 †
Phospholipids				
SFA sum	52.8 (11.3) [a]	54.1 (11.3)	56.4 (5.9) [b]	0.017 †
Palmitic-16:0	30.6 ± 3.4 [a]	31.7 ± 3.0	33.2 ± 3.0 [b]	0.006 *
Stearic-18:0	19.8 (4.9)	20.1 (6.0)	21.2 (2.1)	0.34 †
Behenic-22:0	0.5 (0.2) [a]	0.6 (0.2) [b,c]	0.8 (0.2) [b,c]	0.015 †
MUFA sum	17.5 (7.3) [a]	15.1 (8.3) [b,c]	13.8 (3.5) [b,c]	<0.001 †
Palmitoleic-16:1*n*-7 [4]	0.9 (0.4) [a]	0.8 (0.2) [b]	0.5 (0.2) [c]	<0.001 †
Oleic-18:1*n*-9	16.7 (7.3) [a]	14.1 (8.1) [b,c]	13.5 (3.4) [b,c]	<0.001 †
PUFA sum	30.0 (4.8)	31.1 (3.8)	29.9 (4.1)	0.74 †
Linoleic-18:2*n*-6	18.0 ± 2.2 [a]	19.2 ± 2.6 [a]	21.0 ± 2.8 [b]	<0.001 *
DHGL-20:3*n*-6	2.8 ± 0.7 [a]	2.5 ± 0.4	2.1 ± 0.5 [b]	<0.001 *
Eicosatrienoic-20:3*n*-3 [5]	8.2 ± 2.2	7.7 ± 2.0	5.6 ± 2.7	0.063 *
Arachidonic-20:4*n*6	5.0 (1.2)	5.3 (1.5)	4.8 (2.3)	0.77 *
Cholesterol Esters				
SFA sum	35.7 (15.5)	35.1 (16.0)	35.7 (13.2)	0.92 †
Palmitic-16:0	33.2 ± 7.7	31.0 ± 7.1	31.2 ± 5.2	0.35 *
Stearic-18:0 [6]	10.4 (12.1)	11.3 (7.0)	12.3 (9.3)	0.96 †
MUFA sum	-	-	-	-
Oleic-18:1*n*-9	28.4 (4.1)	26.3 (8.2)	26.2 (5.7)	0.44 †
PUFA sum	-	-	-	-
Linoleic-18:2*n*-6	35.9 ± 9.5	34.5 ± 10.7	35.2 ± 10.4	0.84 *
Free Fatty Acids				
SFA sum	44.7 (4.1)	46.1 (6.4)	43.2 (6.7)	0.59 †
Myristic-14:0	1.1 (0.2)	1.4 (0.1)	1.1 (0.5)	0.47 *
Palmitic-16:0	30.0 (2.4)	30.0 (3.7)	30.8 (4.5)	0.93 †
Stearic-18:0	14.4 (2.2)	15.4 (2.7)	14.5 (3.4)	0.45 †
MUFA sum	20.9 (4.1)	19.1 (4.6)	19.1 (5.6)	0.22 †
Palmitoleic-16:1*n*-7 [7]	1.7 (0.7)	1.7 (0.5)	1.5 (0.6)	0.46 †
Oleic-18:1*n*-9	19.3 (4.0)	17.9 (3.3)	18.4 (3.4)	0.31 †
PUFA sum	33.5 (3.4)	34.0 (4.1)	34.4 (4.9)	0.68 †
Linoleic-18:2*n*-6	21.7 (3.3)	22.6 (3.3)	24.5 (5.3)	0.14 †
DHGL-20:3*n*-6	3.0 ± 0.6 [a]	2.8 ± 0.6	2.4 ± 2.5 [b]	<0.001 *
Arachidonic-20:4*n*6	6.6 (1.1)	6.5 (3.1)	5.8 (2.0)	0.25 †
DHA-22:6*n*-3	1.9 ± 0.4	1.9 ± 0.5	1.8 ± 0.5	0.51 *
Total FFA (mg/dL)	199.5 (40.0) [a]	100.8 (24.1) [b]	98.8 (29.9) [b]	0.014 †

OBMS: obesity with metabolic syndrome; OB: obesity; AW: Appropriate weight; SFA: saturated fatty acid; MUFA: monounsaturated fatty acid; PUFA: polyunsaturated fatty acid; FFA: free fatty acid; DHGL: Dihomo-gamma-linolenic; DHA: docosahexaenoic acid; * ANOVA; † Kruskal-Wallis test; [1] Data expressed as Averages±standard deviations or medians (interquartile ranges); [2] Different letters between lines show significant differences between groups, according to the Scheffé post-test for parametric variables or the Mann–Whitney U test for nonparametric variables; [3] OBMS $n = 28$, OB $n = 20$, AW $n = 16$; [4] OBMS $n = 28$ OB $n = 25$, AW $n = 8$; [5] OBMS $n = 15$, OB $n = 13$, AW $n = 6$; [6] OBMS $n = 15$, OB $n = 13$, AW $n = 6$; [7] OBMS $n = 27$, OB $n = 19$; AW $n = 8$.

In the PL fraction, total SFAs were present in significantly lower amounts in the OBMS group compared to the AW group. The OBMS group had higher total MUFAs compared to the other two groups (p = 0.001), with no difference between the OB and AW groups (p = 0.05). In particular, palmitoleic-16:1n-7 was higher in OBMS compared to the other two groups (p = 0.001), and time was higher in OB than AW (p = 0.004). With respect to linoleic-18:2n-6, a significantly lower proportion was found in the OBMS and the OB group compared to the AW group (p = 0.001, p = 0.021, respectively). DHGL-20:3n-6 had a significantly higher proportion in the OBMS group compared to the AW group (p = 0.001), with no differences between OB and AW (p = 0.079) (Table 3). In the PL fraction, palmitoleic-16:1n-7 was directly associated with serum TG (Rho = 0.54 p = 0.001) and inversely associated with HDL-C (Rho = −0.43 p = 0.001). DHGL-20:3n-6 correlated directly with the HOMA (Rho = 0.36 p = 0.000) and serum TG (Rho = 0.33 p = 0.001), while linoleic-18:2n-6 correlated inversely with the HOMA (Rho = −0.31 p = 0.002) and serum TG (Rho = −0.29 p = 0.004) and directly with HDL-C (Rho = 0.30 p = 0.003) (Table S1).

In the FFA fraction, total circulating FFAs were significantly greater in the OBMS group, with double the concentration compared to the other groups (p = 0.014). The OB group had the same concentration of total FFAs as the AW group (Table 3). Among PUFAs, DHGL-20:3n-6 was significantly higher in the OBMS group than in the AW group (p = 0.001); with no differences between OB and AW. The DHGL-20:3n-6/linoleic-18:2n-6 ratio was significantly greater in the OBMS and OB groups compared to the AW group (p = 0.001) (Table 4). DHGL-20:3n-6 correlated directly with the HOMA (Rho = 0.36 p = 0.001) and TG (Rho = 0.33 p = 0.001) (Table S1).

Table 4. Ratios of fatty acids in lipid fractions of youth according to the study groups [1].

Ratio of Fatty Acids	OBSM n = 32	OB n = 32	AW n = 32	p *,†
Triglycerides				
16:1/16:0 [3]	0.1 (0.1) [a, 2]	0.1 (0.2)	0.1 (0.1) [b]	0.005 †
18:1/18:0	5.1 ± 1.9	4.4 ± 1.9	4.4 ± 1.8	0.30 †
Phospholipids				
16:1n-7/16:0 [4]	0.03 (0.01) [a]	0.02 (0.01) [b]	0.01 (0.01) [c]	<0.001 †
18:1n-9/18:0	0.8 (0.7) [a]	0.7 (0.7)	0.6 (0.2) [b]	<0.001 †
20:3n-6/18:2n-6	0.2 (0.1) [a]	0.1 (0.0) [b]	0.1 (0.0) [c]	<0.001 †
20:4n6/20:3n6	1.9 (0.7)	2.0 (1.2)	2.3 (1.4)	0,059 †
Cholesterol Esters				
18:1n-9/18:0 [5]	2.3 (2.6)	2.4 (1.7)	2.1 (1.6)	0.94 *
Free Fatty Acids				
16:1/16:0 [6]	0.5 (0.0)	0.6 (0.0)	0.5 (0.0)	0.57 †
18:1n-9/18:0	1.3 (0.4)	1.2 (0.4)	1.3 (0.4)	0.47 †
20:3n-6/18:2n-6	0.1 ± 0.0 [a]	0.1 ± 0.0 [a]	0.1 ± 0.0 [b]	<0.001 *
20:4n6/20:3n6	2.2 (0.8)	2.3 (0.8)	2.5 (1.5)	0.22 †

OBMS: obesity with metabolic syndrome; OB: obesity; AW: Appropriate weight; * ANOVA; † Kruskal-Wallis test; [1] Data expressed as Averages±standard deviations, medians (interquartile ranges); [2] Different letters between lines show significant differences between groups, according to the Scheffé post-test for parametric variables or the Mann–Whitney U test for nonparametric variables; [3] OBMS n = 28, OB n = 20, AW n = 16; [4] OBMS n = 28, OB n = 25, AW n = 18; [5] OBMS n = 15, OB n = 13, AW n = 6; [6] OBMS n = 27, OB n = 19, AW n = 8.

A descriptive multivariate analysis of the HOMA revealed that WC increased the average HOMA by 1.025, total FFAs increased average HOMA by 1.004, and each unit of DHGL-20:3n-6 in FFAs increased the average HOMA by 1.258, while physical activity (METs) and linoleic-18:2n-6 in TG decreased average HOMA by −1.018 and −1.016, respectively. The independent variables explained 62% of the behavior of the HOMA. All relationships observed were significant and remained the same after making adjustments for food consumption variables (Table 5).

Table 5. Multiple linear regression model with explanatory variables of the HOMA index.

Variables	β *	β †	IC †	p †	IFV †
Waist circumference	1.025	1.025	0.008; 0.015	0.000	1.543
Average METs/d	−1.018	−1.018	−0.012; −0.003	0.001	1.278
Linoleic-18:2*n*-6 in TG	−1.016	−1.016	−0.013; −0.001	0.024	1.606
DHGL-20:3*n*-6 in FFA	1.276	1.258	0.028; 0.172	0.007	1.767
Total FFA in mg/dL	1.004	1.004	0.000; 0.003	0.028	1.379

HOMA: The Homeostatic model assessment.* Raw model: R^2: 0.637, ANOVA: $p = 0.0001$, Normality: $p = 0.200$, Colinearity: Inflation factor of the variance (IFV) <5, Durbin Watson: 0.930. Values expressed in HOMA units. † Adjusted for total calories, saturated fat, monounsaturated fat, polyunsaturated fat and simple carbohydrates. Values expressed in HOMA units. Adjusted model: R^2: 0.620, ANOVA: 0.0001, Normality: $p = 0.050$, Colinearity: IFV < 5, Durbin Watson: 0.987.

4. Discussion

This study detected proportions of some FA for youth with OBMS in the TG, PL and FFA fractions that correlated with disturbances of MetS.

In OBMS the TG fraction showed significantly higher concentrations of total SFAs and MUFAs, but a lower concentration of PUFAs. This pattern could be due to accelerated hepatic lipogenesis that results in the incorporation of FAs, such as palmitic-16:0, palmitoleic-16:1*n*-7 and oleic-18:1*n*-9 in VLDL, with a simultaneous decrease in the amount of linoleic-18:2*n*-6 [19].

This study, consistent with that detected previously by others, found high proportions of MUFAs in the OBMS and OB groups [23,24,49]. Palmitoleic-16:1n-7 was directly and significantly associated with serum TG. The palmitoleic-16:1*n*-7/palmitic-16:0 and oleic-18:1*n*-9/stearic-18:0 ratios that could indirectly indicate enzyme activity of delta-9 desaturase were higher in the OBMS group, consistent with other studies [10–12,24] where they have been associated with obesity [10], IR and MetS [12]. The increase in the activity levels of desaturase enzymes in obesity could be related to hyperinsulinemia arising from excess states, as insulin is a potent activator and regulator of delta-6 and delta-9 desaturases [50].

This study found low proportions of PUFAs in the OBMS group. The concentrations of linoleic-18:2*n*-6 in both the TG and PL fractions were correlated directly with HDL-C and inversely with serum TG and the HOMA. These inverse relationships could be explained because reduced availability of PUFAs in cell membranes has been associated with lower fluidity and changes in insulin sensitivity [51].

DHGL-20:3*n*-6, a product of desaturation and elongation of linoleic-18:2n-6, appears at significantly higher percentages in the PL and FFA fractions in the OBMS group than in the AW group; consistent with this finding, the DHGL-20:3*n*-6/linoleic-18:*n*-6 ratio was higher in the OBMS group in both fractions, with similar results as those reported by Okada [11]. DHGL-20:3*n*-6 in the PL and FFA fractions correlated positively and significantly with WC, HOMA and TG, which agrees with other studies that conclude that this FA is associated with greater IR, cardiovascular risk [10,22,24,25] and inflammation [22]. In adults, Kurotani et al. also associated this FA and the DHGL-20:3*n*-6/linoleic-18:2*n*-6 ratio with early markers of IR and DM, such as high levels of C peptide [52]. DHGL-20:3*n*-6 is a precursor of thromboxanes and series 1 prostanoids (anti-inflammatory) via cyclooxygenase; its increase in these young people, without a simultaneous increase in ARA-20:4*n*-6, could indicate a compensatory mechanism associated with increased activity of delta-6 desaturase, which would enhance the anti-inflammatory activity helping to maintain the balance between pro- and anti-inflammatory substances [53].

The main finding in the FFA fraction was that the OBMS group had double the circulating total FFAs of other groups. This finding has been reported by other authors [54,55], in addition to its positive correlations with WC, insulin, HOMA [55], CT and serum TG [54]. The increase in total FFAs suggests that in those who present central obesity, adipocytes increase FA release due to saturation of the storage capacity and stress to the endoplasmic reticulum of visceral adipocytes. This effect diminishes the anti-lipolytic signal of insulin, perpetuating the release of FAs from visceral adipose tissue, which, once in circulation, are lipotoxic and are associated with the development of lipid alterations, IR and MetS [6,55,56].

Given the aforementioned associations, it was investigated whether FAs could explain the link between visceral obesity and insulin resistance in these youth using a multiple linear regression model. It was found that 62% of the HOMA was explained by the increases in total FFAs, DHGL-20:3*n*-6 in FFA and WC, in addition to decreases in linoleic-18:2*n*-6 in TG and the average METs/d.

The OB group presented proportions similar to those of the AW group in DHGL-20:4*n*-6 and in the total amount of circulating FFAs, variables – which in the OBMS group – has been associated with metabolic alterations, especially with IR. However, the OB group, compared to the AW group, presented a greater proportion of SFAs and MUFAs, a lower proportion of PUFAs in the TG fraction, higher values of WC, HOMA and TG and lower proportions of HDL-C, which is consistent with increased lipogenesis and confirms that obesity itself is a disorder that leads to future metabolic abnormalities and probably to NAFLD, if weight gain continues; consequently, the OB youth group should not be considered metabolically healthy. In these obese youth, therapeutic measures necessary to avoid or diminish MetS and NAFLD should be considered, especially in stimulating weight reduction with an increase in physical activity and the adoption of healthy eating habits, among others, as well as encouraging a greater consumption of polyunsaturated fat, a source of Omega 3 FA; if necessary, prescribe the consumption of lipid-lowering agents [57].

Like Waresnjo, this study found no association between circulating FAs and the PA level [12]; however, PA was incorporated as an explanatory variable of the HOMA in the multiple regression model, indicating that certain FAs in the profile and environmental factors influence its value.

In this study, the AW group consumed more calories and fats than the obese groups, results that have been reported by other authors [58,59]; these findings may be due to underestimations in evaluations of self-reported consumption, especially in obese individuals, or, when excess weight is evident, obese individuals decrease food intake. Therefore, current consumption cannot be correlated with nutritional status.

We did not detect a consumption pattern that could explain the differences in the FA profiles among the groups. Qualitative analysis of diets allowed us to establish that these youth did not consume significant omega-3 food sources, such as fish or seed oils, which could explain to some degree the low proportions of these FAs in the different fractions. In any event, to eliminate the effect of consumption on the descriptive model of the HOMA index, an adjustment was made for these variables, and the model was not modified.

This study has some limitations: the 24-h recall does not allow establishing individual associations with biochemical variables because of intra-individual variations in food intake; estimation of desaturase enzymes was performed using an indirect method due to technical difficulties involving their measurement *in vivo*. The diagnostic criteria for NAFLD in youth were not evaluated, which prevents establishing some degree of association with the profile of the fatty acids of the different fractions.

Finally, it is expected that there will be further research involving more complex lipids, such as waxes and eicosanoids, and methodological designs that establish causal relationships between the FA profile and metabolic disturbances that make up MetS, especially in children and youths.

5. Conclusions

This study detected proportions of some FA for youth with OBMS in the TG, PL and FFA fractions that correlated with disturbances of MetS, principally IR. High concentrations of total FFAs, high proportions of palmitic-16:0 in TG, high palmitoleic-16:1*n*-7 and low linoleic-18:2*n*-6 in TG and PL, and high DHGL-20:2*n*-6 in PL and FFAs could all be early markers of IR in youths. The findings further suggest that the connection between FA profiles and metabolic disturbances is associated more with high WC than BMI. The OB group presented greater proportions of SFA and MUFA and lower proportions of PUFA, as well as some higher biochemical values than those youth with AW, suggesting the possibility of developing future metabolic abnormalities if weight gain continues.

Table S1 Correlations between fatty acids of triglycerides, phospholipids, free fatty acids fractions, and cardiovascular risk factors in adolescents.

Acknowledgments: Acknowledgments: Resources were received from *Colciencias* Contract 487 (2012) and from the Universidad de Antioquia 2013–2014 through funds from the Committee for Research Development.

Author Contributions: Author Contributions: Claudia Velásquez-Rodríguez designed the study and directed the statistical analysis. Juliana Bermúdez-Cardona conducted the research and performed the statistical analysis. Claudia Velásquez-Rodríguez and Juliana Bermúdez-Cardona wrote the manuscript and are responsible for final content of the article.

Abbreviations

ARA	arachidonic acid
AW	appropriate weight
BMI	Body Mass Index
CE	cholesterol ester
HDL-C	high-density lipoprotein
LDL-C	low-density lipoprotein
DHA	docosahexaenoic acid
DHGL	dihomo-γ-linolenic acid
DM	diabetes mellitus
FA	fatty acid
FFA	free fatty acid
HOMA	Homeostasis Model Assessment
hsCRP	high-sensitivity C-reactive protein
HT	hypertension
IR	insulin resistance
MET	Metabolic equivalent
MetS	metabolic syndrome
MUFA	monounsaturated fatty acid
MVPA	moderate to vigorous physical activity
OBMS	obese with metabolic syndrome
OB	obese
PA	physical activity
PL	phospholipid
PUFA	polyunsaturated fatty acid
SFA	saturated fatty acid
TG	triglyceride
VLDL	very-low-density lipoprotein
VPA	vigorous physical activity
WC	waist circumference

References

1. World Health Organization. *Global Status Report on Noncommunicable Diseases;* Publisher: World Health Organization (WHO), Geneve, Switzerland, 2011.

2. Ng, M.; Fleming, T.; Robinson, M.; Thomson, B.; Graetz, N.; Margono, C.; Mullany, E.C. Global, regional, and national prevalence of overweight and obesity in children and adults during 1980–2013: A systematic analysis for the Global Burden of Disease Study 2013. *Lancet* **2014**, *384*, 766–781. [CrossRef]
3. Rivera, J.Á.; de Cossío, T.G.; Pedraza, L.S.; Aburto, T.C.; Sánchez, T.G.; Martorell, R. Childhood and adolescent overweight and obesity in Latin America: A systematic review. *Lancet. Diabetes Endocrinol.* **2014**, *2*, 321–332. [CrossRef]
4. Eckel, R.H.; Grundy, S.M.; Zimmet, P.Z. The metabolic syndrome. *Lancet* **2005**, *365*, 1415–1428. [CrossRef]
5. Lafontan, M. Adipose tissue and adipocyte dysregulation. *Diabetes Metab.* **2014**, *40*, 16–28. [CrossRef] [PubMed]
6. Shulman, G.I. Ectopic fat in insulin resistance, dyslipidemia, and cardiometabolic disease. *N. Engl. J. Med.* **2014**, *371*, 1131–1141. [CrossRef] [PubMed]
7. Tarantino, G. Spleen: A new role for an old player? *World J. Gastroenterol.* **2011**, *17*, 3776–3784. [CrossRef] [PubMed]
8. Takahashi, Y.; Fukusato, T.; Inui, A.; Fujisawa, T. Nonalcoholic fatty liver disease and nonalcoholic steatohepatitis. *Nihon Rinsho* **2012**, *70*, 1827–1834. [CrossRef] [PubMed]
9. Aguilera, C.M.; Gil-Campos, M.; Cañete, R.; Gil, A. Alterations in plasma and tissue lipids associated with obesity and metabolic syndrome. *Clin. Sci.* **2008**, *114*, 183–193. [CrossRef] [PubMed]
10. Steffen, L.M.; Vessby, B.; Jacobs, D.R.; Steinberger, J.; Moran, A.; Hong, C.-P.; Sinaiko, A.R. Serum phospholipid and cholesteryl ester fatty acids and estimated desaturase activities are related to overweight and cardiovascular risk factors in adolescents. *Int. J. Obes.* **2008**, *32*, 1297–1304. [CrossRef] [PubMed]
11. Okada, T.; Furuhashi, N.; Kuromori, Y.; Miyashita, M.; Iwata, F.; Harada, K. Plasma palmitoleic acid content and obesity in children. *Am. J. Clin. Nutr.* **2005**, *82*, 747–750. [PubMed]
12. Warensjö, E.; Ohrvall, M.; Vessby, B. Fatty acid composition and estimated desaturase activities are associated with obesity and lifestyle variables in men and women. *Nutr. Metab. Cardiovasc. Dis.* **2006**, *16*, 128–136. [CrossRef] [PubMed]
13. Warensjö, E.; Risérus, U.; Vessby, B. Fatty acid composition of serum lipids predicts the development of the metabolic syndrome in men. *Diabetologia* **2005**, *48*, 1999–2005. [CrossRef] [PubMed]
14. Paillard, F.; Catheline, D.; Duff, F.; le Bouriel, M.; Deugnier, Y.; Pouchard, M.; Daubert, J.-C.; Legrand, P. Plasma palmitoleic acid, a product of stearoyl-coA desaturase activity, is an independent marker of triglyceridemia and abdominal adiposity. *Nutr. Metab. Cardiovasc. Dis.* **2008**, *18*, 436–440. [CrossRef] [PubMed]
15. Warensjö, E.; Sundström, J.; Lind, L.; Vessby, B. Factor analysis of fatty acids in serum lipids as a measure of dietary fat quality in relation to the metabolic syndrome in men. *Am. J. Clin. Nutr.* **2006**, *84*, 442–448. [PubMed]
16. Araya, J.; Rodrigo, R.; Pettinelli, P.; Araya, A.V.; Poniachik, J.; Videla, L.A. Decreased liver fatty acid delta-6 and delta-5 desaturase activity in obese patients. *Obesity* **2010**, *18*, 1460–1463. [CrossRef] [PubMed]
17. Nikolaidis, M.G.; Mougios, V. Effects of Exercise on the Fatty-Acid Composition of Blood and Tissue Lipids. *Sport Med.* **2004**, *34*, 1051–1076. [CrossRef]
18. Hodson, L.; Skeaff, C.M.; Fielding, B.A. Fatty acid composition of adipose tissue and blood in humans and its use as a biomarker of dietary intake. *Prog. Lipid Res.* **2008**, *47*, 348–380. [CrossRef] [PubMed]
19. Kotronen, A.; Velagapudi, V.; Yetukuri, L.; Westerbacka, J.; Bergholm, R.; Ekroos, K.; Makkonen, J.; Taskinen, M.-R.; Oresic, M.; Yki-Järvinen, H. Serum saturated fatty acids containing triacylglycerols are better markers of insulin resistance than total serum triacylglycerol concentrations. *Diabetologia* **2009**, *52*, 684–690. [CrossRef] [PubMed]
20. Kishino, T.; Watanabe, K.; Urata, T.; Takano, M.; Uemura, T.; Nishikawa, K.; Mine, Y.; Matsumoto, M.; Ohtsuka, K.; Ohnishi, H.; *et al.* Visceral fat thickness in overweight men correlates with alterations in serum fatty acid composition. *Clin. Chim. Acta* **2008**, *398*, 57–62. [CrossRef] [PubMed]
21. Agudelo, G.; Velásquez, C.; Bedoya, G.; Estrada, A.; Manjarrés, L.M.; Patiño, F. Variations in the prevalence of metabolic syndrome in adolescents according to different criteria used for diagnosis: which definition should be chosen for this age group? *Metab. Syndr. Relat. Disord.* **2014**, *12*, 202–209. [CrossRef] [PubMed]
22. Klein-platat, C.; Drai, J.; Oujaa, M.; Schlienger, J.; Simon, C. Plasma fatty acid composition is associated with the metabolic syndrome and low-grade inflammation in overweight adolescents. *Am. J. Clin. Nutr.* **2005**, *82*, 1178–1184. [PubMed]

23. Gil-Campos, M.; del Carmen Ramírez-Tortosa, M.; Larqué, E.; Linde, J.; Aguilera, C.M.; Cañete, R.; Gil, A. Metabolic syndrome affects fatty acid composition of plasma lipids in obese prepubertal children. *Lipids* **2008**, *43*, 723–732. [CrossRef] [PubMed]
24. Decsi, T.; Csábi, G.; Török, K.; Erhardt, É.; Minda, H.; Burus, I.; Molnár, S.; Molnár, D. Polyunsaturated Fatty Acids in Plasma Lipids of Obese Children With and Without Metabolic Cardiovascular Syndrome. *Lipids* **2000**, *35*, 1179–1184. [CrossRef] [PubMed]
25. Elizondo, L.; Serrano, M.; Ugalde, P.; Cuello, C.; Borbolla, J. Plasma phospholipid fatty acids in obese male and female Mexican children. *Ann. Nutr. Metab.* **2010**, *57*, 234–241. [CrossRef] [PubMed]
26. De Onis, M.; Onyango, A.W.; Borghi, E.; Siyam, A.; Siekmann, J. Development of a WHO growth reference for school-aged children and adolescents. *Bull. World Health Organ.* **2007**, *85*, 660–667. [CrossRef] [PubMed]
27. Ford, E.S.; Li, C.; Cook, S.; Choi, H.K. Serum concentrations of uric acid and the metabolic syndrome among US children and adolescents. *Circulation* **2007**, *115*, 2526–2532. [CrossRef] [PubMed]
28. Lohman, T.; Roche, A.; Martorell, F. *Anthropometric standardization reference manual.*; Human Kinetics Books: Champaign, IL, USA, 1988.
29. Fernandez, J.; Redden, D.; Pietrobelli, A.; Allison, D. Waist circumference percentiles in nationally representative samples of African-American, European-American, and Mexican-American children and adolescents. *J. Pediatr.* **2004**, *145*, 439–444. [CrossRef] [PubMed]
30. Food and Nutrition Board; Institute of Medicine. *Dietary Reference Intakes. Application in Dietary Assessment*; National Academy Press: Washington DC, 2000.
31. Manjarrés, L. Métodos para precisar la recolección de la ingesta dietética en estudios poblacionales. *Perspect. Nutr. Humana* **2007**, *9*, 155–163.
32. Manjarrés, L.; Manjarrés, S. *Programa de Evaluación de Ingesta Dietética EVINDI v4*; Colombia Universidad de Antioquia. Escuela de Nutrición y Dietética: Medellín, Colombia, 2008.
33. Pate, R.R.; Ross, R.; Trost, S.G.; Sirard, J.R.; Dowda, M. Validation of a 3-Day Physical Activity Recall Instrument in Female Youth Recall Instrument in Female Youth. *Pediatr. Exerc. Sci.* **2003**, *15*, 257–265.
34. Dowda, M.; Saunders, R.; Hastings, L.; Gay, J.; Evans, A. Physical activity and sedentary pursuits of children living in residential children's homes. *J. Phys. Act. Health* **2009**, *6*, 195–202. [PubMed]
35. Ainsworth, B.E.; Haskell, W.L.; Whitt, M.C.; Irwin, M.L.; Swartz, A.N.N.M.; Strath, S.J.; Brien, W.L.O.; Bassett, D.R.; Schmitz, K.H.; Emplaincourt, P.O.; *et al.* Compendium of Physical Activities: An MET intensities. *Med. Sci. Sport. Exerc.* **2000**, *32*, S498–S504. [CrossRef]
36. Gomez, L.F.; Parra, D.C.; Lobelo, F.; Samper, B.; Moreno, J.; Jacoby, E.; Lucumi, D.I.; Matsudo, S.; Borda, C. Television viewing and its association with overweight in Colombian children: results from the 2005 National Nutrition Survey: A cross sectional study. *Int. J. Behav. Nutr. Phys. Act.* **2007**, *4*. [CrossRef] [PubMed]
37. Marshall, W.; Tanner, J. Variations in pattern of pubertal changes in girls. *Arch. Dis. Child.* **1969**, *44*, 291–303. [CrossRef] [PubMed]
38. Marshall, W.; Tanner, J. Variations in the pattern of pubertal changes in boys. *Arch. Dis. Child.* **1970**, *45*, 13–23. [CrossRef] [PubMed]
39. National High Blood Pressure Education Program Working Group on High Blood Pressure in Children and Adolescents The fourth report on the diagnosis, evaluation, and treatment of high blood pressure in children and adolescents. *Pediatrics* **2004**, *114*, 555–577.
40. National Cholesterol Education Program Third Report of the National Cholesterol Education Program (NCEP) Expert Panel on Detection, Evaluation, and Treatment of High Blood Cholesterol in Adults (Adult Treatment Panel III) final report. *Circulation* **2002**, *106*, 3143–3421.
41. Lee, J.M.; Okumura, M.J.; Davis, M.M.; Herman, W.H.; Gurney, J.G. Prevalence and determinants of insulin resistance among U.S. adolescents: a population-based study. *Diabetes Care* **2006**, *29*, 2427–2432. [CrossRef] [PubMed]
42. Yin, J.; Li, M.; Xu, L.; Wang, Y.; Cheng, H.; Zhao, X.; Mi, J. Insulin resistance determined by Homeostasis Model Assessment (HOMA) and associations with metabolic syndrome among Chinese children and teenagers. *Diabetol. Metab. Syndr.* **2013**, *5*, 71. [CrossRef] [PubMed]
43. Myers, G.L.; Rifai, N.; Tracy, R.P.; Roberts, W.L.; Alexander, R.W.; Biasucci, L.M.; Catravas, J.D.; Cole, T.G.; Cooper, G.R.; Khan, B.V.; *et al.* CDC/AHA Workshop on Markers of Inflammation and Cardiovascular Disease: Application to Clinical and Public Health Practice: report from the laboratory science discussion group. *Circulation* **2004**, *110*, e545–e549. [CrossRef] [PubMed]

44. Folch, J.; Lees, M.; Stannley, S. A simple method for the isolation and purification of total lipid from animal tissues. *J. Biol. Chem.* **1957**, *226*, 497–509. [PubMed]
45. Agren, J.; Julkunen, A.; Penttila, I. Rapid separation of serum lipids for fatty acid analysis by a single aminopropyl column. *J. Lipid Res.* **1992**, *33*, 1871–1876. [PubMed]
46. Kaluzny, M.; Duncan, L.; Merrit, M.; Epps, D. Rapid separation of lipid classes in high yield and purity using bonded phase columns. *J. Lipid Res.* **1985**, *26*, 135–140. [PubMed]
47. Kang, J.X.; Wang, J. A simplified method for analysis of polyunsaturated fatty acids. *BMC Biochem.* **2005**, *6*, 5. [CrossRef] [PubMed]
48. Ntambi, J. Regulation of stearoyl-CoA desaturases and role in metabolism. *Prog. Lipid Res.* **2004**, *43*, 91–104. [CrossRef]
49. Zong, G.; Zhu, J.; Sun, L.; Ye, X.; Lu, L.; Jin, Q.; Zheng, H.; Yu, Z.; Zhu, Z.; Li, H.; Sun, Q.; Lin, X. Associations of erythrocyte fatty acids in the de novo lipogenesis pathway with risk of metabolic syndrome in a cohort study of middle-aged and older Chinese. *Am. J. Clin. Nutr.* **2013**, *98*, 319–326. [CrossRef] [PubMed]
50. Nakamura, M.T.; Nara, T.Y. Structure, function, and dietary regulation of delta6, delta5, and delta9 desaturases. *Annu. Rev. Nutr.* **2004**, *24*, 345–376. [CrossRef] [PubMed]
51. Tremblay, A.J.; Després, J.-P.; Piché, M.-È.; Nadeau, A.; Bergeron, J.; Alméras, N.; Tremblay, A.; Lemieux, S. Associations between the fatty acid content of triglyceride, visceral adipose tissue accumulation, and components of the insulin resistance syndrome. *Metabolism* **2004**, *53*, 310–317. [CrossRef] [PubMed]
52. Kurotani, K.; Sato, M.; Ejima, Y.; Nanri, A.; Yi, S.; Pham, N.M.; Akter, S.; Poudel-Tandukar, K.; Kimura, Y.; Imaizumi, K.; Mizoue, T. High levels of stearic acid, palmitoleic acid, and dihomo-γ-linolenic acid and low levels of linoleic acid in serum cholesterol ester are associated with high insulin resistance. *Nutr. Res.* **2012**, *32*, 669–675. [CrossRef] [PubMed]
53. Roke, K.; Ralston, J.C.; Abdelmagid, S.; Nielsen, D.E.; Badawi, A.; El-Sohemy, A.; Ma, D.W.L.; Mutch, D.M. Variation in the *FADS1/2* gene cluster alters plasma *n-6* PUFA and is weakly associated with hsCRP levels in healthy young adults. *Prostaglandins Leukot. Essent. Fatty Acids* **2013**, *89*, 257–263. [CrossRef] [PubMed]
54. Sabin, M.A.; de Hora, M.; Holly, J.M.; Hunt, L.P.; Ford, A.L.; Williams, S.R.; Baker, J.S.; Retallick, C.J.; Crowne, E.C.; Shield, J.P.H. Fasting nonesterified fatty acid profiles in childhood and their relationship with adiposity, insulin sensitivity, and lipid levels. *Pediatrics* **2007**, *120*, e1426–e1433. [CrossRef] [PubMed]
55. Reinehr, T.; Kiess, W.; Andler, W. Insulin sensitivity indices of glucose and free fatty acid metabolism in obese children and adolescents in relation to serum lipids. *Metabolism* **2005**, *54*, 397–402. [CrossRef] [PubMed]
56. Deng, J.; Liu, S.; Zou, L.; Xu, C.; Geng, B.; Xu, G. Lipolysis response to endoplasmic reticulum stress in adipose cells. *J. Biol. Chem.* **2012**, *287*, 6240–6249. [CrossRef] [PubMed]
57. Finelli, C.; Tarantino, G. Is there any consensus as to what diet or lifestyle approach is the right one for NAFLD patients? *J. Gastrointest. Liver Dis.* **2012**, *21*, 293–302.
58. Telford, R.D.; Cunningham, R.B.; Telford, R.M.; Riley, M.; Abhayaratna, W.P. Determinants of childhood adiposity: evidence from the Australian LOOK study. *PLoS ONE* **2012**, *7*, e50014. [CrossRef] [PubMed]
59. Martín-Calvo, N.; Ochoa, M.C.; Marti, A.; Martínez-González, M.Á. Asociación entre los macronutrientes de la dieta y la obesidad en la infancia y adolescencia; un estudio de casos y controles. *Nutr. Hosp.* **2013**, *28*, 1515–1522. [PubMed]

Executive Functioning in Obesity, Food Addiction and Binge-Eating Disorder

Marie Blume *, Ricarda Schmidt and Anja Hilbert

Integrated Research and Treatment Center Adiposity Diseases, Departments of Medical Psychology and Medical Sociology and Psychosomatic Medicine and Psychotherapy, University of Leipzig Medical Center, 04103 Leipzig, Germany; ricarda.schmidt@medizin.uni-leipzig.de (R.S.); anja.hilbert@medizin.uni-leipzig.de (A.H.)

* Correspondence: marie.blume@medizin.uni-leipzig.de

Abstract: This study aimed to investigate food addiction (FA) and binge-eating disorder (BED) in their association to executive dysfunctions in adults with obesity. Data on response inhibition, attention, decision-making, and impulsivity were derived from four groups of adults with obesity: obesity and FA (n = 23), obesity and BED (n = 19), obesity and FA plus BED (FA/BED, n = 23), and a body mass index-, age-, and sex-stratified control group of otherwise healthy individuals with obesity (n = 23, OB), using established computerized neuropsychological tasks. Overall, there were few group differences in neuropsychological profiles. Individuals of the FA group did not differ from the OB group regarding executive functioning. Individuals with BED presented with significantly higher variability in their reaction times and a deficient processing of feedback for performance improvement compared to individuals of the OB group. Strikingly, individuals with FA/BED did not present neuropsychological impairments, but higher levels of depression than all other groups. The results indicated the presence of a BED-specific neuropsychological profile in the obesity spectrum. The additional trait FA was not related to altered executive functioning compared to the OB or BED groups. Future research is needed to discriminate FA and BED further using food-specific tasks.

Keywords: executive function; obesity; binge-eating disorder; food addiction; addictive-like eating

---

1. Introduction

Obesity, defined as an excessive accumulation of body fat (body mass index (BMI) ≥ 30.0 kg/m ^{2}) [1], presents one of the most prevalent health conditions in the Western world [2]. During the last decade, research on the causal and maintaining factors of obesity has focused on executive functioning and neural characteristics [3–5]. Executive functions represent a range of higher cognitive capacities enabling goal-directed behavior including inhibition, cognitive flexibility, planning, or decision-making [6,7]. Importantly, impairments in general executive functions in individuals with obesity, for example, reduced inhibition and planning, were linked to unsuccessful weight-loss related behavior, such as poor dietary quality and less success in weight loss therapies [8,9]. In order to provide targeted treatment options for executive dysfunctions, the specification of neuropsychological profiles in the obesity spectrum is warranted [10].

In this context, a recent review showed substantial similarities between executive functions in obesity and substance use disorder, including increased impulsive decision-making and an attentional bias towards disorder-related stimuli in both conditions [11]. In addition to these neuropsychological abnormalities, several neuroimaging studies documented a considerable overlap between obesity and substance use disorder regarding functional alterations in frontal brain regions and meso-corticolimbic circuits, which are involved in reward processing and decision-making [11–13].

Recent research hypothesized that certain foods, especially high-fat and high-sugar foods, elicit addictive-like behavioral responses in vulnerable individuals characterized by high impulsivity and reward sensitivity through the activation of reward-related brain circuits [12,14–16]. This so-called food addiction (FA) hypothesis has been controversially discussed [15,17–20], since certain aspects of substance use symptomatology, including symptoms of withdrawal or tolerance, have not been demonstrated regarding food [21]. FA is mainly operationalized as a trait based on a self-report questionnaire to assess food-related addictive behavior, the *Yale Food Addiction Scale 2.0* (YFAS 2.0) [22]. Although FA was found in individuals across the weight range, it was often described in the context of obesity, with highly varying prevalence of 6.7–56.8% in samples of treatment-seeking individuals who were overweight or obese [14]. Two recent studies specifically investigated alterations in executive functioning in individuals with obesity and trait FA, showing that higher versus lower FA severity in obesity was related to poorer decision-making, greater attentional impairments [23], significantly poorer inhibition and cognitive flexibility assessed via self-report questionnaires and a computerized neuropsychological test battery [24]. Individuals with obesity and trait FA, may therefore present with a specific neuropsychological profile in the obesity spectrum.

Likewise, the clinical eating disorder diagnosis of binge-eating disorder (BED) [25] has been associated with addictive-like eating behavior [26,27]. According to the 5th edition of the Diagnostic and Statistical Manual of Mental Disorders (DSM-5) [25], the core feature of BED is represented by recurrent episodes of objective binge eating, which are characterized by a feeling of loss of control over eating while consuming an unambiguously large amount of food in a discrete period of time. BED is not associated with regular inappropriate compensatory behaviors, such as vomiting or excessive exercising [25]. Among treatment-seeking individuals with overweight and obesity, 23.9% presented with comorbid BED [28]. Individuals with BED were repeatedly found to show impairments in executive functioning exceeding those observed in obesity only, including increased impulsivity, reward sensitivity, rash spontaneous behavior, risky decision-making, and reduced inhibition [29–34]. These alterations were found in general executive functioning tasks [30,35,36] as well as in food-related tasks [30,37,38], strengthening the assumption of a specific neuropsychological profile of individuals with obesity and comorbid BED.

Even though trait FA and the diagnosis of BED have a significant number of behavioral symptoms in common (e.g., consumption of large amounts of food, loss of control, continued use despite negative consequences, cravings) and show a comorbidity of 57.0–72.2% in treatment-seeking and population-based samples with obesity [39], no study has yet compared the neuropsychological profiles of individuals with obesity presenting with or without FA and BED.

In the context of executive functions in obesity as described above, we therefore aimed to investigate general executive functions, specifically decision-making, reward sensitivity, cognitive flexibility, inhibition, and cognitive control in four distinct groups of individuals with obesity: those with FA, BED, FA plus BED (FA/BED), and a control group of otherwise healthy individuals with obesity (OB) stratified to the other groups based on age, sex, and BMI. Among the four groups, we assumed that individuals with OB would show the highest levels of executive functioning. For those with FA, we particularly expected poorer decision-making, cognitive control, inhibition, and flexibility than for OB. Furthermore, we assumed that individuals with BED would perform significantly worse than individuals with OB in tasks investigating impulsivity, reward sensitivity, and inhibition. Due to a lack of evidence, no evidence-based hypothesis was derived regarding possible differences on executive functioning between individuals with trait FA and those with BED. However, based on a recent finding that individuals with FA plus BED displayed greater eating disorder and general psychopathology than individuals with BED only [40], we suggested cumulative adverse effects on executive functioning. Thus, individuals with FA/BED were expected to show lower levels of executive functioning than individuals with OB, FA, and BED only.

2. Materials and Methods

2.1. Participants

Adults with obesity were recruited at the time of admission of two outpatient brain-directed psychological treatment studies at the Integrated Research and Treatment Center Adiposity Diseases in Leipzig, Germany (Cognitive remediation therapy for adults with obesity [41]; electroencephalographic neurofeedback training for adults with BED [42]), and were tested prior to the beginning of either intervention. Inclusion and exclusion criteria for both studies were similar. Relatedly, participants included in this study were required to be between 18 and 60 years of age, present with a BMI $\geq$ 35.0 kg/m^2, display sufficient German language skills, and provide informed consent. Exclusion criteria were (1) serious somatic conditions (e.g., neurological disorders, stroke, head injury); (2) serious mental conditions (e.g., psychotic disorder, suicidality, substance use disorder, developmental or intellectual disability); (3) physical, mental, or other inability to participate in assessments (e.g., impediment in hearing, vision, or language); (4) previous or planned bariatric surgery; (5) use of medication that impacts weight or executive functioning (e.g., antipsychotics, sedatives, hypnotics); (6) current psychotherapy regarding weight or eating behavior; (7) current participation in other interventional studies; (8) lack of compliance; and (9) pregnancy or lactation. Individuals eligible for the OB group were required not to display any FA symptoms according to the YFAS 2.0 [22,43] and not to report any objective binge-eating episode during the last three months as determined via clinical interview [44,45]. Individuals eligible for the FA group needed to present with trait FA, according to the YFAS 2.0 [22,43], and were required not to report any objective binge-eating episode during the last three months as determined via clinical interview [44,45]. Individuals eligible for the BED group were required to present with the DSM-5 diagnosis of BED assessed with a clinical interview [44,45] and not to present with trait FA according to the YFAS 2.0 [22,43]. Individuals eligible for the FA/BED group had to present with trait FA, according to the YFAS 2.0 [22,43], and with the DSM-5 diagnosis of BED assessed with a clinical interview [44,45].

2.2. Ethics and Procedure

Both studies were approved by the Ethical Committee of Leipzig University Medical Center (256-15-13072015, 143-15-20042015) and carried out in accordance with the Declaration of Helsinki. Within the two mentioned treatment studies, all participants were screened for eligibility using a standardized telephone interview. All eligible participants were invited to a baseline in-person diagnostic session. At the beginning of the diagnostic session, informed consent was obtained, followed by a series of neuropsychological tasks (see below). BMI was calculated based on participants' weight (in kg) and height (in cm) which were objectively measured using calibrated instruments at the end of the diagnostic session. The diagnostic sessions were standardized and conducted by trained staff. All participants were asked to refrain from eating at least 2 h prior to testing, in order to avoid any uncontrolled confounding effects of hunger or satiety on executive functioning.

2.3. Sample

Between November 2015 and April 2018, a total of n = 1082 individuals registered with an interest in one of the two brain-directed treatment studies, of whom a total of n = 258 were eligible and included in one of these brain-directed treatment studies. All n = 258 individuals participated in the baseline diagnostic session. For the present study, a convenience sample out of this study population was used, consisting of n = 23 individuals with trait FA based on the YFAS 2.0 [22,43], n = 19 with the DSM-5 diagnosis of BED based on clinical interview [44,45], and n = 23 individuals characterized by trait FA and BED (FA/BED). Out of n = 85 individuals eligible for the OB group, a total of n = 23 otherwise healthy individuals with obesity were stratified to the mean scores of the other groups regarding age, BMI, sex, and education.

2.4. Measures

2.4.1. Eating Disorder Examination

The diagnosis of BED according to DSM-5 [25] was derived from the diagnostic items of the validated German version of the Eating Disorder Examination interview (EDE 17.0D) [44,45]. According to DSM-5, the following severity levels of BED were determined: mild (1–3 objective binge-eating episodes per week), moderate (4–7 objective binge-eating episodes per week), severe (8–13 objective binge-eating episodes per week), and extreme (≥14 objective binge-eating episodes per week). The EDE has high interrater reliability ($r \geq 0.90$) [46].

2.4.2. Yale Food Addiction Scale

The validated German version of the 35-item self-report Yale Food Addiction Scale 2.0 (YFAS 2.0; $\alpha = 0.914$) [22,43] was used to determine FA. Participants were instructed to indicate how often they experienced addictive-like behavior towards food over the last year, with responses ranging from 0 (never) to 7 (every day). A total score was calculated by adding up all DSM-5 symptoms for addiction, ranging from 0 to 11. Scores ≥ 2 in combination with clinically significant distress indicate the presence of FA, with higher scores representing more severe FA: mild (2–3 symptom scores), moderate (4–5 symptom scores), and severe (≥6 symptom scores).

2.4.3. Eating Disorder Examination-Questionnaire

The validated German version of the short 8-item version of the Eating Disorder Examination-Questionnaire (EDE-Q8; $\alpha = 0.766$) [47] was used to evaluate participants' global eating disorder psychopathology. A mean score, ranging from 0 to 6, was calculated, with higher scores indicating greater eating disorder psychopathology.

2.4.4. Patient Health Questionnaire-Depression Scale

The validated German version of the 9-item Patient Health Questionnaire-Depression Scale (PHQ-9; $\alpha = 0.813$) [48,49] was administered to assess the level of depression based on the DSM-5 criteria for depression. Items were scored on a 0 (not at all) to 3 (almost every day) scale. Participants' sum scores were computed, ranging from 0 to 27, with higher scores representing more severe depression. Scores < 5 indicate no depressive symptoms, scores between 5 and 10 a mild depression, and scores > 10 a major depression [48,49].

2.5. Neuropsychological Assessment

2.5.1. Iowa Gambling Task

The computerized version of the Iowa Gambling Task (IGT) [50] was used to assess decision-making under uncertainty and complexity. The IGT requires participants to choose 100 times from four possible card decks (A, B, C, and D), aiming at winning the highest possible amount of virtual money. Each card deck contains profits and losses of different amounts. In the long term, choosing from card decks A and B will result in overall long-term loss (disadvantageous decks), whereas choosing cards from card decks C and D will result in overall long-term gain (advantageous decks). Performance in the IGT was determined by the total net score, calculated by subtracting the total number of disadvantageous choices from the total number of advantageous choices. Additionally, a learning effect across the net score of the five consecutive blocks of 20 cards was considered.

2.5.2. Delay Discounting Task

The computerized version of the Delay Discounting Task (DDT) [51], provided by the test software Millisecond [52] was used to determine the individual discounting rate of delayed rewards, which represents a measure of impulsive decision-making [51]. In this paradigm participants were instructed to choose between a standard amount of money (10 EUR) with different temporal delays (0, 2, 30, 180, and 365 days) or a variable amount (0–10 EUR) with no delay, until an indifference point for each delay was found or until the maximum number of trials (30) has been run for each delay. Five indifference points were calculated, where the immediate reward and delayed reward were equal in terms of subjective value. To determine performance in the DDT, the five indifference points were used to calculate the area under the curve (AUC) [53]. The AUC may range from 0 to 1 with greater AUC values being associated with less discounting of delayed rewards, i.e., less impulsivity [53].

2.5.3. Go/No Go

The computerized version of the visual Go/No Go paradigm [54], provided by the Vienna Test System [55], was used to assess inhibitory control. The visual Go/No Go paradigm required participants to determine whether a stimulus required a reaction or an inhibition. Therefore, 202 triangles were shown on the screen, which required a fast response, while a total of 48 circles appeared randomly in-between, indicating that no response should be given. Performance in the Go/No Go paradigm was determined by the number of commission errors (false positive responses towards a No Go trial), with more commission errors suggesting diminished inhibitory control [56].

2.5.4. Wisconsin Card Sorting Test

The computerized version of the Wisconsin Card Sorting Test (WCST) [57] was used as a measure of cognitive flexibility. The WCST required participants to sort each of maximally 128 cards according to three possible principles or rules (e.g., shape, color, or number), which were unknown to the participant, but would become apparent via feedback during the trials. After 10 consecutively and correctly sorted cards the rule changed suddenly and without warning. The participant then had to generate solutions and use the feedback to adapt to the new rule. Performance on the WCST was measured with the percentage of perseverative errors, which represent a tendency to perseverate on the previous rule, and the learning to learn score, which represents the average growth of conceptual efficiency during the test (average difference in percent errors between successive categories). The learning to learn score can only be calculated if participants have completed at least three categories or completed two categories and attempted a third. The learning to learn score can obtain positive and negative values, with positive scores indicating enhanced efficiency across consecutive categories, presumably because of learning [57].

2.5.5. Alertness

Alertness and the variability in early attentional processes was assessed with a computerized perception and attention functions battery (WAFA) [58], provided by the Vienna Test System [55]. To assess visual intrinsic alertness, participants were required to look at a fixation cross at the center of the screen and press a button as fast as possible when a target stimulus, a circle, appeared. For the assessment of phasic alertness, an auditory cue appeared shortly before the visual stimulus, preparing the participant for next execution of the reaction. Performance in intrinsic and phasic alertness was reported as log-transformed mean reaction time, with higher scores indicating longer reaction times and therefore less alertness [58]. Variability in performance in intrinsic and phasic alertness was reported as a measure of dispersion, with higher scores indicating greater variability in intrinsic or phasic alertness.

2.6. Statistical Procedure

Statistical analyses were performed using IBM SPSS Statistics version 24 (IBM Corp. Released 2016. IBM SPSS Statistics for Windows, Version 24.0. Armonk, NY: IBM Corp). All tests were two-tailed and considered significant when p values were <0.05. Since the domains of executive functioning are distinct and based on single measures, adjusting for multiple testing was not necessary, except for the computerized alertness task (WAFA) where four outcome measures were used. The p value for testing group differences in the WAFA was therefore adjusted to $p = 0.05/4 = 0.0125$. For the comparison of groups regarding socio-demographic and clinical variables, univariate analyses of variance (ANOVAs) were calculated for continuous variables and Chi-square tests (X^2) for categorical variables. The prerequisites for performing the tests (normal distribution and homogeneity of variance) were tested with the Shapiro-Wilk and Levene tests. When prerequisites were not met, Welch ANOVA was used, because of its robustness against violations of the assumption of homogeneity of variances [59]. In case of significance and homogeneity of variances, the Bonferroni post-hoc test was used to determine pair-wise differences; in case of violation of homogeneity of variances the Games-Howell post-hoc test was used. For Welch ANOVA, estimated omega squared (est. ω^2) was calculated for which $\omega^2 \geq 0.01$ is considered a small effect, $\omega^2 \geq 0.06$ a moderate, and $\omega^2 \geq 0.14$ a large effect [60]. For mean differences in post-hoc tests Cohen's d was calculated, with $d \geq 0.2$ being considered a small effect, $d \geq 0.5$ a moderate, and $d \geq 0.8$ a large effect [61]. In the present study, a power of ≥ 0.75 was observed to detect moderate and ≥ 0.95 to detect large group differences in ANOVAs (two-tailed $p < 0.05$).

3. Results

3.1. Sample

As depicted in Table 1, groups did not differ in socio-demographic characteristics. Significant differences between groups were found in eating disorder psychopathology and depression. For eating disorder psychopathology, post-hoc tests did not reach significance. The FA/BED group showed significantly more depressive symptoms compared to the OB group (5.17, 95% Confidence interval (CI) (1.86, 8.49), $p \leq 0.001$). Significantly more individuals of the FA/BED group presented with severe FA compared to the FA group, where there were more cases of mild FA. The FA/BED group did not differ significantly regarding BED severity from the BED group.

Table 1. Sociodemographic characteristics.

Variable	Obesity Only $n = 23$	Food Addiction $n = 23$	Binge-Eating Disorder $n = 19$	Food Addiction Plus Binge-Eating Disorder $n = 23$	Test			Effect Size
	M (SD)	*M (SD)*	*M (SD)*	*M (SD)*	*F*	*df*	*p*	*Est.* ω^2
Age (years)	40.48 (10.85)	43.39 (10.35)	38.84 (9.43)	37.53 (10.12)	1.38	3, 84	0.254	0.013
Body mass index (kg/m^2)	42.84 (4.76)	44.14 (6.59)	41.92 (5.25)	42.23 (6.13)	0.64	3, 84	0.589	−0.012
	n	*n*	*n*	*n*	χ^2	*df*	*p*	
Sex (female/male)	17/6	18/5	14/5	16/7	0.45	3	0.930	
Education (low/middle/high) [1]	3/11/9	3/16/4	1/7/11	4/10/9	8.50	6	0.203	
	M (SD)	*M (SD)*	*M (SD)*	*M (SD)*	*F*	*df*	*p*	*Est.* ω^2
Eating disorder psychopathology (EDE-Q8)	3.59 (0.98) ^{a}	4.20 (0.80) ^{a}	3.55 (1.03) ^{a}	4.36 (1.20) ^{a}	3.92	3, 84	0.011	0.091
Depression (PHQ-D)	5.00 (3.47) ^{a}	7.71 (3.80) ^{a,b}	7.99 (5.27) ^{a,b}	10.17 (4.10) ^{b}	5.98	3, 84	0.001	0.145
	n	*n*	*n*	*n*	χ^2	*df*	*p*	
FA severity (mild/moderate/severe)	-	9/10/4	-	0/6/17	18.05	2	<0.001	
BED severity (mild/moderate/severe)	-	-	14/5/0	16/4/3	2.89	2	0.236	

Note. M: mean, SD: standard deviation, df: degrees of freedom, FA: food addiction, BED: binge-eating disorder, BMI: body mass index, PHQ-D: Patient Health Questionnaire-Depression Scale, EDE-Q8: short version of the Eating Disorder Examination-Questionnaire ^{a,b} Different superscripts denote significant differences in post-hoc comparisons with Bonferroni corrections. [1] In Germany, secondary school is subdivided into three tracks: lower $\leq$ 9 years of education, middle = 10 years of education, high $\geq$ 12 years of education.

3.2. Neuropsychological Assessment

In the WAFA, groups differed significantly in the variability to react to a cued target (measure of dispersion phasic alertness), see Table 2, with individuals with BED showing significantly more variability in reaction times than individuals with OB (0.88, 95% CI [0.13, 1.63], $p = 0.018$, $d = 1.12$). Significant group differences were furthermore observed in the growth of conceptual efficiency in the WCST (learning to learn score), indicating that individuals with BED showed significantly less growth of conceptual efficiency in learning compared to individuals with OB (−3.47, 95% CI [−6.92, −0.01], $p = 0.049$, $d = -0.85$). Regarding decision-making, all groups improved their net score over the five consecutive blocks of the IGT, as depicted in Figure 1. Although descriptive data of the IGT net score seem to differ substantially, no significant group differences were found and only a small effect size was observed (see Table 2), suggesting that trait FA and BED diagnosis were not associated with altered decision-making in individuals with obesity. In addition, groups did not differ in their mean reaction time (intrinsic and phasic) and variability to react to un-cued visual targets (measure of dispersion intrinsic alertness) in the WAFA, the amount of perseverative errors in the WCST, and the amount of commission errors in the Go/No Go task (see Table 2), indicating that trait FA and BED were not associated with altered attention, cognitive flexibility, and inhibition in individuals with obesity.

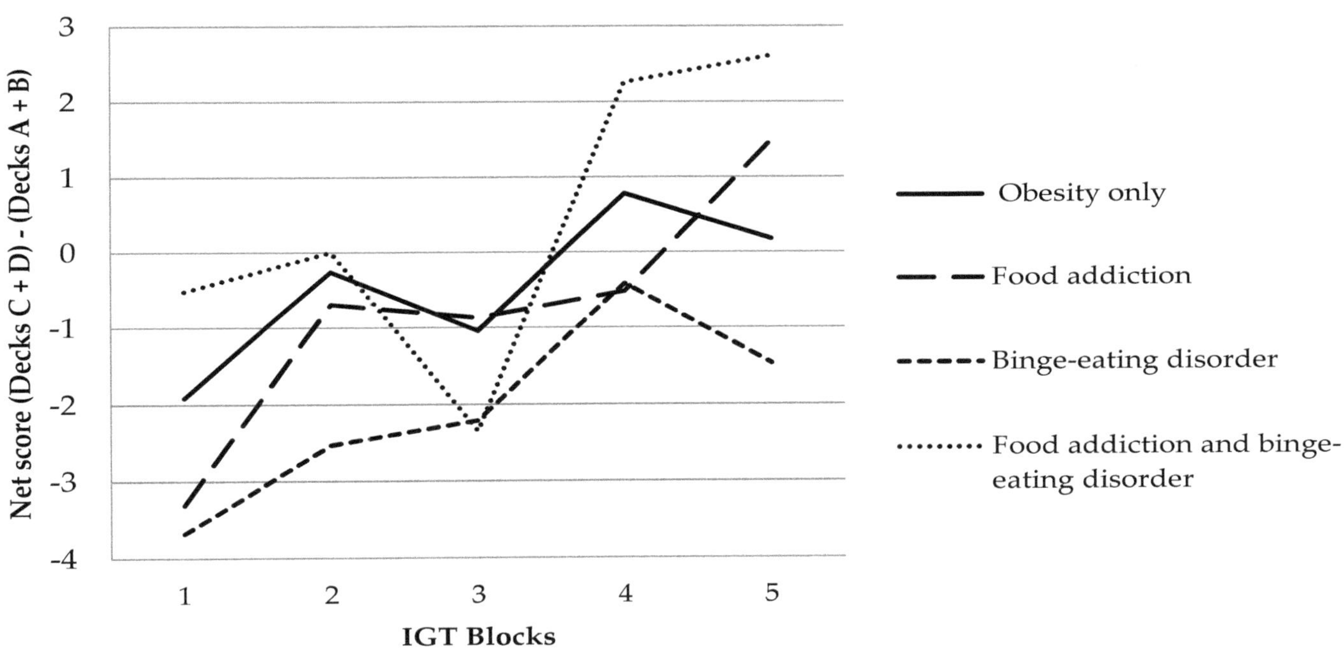

Figure 1. Iowa Gambling Task (IGT) learning effect across five consecutive blocks.

Table 2. Performance on neuropsychological assessments.

Variable		Obesity Only $n = 23$	Food Addiction $n = 23$	Binge-Eating-Disorder $n = 19$	Food Addiction plus Binge-Eating Disorder $n = 23$	Welch ANOVA			Effect Size
		M (SD)	*M (SD)*	*M (SD)*	*M (SD)*	*F*	*df*	*p*	*Est.* ω^2
IGT	Net score	−2.26 (32.78)	−3.91 (32.18)	−10.32 (39.36)	2.00 (35.17)	0.37	3, 46	0.773	−0.022
DDT	Area under the curve	0.47 (0.32)	0.31 (0.26)	0.54 (0.26)	0.46 (0.24)	2.80	3, 46	0.050	0.058
Go/No Go	Commission errors	11.61 (5.98)	11.39 (7.88)	9.74 (6.06)	12.52 (7.22)	0.64	3, 46	0.591	−0.012
WCST	Perseverative errors	17.70 (6.67)	17.40 (8.38)	14.31 (4.75)	18.38 (8.28)	2.02	3, 46	0.125	0.034
	Learning to learn [1]	2.01 (4.22) [a]	0.88 (6.60) [a, b]	−1.45 (3.90) [b]	3.70 (10.08) [a, b]	2.94	3, 40	0.045	0.069
WAFA	Mean reaction time intrinsic in ms	254.22 (45.69)	264.61 (45.02)	265.37 (43.22)	266.00 (72.05)	0.30	3, 46	0.824	−0.024
	Mean reaction time phasic in ms	253.78 (57.09)	242.04 (61.98)	223.63 (88.57)	249.00 (95.92)	0.56	3, 45	0.642	−0.015
	Measure of dispersion intrinsic	1.18 (0.67)	1.24 (0.11)	1.18 (0.06)	1.28 (0.39)	2.53	3, 45	0.069	0.050
	Measure of dispersion phasic	1.41 (0.18) [a]	1.56 (0.50) [a, b]	2.29 (1.15) [b]	1.79 (1.02) [a, b]	4.80	3, 37	0.006	0.115

Note. M: mean, SD: standard deviation, df: degrees of freedom, IGT: Iowa Gambling Task, DDT: Delay Discounting Task, WAFA: Perception and attention functions battery alertness, WCST: Wisconsin Card Sorting Task, ms: milliseconds. [a,b] Different superscripts denote significant differences in post-hoc comparisons with Games-Howell corrections. [1] Sample size for learning to learn score $n = 79$ ($n = 22$ obesity only, $n = 19$ food addiction, $n = 18$ binge-eating disorder, $n = 20$ food addiction plus binge-eating disorder).

4. Discussion

The present study aimed at investigating the associations of trait FA and the DSM-5 diagnosis of BED regarding executive functions in adults with obesity. It was found that individuals with BED showed lower executive functioning, characterized by a higher variability in reaction times and less feedback integration, compared to otherwise healthy individuals with obesity. Contrary to expectations, there were no differences in executive functioning among individuals with FA, FA/BED, and obesity only. The results thus suggest a BED-specific, but not a FA-specific, neuropsychological profile in individuals with obesity. The combined presentation of trait FA and BED was not associated with greater impairments in executive functioning compared to their single presentations.

The fact that individuals with obesity and BED displayed a significantly higher variability in their reaction times compared to the OB group is similar to findings showing a high variability in reaction times in ADHD [62]. ADHD is highly comorbid to obesity and BED and is associated with comparable neuronal processes [62–64]. In ADHD, it is usually believed that the variability of response times reflects occasional gaps in attention [62], which could be related to high distractibility, making an attentional shift and the detection of task-irrelevant stimuli, for example, food cues, more likely. Another result was the significant and medium-sized difference between the BED and the OB group in the learning to learn score in the WCST, in accordance with recent research [37]. The negative learning to learn score indicated that individuals with BED became less rather than more efficient on consecutive trials of the WCST [57]. Hypothetically, this could be caused by an inability to appropriately integrate the feedback in order to improve performance, as previously evidenced in BED [29]. Transferred into everyday life, the deficient processing of feedback to improve performance could be related to a lack of feedback integration in daily learning, such as feedback given by one's own body after an objective binge-eating episode in order to prevent such an episode from occurring again, leaving an individual without control [65]. In this context, it is worth noting that the BED group did not display heightened depressive symptoms compared to the OB and FA group. Observed differences between the BED and OB group can therefore not be attributed to increased general psychopathology, but were related to BED diagnosis.

Contrary to the two previous studies investigating executive functions in individuals with trait FA [23,24], demonstrating that higher versus lower FA severity in obesity was related to poorer decision-making, inhibition, and cognitive flexibility, no other performance score reached significance in the present study. The hypothesis that individuals with obesity and FA may present with a specific neuropsychological profile in the obesity spectrum was therefore not supported in this clinical treatment-seeking sample. It is of note, however, that the FA group mostly presented with mild and moderate FA symptomatology only, allowing to speculate that FA severity was not high enough to be accompanied by cognitive impairments in this sample. On the other hand, this result could also reflect the assumption that BED, as a clinical eating disorder diagnosis, is associated with more cognitive impairments than subjective trait FA.

The hypothesis of cumulative effects on executive dysfunctions in individuals with FA plus BED was not confirmed in the present study, since the FA/BED group did not display lower performance compared to the OB, FA, or BED group in any of the tasks under investigation. Notably, the FA/BED group reported considerably more depressive symptoms compared to the OB group, with an average in the range of a major depression [48,49], and thus contradicts neuropsychological evidence of impaired executive functioning in individuals with depression [66]. However, the underlying mechanisms of this finding cannot currently be identified. Therefore, this result needs replication in larger, independent samples of individuals with FA/BED.

4.1. Methodological Considerations

When interpreting the results several strength and limitations have to be mentioned. First, using well-established measures, the diagnosis of BED was derived from an expert interview, the EDE 17.0D [44,45], and trait FA was assessed via the established self-questionnaire YFAS 2.0 [22,43]. Second, the OB group was stratified to the other groups and groups were mutually exclusive regarding trait FA and objective binge-eating episodes. Third, executive functioning was measured with established, standardized, and computerized tasks. Critically, the relatively small group sizes have to be mentioned, as only medium-to-large-sized effects could be detected with adequate power. Additionally, there might be an assessment bias across diagnostic groups, as FA was assessed with a self-administered questionnaire, while BED diagnosis was made by clinical expert interview, suggesting that trait FA and BED mirror different levels of clinical severity. Furthermore, no food-specific tasks were used. Various studies have shown a stronger association between executive functions in food-related tasks in relation to binge-eating behavior [30,38]. Lastly it is important to note that the design of this study was cross-sectional; therefore, causal conclusions about the direction of observed effects are not indicated.

4.2. Implications and Future Directions

The current study identified greater executive dysfunctions in individuals with obesity and comorbid BED compared to those with obesity only. Clinically, the assessment of eating disorder symptomatology, specifically a diagnosis of BED, seems therefore indicated in individuals with obesity. In these individuals, an increase in neuropsychological impairments is likely to interfere with standard treatment options [8,9] and may thus constitute a specific target for intervention, for example, via cognitive remediation therapy [41]. Based on this study's results, an in-depth investigation in the variability of reaction times (alertness tasks) is indicated, especially considering the effects of food stimuli, as current research points to an increased attentional bias towards food cues in individuals with BED e.g., [66,67].

Regarding trait FA, this study revealed no impairments in executive functioning other than a tendency towards higher choice-impulsivity, which could be related to the high proportion of individuals characterized by low FA severity in the FA group. Studies investigating executive functions in individuals with obesity and more severe FA are therefore needed. Alternatively, it could be argued that similarities in executive functioning between individuals with obesity plus trait FA and individuals with substance use disorder as recently shown [12] only manifest on a neurobiological [12] and not on a neuropsychological level. To further differentiate these aspects of addictive-like eating behavior, future research is warranted to specifically investigate neuronal and neuropsychological overlaps and distinctive features between trait FA and substance use disorder, especially in the context of disorder-related stimuli (e.g., food stimuli).

It was surprising that the observed large differences in attentional variability and conceptual learning between the BED and OB group did not manifest in the FA/BED group, particularly as this group presented as the most impaired group concerning mental health, with more depressive symptoms than the OB group. The assessment of trait FA in individuals with versus without BED may therefore be helpful to determine identify individuals at risk for greater mental health impairment and in need of more intensive treatment. Further research into the neuropsychological characteristics of individuals with FA plus BED is however warranted, preferably using larger samples and a longitudinal study design in order to evaluate the effects of trait FA plus BED on weight trajectories and treatment outcome in individuals with obesity.

Author Contributions: Conceptualization, M.B., R.S. and A.H.; methodology, M.B., R.S. and A.H.; software, M.B. and A.H.; formal analysis, M.B. investigation, M.B.; resources, A.H.; data curation, M.B.; writing—original draft preparation, M.B.; writing—review and editing, M.B., R.S. and A.H.; visualization, M.B.; supervision, R.S. and A.H.; project administration, M.B. and A.H.; funding acquisition, A.H.

Acknowledgments: The authors would like to thank Claudia Hübner, Helen Eißner, Ronja Runge, Annika Kleinschmitt, Robert Kratzer, Fabrice Sigleur, Eva Stenger, Johanna Müller, Eileen Lashani, Nikolas Verfuß, Anne-Sophie Pelzl, Anna-Maria Hoffmann, Sabrina Höft, Jenny Kaiser-Baumgärtner and Sarah-Verena Schmieger for their assistance in data collection.

References

1. World Health Organization [WHO]. Obesity and Overweight: Fact Sheet. Available online: http://www.who.int/mediacentre/factsheets/fs311/en/ (accessed on 30 July 2017).
2. NCD Risk Factor Collaboration (NCD-RisC). Worldwide trends in body-mass index, underweight, overweight, and obesity from 1975 to 2016: A pooled analysis of 2416 population-based measurement studies in 128·9 million children, adolescents, and adults. *Lancet* **2017**, *390*, 2627–2642. [CrossRef]
3. Horstmann, A. It wasn't me; it was my brain-Obesity-associated characteristics of brain circuits governing decision-making. *Physiol. Behav.* **2017**, *176*, 125–133. [CrossRef] [PubMed]
4. Makaronidis, J.M.; Batterham, R.L. Obesity, body weight regulation and the brain: Insights from fMRI. *Br. J. Radiol.* **2018**. [CrossRef] [PubMed]
5. Yang, Y.; Shields, G.S.; Guo, C.; Liu, Y. Executive function performance in obesity and overweight individuals: A meta-analysis and review. *Neurosci. Biobehav. Rev.* **2018**, *84*, 225–244. [CrossRef] [PubMed]
6. Shallice, T. *From Neuropsychology to Mental Structure*, 1st ed.; Cambridge University Press: Cambridge, England, 1988; ISBN 978-0-521-31360-5.
7. Stuss, D.T.; Benson, D.F. *The Frontal Lobes*; Raven Press: New York, NY, USA, 1986; ISBN 978-0-88167-153-7.
8. Wyckoff, E.P.; Evans, B.C.; Manasse, S.M.; Butryn, M.L.; Forman, E.M. Executive functioning and dietary intake: Neurocognitive correlates of fruit, vegetable, and saturated fat intake in adults with obesity. *Appetite* **2017**, *111*, 79–85. [CrossRef] [PubMed]
9. Brockmeyer, T.; Hamze Sinno, M.; Skunde, M.; Wu, M.; Woehning, A.; Rudofsky, G.; Friederich, H.-C. Inhibitory control and hedonic response towards food interactively predict success in a weight loss programme for adults with obesity. *Obes. Facts* **2016**, *9*, 299–309. [CrossRef] [PubMed]
10. Jones, A.; Hardman, C.A.; Lawrence, N.; Field, M. Cognitive training as a potential treatment for overweight and obesity: A critical review of the evidence. *Appetite* **2017**, *124*, 50–67. [CrossRef] [PubMed]
11. Michaud, A.; Vainik, U.; Garcia-Garcia, I.; Dagher, A. Overlapping neural endophenotypes in addiction and obesity. *Front. Endocrinol.* **2017**, *8*, 127. [CrossRef]
12. Lindgren, E.; Gray, K.; Miller, G.; Tyler, R.; Wiers, C.E.; Volkow, N.D.; Wang, G.-J. Food addiction: A common neurobiological mechanism with drug abuse. *Front. Biosci. Landmark Ed.* **2018**, *23*, 811–836.
13. Jauch-Chara, K.; Oltmanns, K.M. Obesity—A neuropsychological disease? Systematic review and neuropsychological model. *Prog. Neurobiol.* **2014**, *114*, 84–101. [CrossRef]
14. Burrows, T.; Kay-Lambkin, F.; Pursey, K.; Skinner, J.; Dayas, C. Food addiction and associations with mental health symptoms: A systematic review with meta-analysis. *J. Hum. Nutr. Diet.* **2018**, *31*, 544–572. [CrossRef] [PubMed]
15. Gordon, E.L.; Ariel-Donges, A.H.; Bauman, V.; Merlo, L.J. What is the evidence for "food addiction?" a systematic review. *Nutrients* **2018**, *10*, 477. [CrossRef] [PubMed]
16. Smith, D.G.; Robbins, T.W. The neurobiological underpinnings of obesity and binge eating: A rationale for adopting the food addiction model. *Biol. Psychiatry* **2013**, *73*, 804–810. [CrossRef] [PubMed]
17. Davis, C. A commentary on the associations among "food addiction", binge eating disorder, and obesity: Overlapping conditions with idiosyncratic clinical features. *Appetite* **2017**, *115*, 3–8. [CrossRef] [PubMed]
18. Gearhardt, A.N.; Corbin, W.R.; Brownell, K.D. Preliminary validation of the yale food addiction scale. *Appetite* **2009**, *52*, 430–436. [CrossRef] [PubMed]
19. Lacroix, E.; Tavares, H.; von Ranson, K.M. Moving beyond the "eating addiction" versus "food addiction" debate: Comment on Schulte et al. (2017). *Appetite* **2018**, *130*, 286–292. [CrossRef] [PubMed]
20. Schulte, E.M.; Potenza, M.N.; Gearhardt, A.N. A commentary on the "eating addiction" versus "food addiction" perspectives on addictive-like food consumption. *Appetite* **2017**, *115*, 9–15. [CrossRef] [PubMed]
21. Hilbert, A. *Binge-Eating Disorder*; Psychiatric Clinics of North America in Press: Amsterdam, The Netherlands, 2002.
22. Gearhardt, A.N.; Corbin, W.R.; Brownell, K.D. Development of the yale food addiction scale version 2.0. *Psychol. Addict. Behav.* **2016**, *30*, 113–121. [CrossRef]
23. American Psychiatric Association. *DSM-5: Diagnostic and Statistical Manual of Mental Disorders*, 5th ed.; American Psychiatric Publishing: Arlington, VA, USA, 2013.

24. Steward, T.; Mestre-Bach, G.; Vintró-Alcaraz, C.; Lozano-Madrid, M.; Agüera, Z.; Fernández-Formoso, J.A.; Granero, R.; Jiménez-Murcia, S.; Vilarrasa, N.; García-Ruiz-de-Gordejuela, A.; et al. Food addiction and impaired executive functions in women with obesity. *Eur. Eat. Disord. Rev.* **2018**, *26*, 574–584. [CrossRef]
25. Rodrigue, C.; Ouellette, A.-S.; Lemieux, S.; Tchernof, A.; Biertho, L.; Bégin, C. Executive functioning and psychological symptoms in food addiction: A study among individuals with severe obesity. *Eat. Weight Disord.* **2018**, *23*, 469–478. [CrossRef]
26. Cassin, S.E.; von Ranson, K.M. Is binge eating experienced as an addiction? *Appetite* **2007**, *49*, 687–690. [CrossRef] [PubMed]
27. Davis, C.; Mackew, L.; Levitan, R.D.; Kaplan, A.S.; Carter, J.C.; Kennedy, J.L. Binge eating disorder (BED) in relation to addictive behaviors and personality risk factors. *Front. Psychol.* **2017**, *8*, 579. [CrossRef] [PubMed]
28. Ricca, V.; Castellini, G.; Lo Sauro, C.; Ravaldi, C.; Lapi, F.; Mannucci, E.; Rotella, C.M.; Faravelli, C. Correlations between binge eating and emotional eating in a sample of overweight subjects. *Appetite* **2009**, *53*, 418–421. [CrossRef] [PubMed]
29. Córdova, M.E.; Schiavon, C.C.; Busnello, F.M.; Reppold, C.T. Nutritional and neuropsychological profile of the executive functions on binge eating disorder in obese adults. *Nutr. Hosp.* **2017**, *34*, 1448–1454. [CrossRef] [PubMed]
30. Giel, K.E.; Teufel, M.; Junne, F.; Zipfel, S.; Schag, K. Food-related impulsivity in obesity and binge eating disorder—A Systematic update of the evidence. *Nutrients* **2017**, *9*, 1170. [CrossRef] [PubMed]
31. Kollei, I.; Rustemeier, M.; Schroeder, S.; Jongen, S.; Herpertz, S.; Loeber, S. Cognitive control functions in individuals with obesity with and without binge-eating disorder. *Int. J. Eat. Disord.* **2018**, *51*, 233–240. [CrossRef] [PubMed]
32. Leehr, E.J.; Schag, K.; Dresler, T.; Grosse-Wentrup, M.; Hautzinger, M.; Fallgatter, A.J.; Zipfel, S.; Giel, K.E.; Ehlis, A.-C. Food specific inhibitory control under negative mood in binge-eating disorder: Evidence from a multimethod approach. *Int. J. Eat. Disord.* **2018**, *51*, 112–123. [CrossRef]
33. Manasse, S.M.; Forman, E.M.; Ruocco, A.C.; Butryn, M.L.; Juarascio, A.S.; Fitzpatrick, K.K. Do executive functioning deficits underpin binge eating disorder? A comparison of overweight women with and without binge eating pathology. *Int. J. Eat. Disord.* **2015**, *48*, 677–683. [CrossRef]
34. Svaldi, J.; Naumann, E.; Biehl, S.; Schmitz, F. Impaired early-response inhibition in overweight females with and without binge eating disorder. *PLoS ONE* **2015**, *10*, e0133534. [CrossRef]
35. Kessler, R.M.; Hutson, P.H.; Herman, B.K.; Potenza, M.N. The neurobiological basis of binge-eating disorder. *Neurosci. Biobehav. Rev.* **2016**, *63*, 223–238. [CrossRef]
36. Schag, K.; Schönleber, J.; Teufel, M.; Zipfel, S.; Giel, K.E. Food-related impulsivity in obesity and binge eating disorder—A systematic review: Food-related impulsivity. *Obes. Rev.* **2013**, *14*, 477–495. [CrossRef]
37. Balodis, I.M.; Grilo, C.M.; Potenza, M.N. Neurobiological features of binge eating disorder. *CNS Spectr.* **2015**, *20*, 557–565. [CrossRef] [PubMed]
38. Kittel, R.; Brauhardt, A.; Hilbert, A. Cognitive and emotional functioning in binge-eating disorder: A systematic review. *Int. J. Eat. Disord.* **2015**, *48*, 535–554. [CrossRef] [PubMed]
39. Davis, C.; Curtis, C.; Levitan, R.D.; Carter, J.C.; Kaplan, A.S.; Kennedy, J.L. Evidence that "food addiction" is a valid phenotype of obesity. *Appetite* **2011**, *57*, 711–717. [CrossRef] [PubMed]
40. Gearhardt, A.N.; White, M.A.; Masheb, R.M.; Morgan, P.T.; Crosby, R.D.; Grilo, C.M. An examination of the food addiction construct in obese patients with binge eating disorder. *Int. J. Eat. Disord.* **2012**, *45*, 657–663. [CrossRef] [PubMed]
41. Hilbert, A.; Blume, M.; Petroff, D.; Neuhaus, P.; Smith, E.; Hay, P.J.; Hübner, C. Group cognitive remediation therapy for adults with obesity prior to behavioural weight loss treatment: Study protocol for a randomised controlled superiority study (CRT study). *BMJ Open* **2018**, *8*, e022616. [CrossRef] [PubMed]
42. Blume, M.; Schmidt, R.; Schmidt, J.; Martin, A.; Hilbert, A. German Clinical Trials Register: EEG Neurofeedback for Adults with Binge-Eating Disorder. Available online: https://www.drks.de/drks_web/navigate.do?navigationId=trial.HTML&TRIAL_ID=DRKS00010496 (accessed on 7 August 2018).
43. Meule, A.; Müller, A.; Gearhardt, A.N.; Blechert, J. German version of the Yale Food Addiction Scale 2.0: Prevalence and correlates of "food addiction" in students and obese individuals. *Appetite* **2017**, *115*, 54–61. [CrossRef] [PubMed]
44. Fairburn, C.G.; Cooper, Z.; O'Connor, M. *Eating Disorder Examination (17.0D)*; Guilford Press: New York, NY, USA, 2014.

45. Hilbert, A.; Tuschen-Caffier, B. *Eating Disorder Examination. Deutschsprachige Übersetzung*, 2nd ed.; Deutsche Gesellschaft für Verhaltensterapie: Tübingen, Germany, 2016; ISBN 978-3-87159-411-3.
46. Berg, K.C.; Peterson, C.B.; Frazier, P.; Crow, S.J. Psychometric evaluation of the eating disorder examination and eating disorder examination-questionnaire: A systematic review of the literature. *Int. J. Eat. Disord.* **2012**, *45*, 428–438. [CrossRef]
47. Kliem, S.; Mößle, T.; Zenger, M.; Strauß, B.; Brähler, E.; Hilbert, A. The eating disorder examination-questionnaire 8: A brief measure of eating disorder psychopathology (EDE-Q8). *Int. J. Eat. Disord.* **2016**, *49*, 613–616. [CrossRef]
48. Gräfe, K.; Zipfel, S.; Herzog, W.; Löwe, B. Screening psychischer Störungen mit dem "Gesundheitsfragebogen für Patienten (PHQ-D)". *Diagnostica* **2004**, *50*, 171–181. [CrossRef]
49. Spitzer, R.L.; Kroenke, K.; Williams, J.B. Validation and utility of a self-report version of PRIME-MD: The PHQ primary care study. Primary Care Evaluation of Mental Disorders. Patient Health Questionnaire. *JAMA* **1999**, *282*, 1737–1744. [CrossRef] [PubMed]
50. Bechara, A.; Damasio, A.R.; Damasio, H.; Anderson, S.W. Insensitivity to future consequences following damage to human prefrontal cortex. *Cognition* **1994**, *50*, 7–15. [CrossRef]
51. Richards, J.B.; Zhang, L.; Mitchell, S.H.; de Wit, H. Delay or probability discounting in a model of impulsive behavior: Effect of alcohol. *J. Exp. Anal. Behav.* **1999**, *71*, 121–143. [CrossRef] [PubMed]
52. Millisecond. *Inquisit (Version 4)*, Windows; Millisecond Software: San Francisco, CA, USA, 2015.
53. Myerson, J.; Green, L.; Warusawitharana, M. Area under the curve as a measure of discounting. *J. Exp. Anal. Behav.* **2001**, *76*, 235–243. [CrossRef] [PubMed]
54. Kaiser, S.; Aschenbrenner, S.; Pfüller, U.; Roesch-Ely, D.; Weisbrod, M. *Wiener Testsystem: Response Inhibition*, Schuhfried: Mödling, Germany, 2015.
55. Schuhfried Gmbh. *Vienna Test System*, Windows; Schuhfried Gmbh: Mödling, Austria, 2015.
56. Lezak, M.D.; Howieson, D.B.; Bigler, E.D.; Tranel, D. *Neuropsychological Assessment*; Oxford University Press: Oxford, NY, USA, 2012; ISBN 978-0-19-539552-5.
57. Heaton, R.K.; Chelune, G.J.; Talley, J.L.; Kay, G.G.; Curtiss, G. *Wisconsin Card Sorting Test Manual*; Psychological Assessment Resources, Inc.: Odessa, FL, USA, 1993.
58. Sturm, W. *Wiener Testsystem: Wahrnehmungs- und Aufmerksamkeitsfunktionen*, Schuhfried: Mödling, Austria, 2015.
59. Lix, L.M.; Keselman, J.C.; Keselman, H.J. Consequences of assumption violations revisited: A quantitative review of alternatives to the one-way analysis of variance f test. *Rev. Educ. Res.* **1996**, *66*, 579–619. [CrossRef]
60. Keppel, G. *Design and Analysis: A Researcher's Handbook*, 3rd ed.; Prentice Hall: Upper Saddle River, NJ, USA, 1991.
61. Cohen, J. *Statistical Power Analysis for the Behavioral Sciences*, 2nd ed.; Lawrence Erlbaum Associates: New York, NY, USA, 1988.
62. Tamm, L.; Narad, M.E.; Antonini, T.N.; O'Brien, K.M.; Hawk, L.W.; Epstein, J.N. Reaction time variability in ADHD: A review. *Neurotherapeutics* **2012**, *9*, 500–508. [CrossRef]
63. Cortese, S.; Bernardina, B.D.; Mouren, M.-C. Attention-deficit/hyperactivity disorder (adhd) and binge eating. *Nutr. Rev.* **2007**, *65*, 404–411. [CrossRef]
64. Voon, V. Cognitive biases in binge eating disorder: The hijacking of decision making. *CNS Spectr.* **2015**, *20*, 566–573. [CrossRef]
65. Restivo, M.R.; McKinnon, M.C.; Frey, B.N.; Hall, G.B.; Syed, W.; Taylor, V.H. The impact of obesity on neuropsychological functioning in adults with and without major depressive disorder. *PLoS ONE* **2017**, *12*, e0176898. [CrossRef]
66. Schmidt, R.; Lüthold, P.; Kittel, R.; Tetzlaff, A.; Hilbert, A. Visual attentional bias for food in adolescents with binge-eating disorder. *J. Psychiatr. Res.* **2016**, *80*, 22–29. [CrossRef] [PubMed]
67. Sperling, I.; Baldofski, S.; Lüthold, P.; Hilbert, A. Cognitive food processing in binge-eating disorder: An eye-tracking study. *Nutrients* **2017**, *9*, 903. [CrossRef] [PubMed]

Permissions

All chapters in this book were first published by MDPI; hereby published with permission under the Creative Commons Attribution License or equivalent. Every chapter published in this book has been scrutinized by our experts. Their significance has been extensively debated. The topics covered herein carry significant findings which will fuel the growth of the discipline. They may even be implemented as practical applications or may be referred to as a beginning point for another development.

The contributors of this book come from diverse backgrounds, making this book a truly international effort. This book will bring forth new frontiers with its revolutionizing research information and detailed analysis of the nascent developments around the world.

We would like to thank all the contributing authors for lending their expertise to make the book truly unique. They have played a crucial role in the development of this book. Without their invaluable contributions this book wouldn't have been possible. They have made vital efforts to compile up to date information on the varied aspects of this subject to make this book a valuable addition to the collection of many professionals and students.

This book was conceptualized with the vision of imparting up-to-date information and advanced data in this field. To ensure the same, a matchless editorial board was set up. Every individual on the board went through rigorous rounds of assessment to prove their worth. After which they invested a large part of their time researching and compiling the most relevant data for our readers.

The editorial board has been involved in producing this book since its inception. They have spent rigorous hours researching and exploring the diverse topics which have resulted in the successful publishing of this book. They have passed on their knowledge of decades through this book. To expedite this challenging task, the publisher supported the team at every step. A small team of assistant editors was also appointed to further simplify the editing procedure and attain best results for the readers.

Apart from the editorial board, the designing team has also invested a significant amount of their time in understanding the subject and creating the most relevant covers. They scrutinized every image to scout for the most suitable representation of the subject and create an appropriate cover for the book.

The publishing team has been an ardent support to the editorial, designing and production team. Their endless efforts to recruit the best for this project, has resulted in the accomplishment of this book. They are a veteran in the field of academics and their pool of knowledge is as vast as their experience in printing. Their expertise and guidance has proved useful at every step. Their uncompromising quality standards have made this book an exceptional effort. Their encouragement from time to time has been an inspiration for everyone.

The publisher and the editorial board hope that this book will prove to be a valuable piece of knowledge for researchers, students, practitioners and scholars across the globe.

List of Contributors

María F. Rabito-Alcón and José I. Baile
Department of Psychology, Open University of Madrid (UDIMA), 28400 Madrid, Spain

Johan Vanderlinden
Campus Kortenberg, Universitair Psychiatrisch (Centrum KU Leuven), 3070 Kortenberg, Belgium

Monika Bucharová, Andrea Malá and Jiří Kantor
Palacky University Evidence-Based Education Working Team: Mentee Centre, and Institute of Special Education Studies, Faculty of Education, Palacky University, 779 00 Olom uc, Czech Republic

Zuzana Svobodová
Czech National Centre for Evidence-Based Healthcare and Knowledge Translation (Cochrane Czech Republic, Czech Evidence-Based Healthcare Centre: Joanna Briggs Institute Centre of Excellence, Masaryk University GRADE Centre), Institute of Biostatistics and Analyses, Faculty of Medicine, Masaryk University, Kamenice 3, 625 00 Brno, Czech Republic

Tracy Burrows, Janelle Skinner, Rebecca McKenna and Megan Rollo
School of Health Sciences, Faculty of Health and Medicine, University of Newcastle, Callaghan 2308, Australia
Priority Research Centre for Physical Activity and Nutrition, University of Newcastle, Callaghan 2308, Australia

Marta Stelmach-Mardas
Department of Epidemiology, German Institute of Human Nutrition, Potsdam-Rehbruecke, Arthur-Scheunert-Allee 114-116, Nuthetal 14558, Germany
Department of Pediatric Gastroenterology and Metabolic Diseases, Poznan University of Medical Sciences, Szpitalna Str 27/33, Poznan 60-572, Poland

Jarosław Walkowiak
Department of Pediatric Gastroenterology and Metabolic Diseases, Poznan University of Medical Sciences, Szpitalna Str 27/33, Poznan 60-572, Poland

Marta Plichta, Marzena Jezewska-Zychowicz and Jerzy Gębski
Department of Organization and Consumption Economics, Faculty of Human Nutrition and Consumer Sciences, Warsaw University of Life Sciences (SGGWWULS), 159C Nowoursynowska Street, 02-787 Warsaw, Poland

Arturo Pujia, Yvelise Ferro, Elisa Mazza, Samantha Maurotti, Cristina Russo and Tiziana Montalcini
Department of Medical and Surgical Science, University Magna Grecia, Catanzaro 88100, Italy

Carmine Gazzaruso
Clinical Institute "Beato Matteo", Vigevano 27029, Italy

Veronica Lazzaro
Department of Health Science, University Magna Grecia, Catanzaro 88100, Italy

Stefano Romeo
Department of Medical and Surgical Science, University Magna Grecia, Catanzaro 88100, Italy
Department of Molecular and Clinical Medicine, University of Gothenburg, Gothenburg 40530, Sweden

Martina Nitsch, Tanja Adamcik, Stefanie Kuso and Karin Waldherr
FernFH Distance Learning University of Applied Sciences, Ferdinand Porsche Ring 3, 2700 Wiener Neustadt, Austria

Michael Zeiler
Department for Child and Adolescent Psychiatry, Medical University of Vienna, Waehringer Guertel 18-20, 1090 Vienna, Austria

Sabri Ahmed Rial, Karl-F. Bergeron and Catherine Mounier
BioMed Research Center, Biological Sciences Department, University of Quebec at Montreal, Montreal, QC H2X 1Y4, Canada

Antony D. Karelis
Department of Exercise Science, University of Quebec at Montreal, Montreal, QC H2X 1Y4, Canada

Věra Olišarová, Valérie Tóthová, Sylva Bártlová, František Dolák, Dita Nováková and Lenka Šedová
Institute of Nursing, Midwifery and Emergency Care, Faculty of Health and Social Sciences, University of South Bohemia in Ceske Budejovice, J. Boreckeho 1167/27, 370 05 Ceske Budejovice, Czech Republic

Alena Kajanová
Institute of Social and Special-paedagogical Sciences, Faculty of Health and Social Sciences, University of South Bohemia in Ceske Budejovice, J. Boreckeho 1167/27, 370 05 Ceske Budejovice, Czech Republic

Radka Prokešová
Institute of Legal Branches, Management and Economics, Faculty of Health and Social Sciences, University of South Bohemia in Ceske Budejovice, J. Boreckeho 1167/27, 370 05 Ceske Budejovice, Czech Republic

Nikul K. Soni, Alastair B. Ross, Nathalie Scheers, Otto I. Savolainen, Britt G. Gabrielsson and Ann-Sofie Sandberg
Division of Food and Nutrition Science, Department of Biology and Biological Engineering, Chalmers University of Technology, Gothenburg SE-41296, Sweden

Intawat Nookaew
Division of Systems and Synthetic Biology, Department of Biology and Biological Engineering, Chalmers University of Technology, Gothenburg SE-412 96, Sweden
Department of Biomedical Informatics, College of Medicine, University of Arkansas for Medical Sciences, Little Rock, AR 72204, USA

Jennifer Martin-Biggers, Virginia Quick and Carol Byrd-Bredbenner
Department of Nutritional Sciences, Rutgers University, 26 Nichol Avenue, New Brunswick, NJ 08901, USA

Kim Spaccarotella
Department of Biological Sciences, Kean University, 1000 Morris Avenue, Union, NJ 07082, USA

Henry Kewen Lu
School of Medicine, Western Sydney University, Penrith NSW 2751, Australia

Phillipa Hay
Translational Health Research Institute (THRI), School of Medicine, Western Sydney University, Locked Bag 1797, Penrith NSW 2751, Australia
Centre for Health Research and School of Medicine, The University of Western Sydney, Locked Bag 1797, Penrith NSW 2751, Australia

Haider Mannan
School of Medicine, Western Sydney University, Penrith NSW 2751, Australia
Translational Health Research Institute (THRI), School of Medicine, Western Sydney University, Penrith NSW 2751, Australia

James M. Kasper and Noelle C. Anastasio
Center for Addiction Research, University of Texas Medical Branch, Galveston, TX 77555, USA
Department of Pharmacology and Toxicology, University of Texas Medical Branch, Galveston, TX 77555, USA

Ara 13
Center for Addiction Research, University of Texas Medical Branch, Galveston, TX 77555, USA

Ashley E. Smith
Center for Addiction Research, University of Texas Medical Branch, Galveston, TX 77555, USA
Department of Neuroscience, Cell Biology and Anatomy, University of Texas Medical Branch, Galveston, TX 77555, USA

Jonathan D. Hommel
Center for Addiction Research, University of Texas Medical Branch, Galveston, TX 77555, USA
Department of Neuroscience, Cell Biology and Anatomy, University of Texas Medical Branch, Galveston, TX 77555, USA
Department of Pharmacology and Toxicology, University of Texas Medical Branch, Galveston, TX 77555, USA

Jessica A. Roekenes and Jessica Swinbourne
The Boden Institute of Obesity, Nutrition, Exercise & Eating Disorders, Sydney Medical School, Charles Perkins Centre, The University of Sydney, NSW 2006, Australia

Amanda Sainsbury
The Boden Institute of Obesity, Nutrition, Exercise & Eating Disorders, Sydney Medical School, Charles Perkins Centre, The University of Sydney, NSW 2006, Australia
School of Psychology, Faculty of Science, The University of Sydney, NSW 2006, Australia

Dhiordan C. da Silva and Margareth da S. Oliveira
Faculty of Psychology, Pontifical Catholic University of Rio Grande do Sul, Av. Ipiranga 6681, Porto Alegre/ RS, CEP 90619-900, Brazil

Felipe Q. da Luz
The Boden Institute of Obesity, Nutrition, Exercise & Eating Disorders, Sydney Medical School, Charles Perkins Centre, The University of Sydney, NSW 2006, Australia
School of Psychology, Faculty of Science, The University of Sydney, NSW 2006, Australia
Faculty of Psychology, Pontifical Catholic University of Rio Grande do Sul, Av. Ipiranga 6681, Porto Alegre/ RS, CEP 90619-900, Brazil
CAPES Foundation, Ministry of Education of Brazil, Brasília, DF 70040-020, Brazil

Stephen Touyz
Faculty of Science, School of Psychology, the University of Sydney, Camperdown, NSW 2006, Australia

Juliana Bermúdez-Cardona and Claudia Velásquez-Rodríguez
Research Group in Food and Human Nutrition, Universidad de Antioquia (UdeA)

Marie Blume, Ricarda Schmidt and Anja Hilbert
Integrated Research and Treatment Center Adiposity Diseases, Departments of Medical Psychology and Medical Sociology and Psychosomatic Medicine and Psychotherapy, University of Leipzig Medical Center, 04103 Leipzig, Germany

Index

www.ingramcontent.com/pod-product-compliance
Lightning Source LLC
LaVergne TN
LVHW081025210926
848485LV00004B/955

* 9 7 8 1 6 3 9 2 7 6 6 5 3 *